Register Now for (to Your B

MW00845465

SPRINGER PUBLISHING COMPANY
CONNECT™

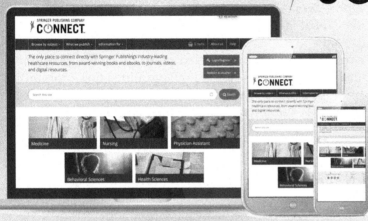

Your print purchase of *Certification in Public Health (CPH) Q&A Exam Review*
includes online access to the contents of your book—increasing accessibility,
portability, and searchability!

Access today at:

**http://connect.springerpub.com/content/book/978-0-8261-6186-4
or scan the QR code at the right with your smartphone
and enter the access code below.**

OM92A3FW

*Scan here for
quick access.*

SPRINGER PUBLISHING COMPANY

View all our products at springerpub.com

Oladele A. Ogunseitan, PhD, MPH, BCES, CPH, holds the University of California (UC) Presidential Chair at UC Irvine where he is a professor and the Founding Chair of the Department of Population Health & Disease Prevention, and professor of social ecology. He earned his professional master of public health degree at UC Berkeley focusing on environmental health and international health. He directs workforce development for the NIH-funded Institute of Clinical and Translational Science; and Training and Empowerment objective for the USAID-funded One Health Workforce–Next Generation. He serves on the Board of Directors of the UC Systemwide Global Health Institute.

Dele served two terms on the inaugural Board of Directors of the Association of Schools and Programs of Public Health. He served on the State of California's Green Ribbon Science Panel and the State's Advisory Committee on Community Protection and Hazardous Waste Reduction. He is co-chair of Apple, Inc.'s Green Chemistry Advisory Board. Dele is an alumni faculty fellow of the Belfer Center for Science and International Affairs at the Kennedy School of Government, Harvard University. He was a Jefferson Science Fellow of the U.S. National Academies of Sciences, Engineering, and Medicine.

Dele served as a Foreign Affairs Officer in the U.S. Department of State's Office of International Health and Biodefence; whence he earned a certificate in Global Health Diplomacy at the U.S. Foreign Service Institute. His honors include a Meritorious Honor Award from the U.S. Department of State for "exceptional teamwork and contributions to the successful achievement of U.S. goals at the third United Nations Environment Assembly, December 2017."

He holds Board Certification in Environmental Science from the American Academy of Environmental Engineers and Scientists. He is certified in Public Health by the National Board of Public Health Examiners.

Certification in Public Health (CPH) Q&A Exam Review

Oladele A. Ogunseitan, PhD, MPH, BCES, CPH

University of California Presidential Chair

Professor of Population Health & Disease Prevention

Professor of Social Ecology

University of California, Irvine

Irvine, California

SPRINGER PUBLISHING COMPANY

Springer Publishing Company, LLC
11 West 42nd Street
New York, NY 10036
www.springerpub.com
http://connect.springerpub.com/home

Acquisitions Editor: David D'Addona
Compositor: diacriTech

ISBN: 978-0-8261-6185-7
ebook ISBN: 978-0-8261-6186-4
DOI: 10.1891/9780826161864

22 23 24 25 / 5 4 3

This book is an independent publication and is not endorsed, sponsored, or otherwise approved by the National Board of Public Health Examiners. The NBPHE is not liable or responsible for any errors, omissions, or timeliness of the information or data available in this book, any individual's negligence in connection with the book, or any other liability resulting from the use or misuse of the book.

The author and the publisher of this Work have made every effort to use sources believed to be reliable to provide information that is accurate and compatible with the standards generally accepted at the time of publication. The author and publisher shall not be liable for any special, consequential, or exemplary damages resulting, in whole or in part, from the readers' use of, or reliance on, the information contained in this book. The publisher has no responsibility for the persistence or accuracy of URLs for external or third-party Internet websites referred to in this publication and does not guarantee that any content on such websites is, or will remain, accurate or appropriate.

Library of Congress Cataloging-in-Publication Data
LCCN: 2019919458

Contact us to receive discount rates on bulk purchases.
We can also customize our books to meet your needs.
For more information please contact: sales@springerpub.com

Publisher's Note: New and used products purchased from third-party sellers are not guaranteed for quality, authenticity, or access to any included digital components.

Printed in the United States of America.

Dedicated to the founding cohorts of public health students, staff, and faculty members at the University of California, Irvine. And to my family.

Contents

Preface

Public health is an ancient practice, but it is a new profession. Many contemporary customs and taboos recognizable in various societies and cultures can be traced back to attempts to codify generalizable knowledge about individual hygiene and population health. Over the past century, there has been rapid evolution of formal education in public health and advances in scientific understanding of the risk factors that produce disease and how to prevent them. The establishment of academic and professional competencies and institutional accreditation advanced the mission of professionalizing public health. However, the pace of population growth on Earth and the increasing recognition that risks to population health transcend geopolitical and social boundaries makes it necessary to develop continuing education schemes for public health academics and professionals, lest we become stale and irrelevant. Board certification through examination beyond institutional degrees and documentation of continuing education are essential components in full professionalization of public health. The National Board of Public Health Examiners established the foundation of this aspect of professionalization through the Certified in Public Health (CPH) credential. This practice workbook is designed to assist all public health enthusiasts who qualify to sit for the CPH examination.

It has been my honor and privilege to be the Founding Chair of the Department of Population Health and Disease Prevention, Program in Public Health, at the University of California, Irvine. In that capacity, I led the design and implementation of our bachelors, masters, and doctoral curricula. Importantly, I taught the graduate course "Foundations of Public Health" for more than a decade. The domain areas covered by the revised CPH examination implemented in 2019 aligned closely with the conceptual framework for the foundations course, which we offer as an introduction to the amazing accomplishments and humbling challenges of public health practice. Many of the questions in this workbook emerged from my course notes and weekly quizzes. Students then proceeded to take courses in specialized topic areas including core courses and concentration courses. It is gratifying to witness the progression of public health away from five narrowly framed subject domains (biostatistics, environmental health, epidemiology, health policy and management, and social and behavioral health) to the more realistic and integrative 10 domains covered in the CPH examination (evidence-based approaches, communication, leadership, law and ethics, biology and human disease risk, collaboration and partnership, program planning and evaluation, program management, policy, health equity and social justice). This workbook of questions and information resources is organized according to the new 10 domain areas. I look forward to the time when our Schools and Programs of Public Health transcend the old five subject areas and organize departments and degree programs in public health around integrative themes similar to the CPH examination. All CPH holders will be very well prepared.

At the University of California, Irvine, we have integrated the CPH examination into the Master of Public Health curriculum. Our experience and student feedback have been very positive. I hope that other institutions will consider this option. This workbook should assist public health students, professors, and practitioners in the workforce to prepare for the CPH examination. Beyond the examination, the workbook can provide an on-the-go refresher for checking the individual status of public health knowledge in the domain areas and for consulting resources to deepen the knowledge. I wish all those with such professional commitments and aspirations all the best.

—*Oladele A. Ogunseitan*

Acknowledgment

I thank the team of editors at Springer Publishing Company, particularly David D'Addona and Jaclyn Shultz for their deftness and patience. This workbook is dedicated to the founding faculty members of the Program in Public Health at the University of California (UC), Irvine. In alphabetical order by last name: Scott Bartell, Zuzana Bic, Tim Bruckner, Cynthia Lakon, Lisa Grant Ludwig, Sharon Stern, David Timberlake, Jun Wu, and Guiyun Yan. I have learnt, and continue to learn, a lot from their dedication, team spirit, and commitment to excellence. They are all cherished pioneers. I also dedicate the workbook to the founding class of MPH students at UC Irvine. They are all "master anteaters" for life and for healthy populations!

1

Evidence-Based Approaches to Public Health

INTRODUCTION

Humans have always tried to explain the causes of illnesses, diseases, and disabilities affecting individuals or populations. Before the discovery and adoption of the "germ" model of disease based on physical pathogenic agents, the "miasma" idea posited that wellness is compromised by human exposure to "bad air" or ill will from the spiritual world potentially under the influence of "bad people." Despite extensive scientific evidence existing to support the germ theory of disease, investigators continue to reveal new understandings of the nature of human existence on the continuum between healthy states to disease states and mortality. Evidence reveals complex interactions between genetics, environment, and risk factors. Yet, we face new threats associated with variability of human behavior and belief systems that threaten to erode the progress in controlling infectious diseases, such as measles, whereby vaccination rates are declining in some communities. Public health is an evidence-based practice. Most reliable evidence is quantitative, whereas other evidence is qualitative. It is essential to master the methodology for producing scientific evidence generated through well-designed studies and surveillance, and to interpret the results for the benefit of policy making and assurance of the health of populations. The questions on evidence-based approaches in public health are designed to examine the mastery of the relevant study-designs, analytical methods, and the interpretation of experimental results and calculations. Practicing with these questions should enable you to

- Interpret results of statistical analyses found in public health studies or reports
- Interpret quantitative or qualitative data following current scientific standards
- Apply common statistical methods for inference
- Apply descriptive techniques commonly used to summarize public data

- Identify the limitations of research results, data sources, or existing practices and programs
- Use statistical packages or software to analyze data
- Synthesize information from multiple data systems or other sources
- Identify key sources of data for epidemiologic or other investigation purposes
- Calculate mortality, morbidity, and health risk factor rates
- Collect valid and reliable quantitative or qualitative data
- Use information technology for data collection, storage, and retrieval
- Illustrate how gender, race, and other demographics affect population health
- Use population health surveillance systems
- Apply evidence-based theories, concepts, and models from a range of social and behavioral disciplines in the development and evaluation of health programs, policies, and interventions

■ QUESTIONS

1. Imagine that you are a behavioral scientist at the Centers for Disease Control and Prevention in Atlanta (CDC). You are responsible for analyzing the behavioral determinants and correlates of an apparent obesity epidemic among children in a rural area of Georgia. Which steps would you NOT want to take in order to best inform your application of theory to understanding this problem?
   A. Research the causes and correlates of obesity within this age and geographical group
   B. Find data on city-, county-, and state-specific rates of childhood obesity to compare the area-specific rates against—so you can discern where there really is a spike in childhood obesity in the target area
   C. Research the demographic characteristics of your target population (e.g., children in the rural area in Georgia)
   D. Interview children in your target population without their parents to understand their own perceptions of factors driving the apparent epidemic

2. Epidemiologists conduct observational and experimental studies. Observation of the exposure and disease status of each study participant has yielded many insights into public health, including John Snow's studies of cholera and drinking water in London, England. The two most common types of observational studies are cohort studies and case–control studies; a third type is cross-sectional studies. The most effective study design for investigating the source of a waterborne disease outbreak is
   A. Case–control study
   B. Prospective cohort study
   C. Retrospective cohort study
   D. Ecological study

3. A fallacy is the use of invalid information or faulty reasoning in reaching a conclusion. Which one of the following epidemiological study designs is most prone to the fallacy of interpreting an aggregate-level association of risk factor and disease for individuals?

   A. Prospective cohort study
   B. Retrospective cohort study
   C. Case–control study
   D. Ecological study

4. A diagnostic test is performed to aid in the detection of disease. Diagnostic tests can also be used to provide prognostic information on people with established disease. The net sensitivity from a sequential disease diagnosis test is equal to the sensitivity of the first test. What is the likely explanation?

   A. Sensitivity of the first test is equal to the sensitivity of the second test.
   B. Sensitivity of the second test is 0%.
   C. Sensitivity of the second test is 100%.
   D. Cannot be determined from the information provided

5. In the United States, the Centers for Disease Control and Prevention publishes annual summaries of domestic foodborne disease outbreaks based on reports provided by state, local, and territorial health departments. In 2016, 839 food-borne disease outbreaks were reported, resulting in 14,259 illnesses, 875 hospitalizations, 17 deaths, and 18 food recalls. Public health officials investigate foodborne outbreaks to control them and to learn how to prevent future occurrence of similar outbreaks. The "attack rate ratio" calculation in the context of a foodborne outbreak requires the following EXCEPT:

   A. Disease status of individuals
   B. Attack rates for foods consumed
   C. Attack rates for foods not consumed
   D. Disease status of the sous chef

6. Public health surveillance through screening programs are fundamental tools in public health. We use data to know where the health burdens are, to signal anomalies and health risks, and to inform actions and interventions that can keep people safer and healthier. The bias of falsely attributing greater survival to early detection of disease in a community with a screening program, compared to a community without such a program, is referred to as

   A. Referral bias
   B. Length bias
   C. Lead time bias
   D. Survival bias

7. Descriptive statistics provide summaries for datasets, which can either represent the population or a sample. The population mean describes the central tendency of a dataset and is an example of a population parameter that can be directly computed from

   A. Convenience sample
   B. Quota sample

C. Complex probability sample
D. Population census

8. Diagnostic tests for diseases are often described in terms of their validity, reliability, sensitivity, and specificity. Positive predictive value is the probability that subjects with a positive screening test truly have the disease. Negative predictive value is the probability that subjects with a negative screening test truly do not have the disease. For a rare disease, the positive predictive value of a screening test increases with

A. Greater disease prevalence
B. Less disease prevalence
C. Less specificity
D. Greater scarcity

9. "Herd immunity" describes a situation in which a sufficient proportion of a population is immune to an infectious disease (through vaccination and/or prior illness) to make its spread from person to person unlikely. Even individuals not vaccinated (such as newborns and those with chronic illnesses) are offered some protection because the disease has little opportunity to spread within the community. The concept of herd immunity is based on the fundamental assumption that

A. The entire population has been vaccinated.
B. Random mixing of vaccinated and unvaccinated individuals occurs.
C. Vaccinated and unvaccinated individuals tend to congregate nonrandomly.
D. A proportion of the population has natural immunity.

10. Experimental study designs can be expensive but they can also yield very informative data. For example, randomized clinical trials (RCTs) are studies in which the participants are randomly assigned into separate groups that compare different exposures (e.g., medical therapies). Random assignment of human participants into treatment groups reduces the likelihood of experimental bias. Nevertheless, RCTs are frequently criticized because of their

A. Poor internal validity
B. Poor external validity
C. Inability to account for confounders
D. Inability to account for self-selection

11. A risk factor, for example, exposure to asbestos fibers, is any attribute, characteristic, or exposure of an individual that increases the likelihood of developing a disease or injury, for example, mesothelioma, a lung disease that may take a long time for symptoms to be detected. Which of the following is a measure of risk assessed from a cohort with a variable length of follow-up time?

A. Incidence
B. Cumulative incidence
C. Incidence density
D. Incidence odds

12. Epidemiologists conduct observational and experimental studies. Observation of the exposure and disease status of each study participant has yielded many insights in public health, including John Snow's studies of cholera and drinking water in London, England. The two most common types of observational studies are cohort studies and case–control studies; cross-sectional studies are also observational. An advantage of the case–control study design in comparison to prospective cohort study design is

   A. Can assess the natural history of disease
   B. Efficient for studying rare exposures
   C. Efficient for studying rare diseases
   D. Less potential for systematic errors

13. Several models of disease causation have been proposed, including the epidemiologic triad or triangle, which consists of an external agent, a susceptible host, and an environment that brings the host and agent together. The causal relationship between an organism and an infectious disease is often

   A. Necessary and sufficient
   B. Necessary but not sufficient
   C. Sufficient but not necessary
   D. Neither sufficient nor necessary

14. The "Global Burden of Disease" project is a public health milestone in its compilation of cause-specific mortality for 282 causes of disease and disability. A cause-specific mortality rate can approximate incidence of disease under the following condition(s):

   A. Disease has a high case fatality rate.
   B. Disease has a low case fatality rate.
   C. Survival from the diseases is long.
   D. Survival from the diseases leads to comorbid conditions.

15. Secondary prevention includes screening for diseases in populations to detect diseases early, and there are now widely used screening tests for breast, cervical, and colorectal cancers, and for diabetes, for which there are effective clinical treatment and disease management options. Sequential screening for disease entails

   A. Rescreening those who initially tested positive
   B. Rescreening those who initially tested negative
   C. Rescreening all subjects
   D. Screening those who have never been screened

16. A diagnostic test is performed to aid in the detection of disease. Diagnostic tests can also be used to provide prognostic information on people with established disease. For example, measurement of hemoglobin A1C in blood is diagnostic for diabetes. If hemoglobin A1C test is assessed by two independent observers, the reliability of the test

   A. Increases with a higher proportion of discordant observations
   B. Increases with a higher proportion of concordant observations

    C. Increases with the same proportion of discordant observations

    D. Should not account for chance agreement between observers

17. Comparing the crude mortality rate of two different populations, for example, in Nigeria compared to the United States, may mask important information needed for designing disease prevention strategies for different age groups and genders. Standardized mortality ratio (SMR) is the ratio between the observed number of deaths in a study population and the number of deaths that would be expected, based on the age- and sex-specific rates in a standard population and the population size of the study population by the same age and sex groups. An SMR higher than 1.0 is indicative of

    A. Higher number of observed cases relative to expected cases

    B. Higher number of expected cases relative to observed cases

    C. Decreased mortality in the study population

    D. Cannot be determined from the information provided

18. The World Health Organization maintains an informational database on outbreaks, epidemics, and pandemics, with specific criteria that define each of these categories relative to the response needed, including source control. An epidemic refers to an increase, often sudden, in the number of cases of a disease above what is normally expected in that population in that area. An outbreak carries the same definition as epidemic, but is often used for a more limited geographic area. If the duration of an infectious disease exceeds the range of the incubation period, then the epidemic curve is not illustrative of a

    A. Common, continuing source outbreak

    B. Common, point source outbreak

    C. Propagated outbreak

    D. Insufficient information

19. Allocation of public health resources to the design and implementation of interventions for diseases such as Alzheimer's or diarrhea requires data on mortality according to age categories. Age-specific mortality rates are essential for this purpose, where the numerator is the number of deaths in each age group and the denominator is the number of persons in the age groups in the population. In comparing death rates between two populations, which method of age-adjustment utilizes age-specific mortality rates from only one population?

    A. Indirect method

    B. Direct method

    C. Directly indirect method

    D. There is not sufficient information to identify the method.

20. There are several potential sources of error in epidemiological studies. Some errors are random, whereas others are systematic. Recall bias is a systematic error caused by differences in the accuracy or completeness of the recollections remembered by study participants regarding events or experiences from the past. Recall bias is a particular concern in which of the following study designs?

    A. Randomized clinical trial

    B. Prospective cohort study

C. Case–control study

D. Ecological study

21. Descriptive epidemiological studies can be used to identify patterns among disease cases and in populations by time, place, and person. Based on these observations, epidemiologists develop hypotheses about the causes of disease patterns and about the factors that increase risk of disease. Epidemiologists can use descriptive epidemiology to generate hypotheses, but only rarely to test those hypotheses. For that, epidemiologists must turn to analytic or experimental epidemiology. Which of the following study designs is more useful for generating a hypothesis rather than testing one?

A. Randomized clinical trial

B. Prospective cohort study

C. Case–control study

D. Ecological study

22. In a case–control study, investigators start by enrolling a group of people already diagnosed with a disease. As a control group, the investigator then enrolls a group of people without the disease. To avoid or minimize bias, the controls from a case–control study should be selected ideally from the

A. General population

B. Population of healthy, nondiseased individuals

C. Population from which the cases had been chosen

D. Hospital setting

23. Several approaches have been developed to detect and minimize bias in epidemiological study designs. For example, a matched case–control design should match pairs on

A. Confounder(s) of interest

B. All possible confounders

C. Main effect and exposure

D. Depends on other epidemiological variables

24. There are several potential sources of error in epidemiological studies. Measurement error can be either random (nonsystematic) or biased (systematic). Identifying the source of error and recognizing its effect on study results is important. Systematic error or bias in an epidemiologic study

A. Is largely due to random sampling

B. Almost always results in a null effect

C. Tends to over- or underestimate the true effect

D. Usually cannot be identified or controlled for

25. The U.S. Centers for Disease Control and Prevention has established an extensive disease surveillance system. Public health surveillance and the essential health data that comes from long-term surveillance are fundamental tools in public health. Surveillance bias is particularly problematic in which of the following study designs?

A. Prospective cohort study
B. Case–control study
C. Cross-sectional study
D. Ecological study

26. A "control" in scientific investigation is defined as an experiment or observation designed to minimize the effects of variables other than the independent variable. In an epidemiological study, a study participant serves as his or her own control in which of the following study designs?

A. Prospective cohort study
B. Retrospective cohort study
C. Case-crossover study
D. Case–control study

27. Tobacco smoking is the major risk factor for lung cancer. In the United States, cigarette smoking is linked to about 80% to 90% of lung cancer deaths. Using other tobacco products, such as cigars or pipes, also increases the risk for lung cancer. Tobacco smoke is a toxic mix of more than 7,000 chemicals. Many are poisons. At least 70 are known to cause cancer in people or animals. The 80% to 90% cited is a measure of

A. Cumulative incidence
B. Proportionate mortality
C. Case-fatality rate
D. Attributable fraction (AF)

28. Several models of disease causation have been proposed, including the epidemiologic triad or triangle, which consists of an external risk factor (e.g., pathogen), a susceptible host, and an environment that connects the host and risk factor. Spurious associations between risk factors and disease can occur because of the following EXCEPT:

A. Are due to an actual difference in risk between groups
B. Can occur by chance
C. Can occur as a result of systematic error or bias
D. Can occur from limitations of a study design

29. There are several potential sources of error in epidemiological studies. For example, recall bias is a systematic error caused by differences in the accuracy or completeness of information by study participants who may not fully remember past experiences. Poor recall of past exposure that is approximately equal in cases and controls

A. Is a form of nondifferential misclassification
B. Is a form of differential misclassification
C. Tends to overestimate the true effect
D. Tends to underestimate the true effect

30. Subtle differences in genetic factors cause people to respond differently when exposed to the same environmental agent. For example, genetic polymorphisms

in the cytochrome P450 profile of liver enzymes may influence the metabolism of toxic compounds. Therefore, some individuals possess a low risk for developing a disease through an environmental exposure, whereas others are much more susceptible. Which of the following study designs can be used in differentiating genetic from environmental influences on disease?

A. Adoption design
B. Classic triplet design
C. Classic quartet design
D. Design comparing those with a plus and minus family history of disease

31. The probability value (p value) is used extensively in statistical hypothesis testing. Which of the following is the best interpretation of a p value <.05?

A. The probability that the null hypothesis is true is <5%.
B. The probability of a type I error is <5%.
C. The probability of a type II error is <5%.
D. Results at least as extreme as the observed data are unlikely to have occurred if the null hypothesis is true.

32. Knowing whether to accept or reject a null hypothesis is very important in the interpretation of study designs that use statistical analysis. The best definition for statistical "power" is

A. The probability of rejecting the null hypothesis given that the null hypothesis is true
B. The probability of rejecting the null hypothesis given that the null hypothesis is false
C. The probability of not rejecting the null hypothesis given that the null hypothesis is true
D. The probability of not rejecting the null hypothesis given that the null hypothesis is false

33. Statistical power is defined as the probability that a study will detect an effect when there is an effect there to be detected (rejection of a null hypothesis). There is a quantitative relationship between statistical power and error. Type I error is falsely rejecting a true null hypothesis. Type II error is failing to reject a false null hypothesis. Imagine that you are testing a hypothesis with a type I error rate of 5% and the type II error rate of 10%. What is the statistical power of the test?

A. 90%
B. 95%
C. 97.5%
D. Not enough information is provided to calculate the statistical power

The following scenario applies to Questions 34, 35, and 36.

Scenario
Globally, in 2012, 2.2 million deaths were attributable to high blood glucose, and in 2016, about 1.6 million people died because of diabetes. Imagine that you work for the International Diabetes Association and are in charge of a

program on nutritional intervention. You recruit 100 currently obese individuals and offer them the opportunity to participate in a nutritional intervention study; 10 participants agree and initially start dieting. After 6 months, three of the participants have returned to excessive caloric intake. After 12 months, a total of five participants have returned to excessive caloric intake. The dieting program's Internet advertisements claim that "80% of our customers lose weight and stay on the diet for at least one year" after starting the intervention.

34. Which of the following probability distributions is most appropriate for representing the number of people in the dieting study that return to excessive caloric intake within 1 year?

A. Binomial
B. Poisson
C. Normal
D. Lognormal

35. The confidence interval defines the upper and lower boundaries within which the true value of a measured parameter will be. Based on the results of the intervention study, which of the following is the most appropriate 95% confidence interval for the probability that a person will successfully maintain the nutritional intervention for at least 6 months after the program starts?

A. (0.70, 1.86)
B. (0.28, 1.44)
C. (0.35, 0.93)
D. (0.56, 2.88)

36. It is important to ensure that the results of epidemiological studies are interpreted correctly in public health communication campaigns. Otherwise, the public is confused and mistrust arises. Which of the following statements best compares the nutritional intervention study results to the advertised claim?

A. Fewer participants successfully quit smoking than expected, so the advertised claim is unlikely to be true.
B. More participants successfully quit smoking than expected, so the advertised claim is unlikely to be true.
C. Fewer participants successfully quit smoking than expected, but not so few that the advertised claim is demonstrably false.
D. More participants successfully quit smoking than expected, but not so many that the advertised claim is demonstrably false.

37. "Normal distribution" defines an ideal population in which arrangement of measures of specific attributes is distributed in a symmetric bell curve. The mean, median, and mode of a normally distributed population are identical. Which of the following conditions is sufficient for the sampling distribution of the arithmetic mean to be approximately normal?

A. The sample size is small.
B. The population values have a normal distribution.
C. The population values have a binomial distribution.
D. The population size has a Poisson distribution.

38. Childhood leukemia, a hematological malignancy, is the most common form of childhood cancer, representing 29% of cancers in children aged 0 to 14 years in 2018. Imagine that you work in the State Department of Public Health, and 12 cases of childhood leukemia were diagnosed during a 10-year period. Assume that there are 12,000 children in the town throughout this 10 years, and that the national incidence rate of childhood leukemia is five cases per 10,000 person-years. What is the 95% confidence interval for the standardized morbidity ratio?

    A. (10.3, 34.9)
    B. (1.03, 3.49)
    C. (1.08, 5.36)
    D. (5.17, 17.5)

39. Statistical power is defined as the probability that a study will detect an effect when there is an effect there to be detected (rejection of a null hypothesis). Which of the following actions increases the statistical power of a hypothesis testing exercise?

    A. Increase the confidence level
    B. Decrease the sample size
    C. Decrease the confidence level
    D. Keep the sample size the same

The following scenario applies to Questions 40, 41, 42, 43, 44, and 45.

Scenario
The American Diabetes Association hosts on its website a "Body Mass Index (BMI) Calculator." BMI is defined as an individual's weight divided by the square of the individual's height. BMI appears to be strongly correlated with various metabolic and disease outcomes such as diabetes. Imagine that you work in the Student Wellness Office in charge of physical fitness, and you measured the following BMI values (in kg/m^2) for a random sample of university students: 20, 28, 28, 21, 24, 21, 30, 19, 22, 21. Obesity is often defined by a BMI of 30 or above, and overweight is defined by a BMI of at least 25 but less than 30. Underweight is defined by a BMI of less than 18.5.

40. Which of the following is a valid sample median for body mass index (BMI)?

    A. 28.0
    B. 21.5
    C. 21.0
    D. 24.5

41. Based on the sample, which of the following is the best 95% confidence interval for the mean body mass index (BMI) among college students?

    A. (14.7, 32.1)
    B. (15.8, 31.0)
    C. (20.6, 26.2)
    D. (21.0, 25.8)

42. If body mass index (BMI) is normally distributed among college students, what proportion of college students is expected to be obese based on the sample mean and sample variance?

    A. 4.5%
    B. 6.2%
    C. 10%
    D. 90%

43. Suppose that the body mass index (BMI) values in the sample were self-reported, and that another study suggests that 30% of overweight and obese college students self-report a normal BMI. If there are no other inaccuracies in self-reporting, what are the sensitivity and specificity of self-reports of overweight and obese (BMI ≥25) among college students?

    A. Sensitivity of 30% and specificity of 100%
    B. Sensitivity of 70% and specificity of 70%
    C. Sensitivity of 70% and specificity of 100%
    D. Sensitivity of 100% and specificity of 70%

44. How does the information described in Question 43 affect the interpretation of the previously calculated confidence interval for the mean body mass index (BMI) among college students?

    A. The confidence interval is still appropriate.
    B. The confidence interval is likely too low.
    C. The confidence interval is likely too high.
    D. The confidence interval is exponential.

45. What information is sufficient to calculate the positive predictive value for self-reports of body mass index (BMI) ≥25?

    A. The proportion of college students with BMI ≥25, and the proportion of college students that self-report as having BMI ≥25
    B. The proportion of college students with BMI <25, and the proportion of college students that self-report as having BMI <25
    C. The sensitivity and specificity of self-reports for BMI ≥25, and the prevalence of BMI ≥25
    D. The proportion of college students with BMI = 25, and the proportion of college students that self-report as having BMI = 25

The following scenario applies to Questions 46, 47, 48, and 49.

Scenario
In 2015, 84.1 million people in the United States had prediabetes, a condition that may be reversed by limiting sugar intake among other interventions. Imagine that you work for the International Diabetes Association, and you have recruited 50 prediabetic patients to undergo a nutritional intervention. Fasting blood sugar concentrations are measured for each participant at the start of the intervention and again after 1 month. At the start of the intervention, the mean fasting blood sugar concentration was 120 mg/dL (sample variance of 50 mg^2/dL^2). After 1 month, the mean fasting blood sugar concentration was 100 mg/dL (sample variance of 40 mg^2/dL^2).

46. What is the 95% confidence interval for the mean fasting blood sugar concentration 1 month after physical activity intervention?

    A. (9.82, 10.18) mg/dL
    B. (98.2, 101.8) mg/dL
    C. (99.8, 100.2) mg/dL
    D. The confidence interval cannot be determined from the information provided.

47. Regarding the physical activity intervention, what is the 95% confidence interval for the average decrease in fasting blood sugar concentration?

    A. (17.3, 22.7) mg/dL
    B. (18.1, 21.9) mg/dL
    C. (19.6, 20.4) mg/dL
    D. Cannot be determined from the information provided

48. Which of the following probability distributions is the most reasonable assumption for describing the sample variance at the start of the physical activity intervention?

    A. Poisson
    B. Binomial
    C. Lognormal
    D. Chi-square

49. In the United States, in 2015, 9.4% (30.3 million people) of the population had diabetes. Another 84.1 million people had prediabetes, a condition that may be reversed by limiting sugar intake among other interventions. Fasting blood sugar analysis measures blood sugar after not eating overnight. A fasting blood sugar of 100 mg/dL (5.6 mmol/L) is considered normal; 100 to 125 mg/dL (5.6–6.9 mmol/L) is indicative of prediabetes; and 126 mg/dL (7 mmol/L) or higher on two separate tests is a confirmatory diagnosis for diabetes. Assume that the sampling variance for the fasting blood sugar concentration will be the same at 2 months after the physical activity intervention as it was at 1 month, and that all participants remain enrolled in the study. For a two-tailed test of the null hypothesis that the mean blood sugar concentration is 100 mg/dL after 2 months, how small a difference between the null hypothesis and the sample mean can be detected with 95% confidence and 80% power?

    A. 2.6 mg/dL
    B. 25.5 mg/dL
    C. 4.1 mg/dL
    D. 5.0 mg/dL

50. Tobacco smoking is the top risk factor for lung cancer. In the United States, cigarette smoking is linked to about 80% to 90% of lung cancer deaths. Using other tobacco products such as cigars or pipes also increases the risk for lung cancer. Tobacco smoke is a toxic mix of more than 7,000 chemicals with at least 70 known to cause cancer in people or animals. A cohort study examined the association between smoking and lung cancer after following 800 smokers and

1,200 nonsmokers for 15 years. At the conclusion of the study, the investigators found a risk ratio (RR) = 15. Which of the following would be the best interpretation of this RR?

A. There were 15 more cases of lung cancer in the smokers.
B. Smokers had 15 times the risk of lung cancer compared to nonsmokers.
C. Smokers had 15% more lung cancers compared to nonsmokers.
D. Smokers had 15 times more risk of lung cancer than nonsmokers.

51. Theoretical frameworks that support public health interventions against risk-taking behaviors such as inhaling tobacco smoke often begin with intrapersonal predispositions. These are followed by multiple levels of aggregation which begin with

A. Individuals
B. Interpersonal relationships
C. Community norms
D. Institutional policies

52. The National Commission for Health Education Credentialing (NCHEC) provides guidelines for academic and professional competencies in health education. The following important events are relevant to the professionalization of health education and health behavior, EXCEPT

A. The LaLonde Report
B. The Declaration of Alma Ata
C. Healthy People 2020
D. The Human Biome Project

53. Individual-level theories of behavior change (e.g., Health Behavior Theory) were modified based on scientific research to include additional levels of theoretical frameworks such as the Social-Ecological Model for which one of the following reasons:

A. Because reliance on individual-level theories of behavior change was not considered valid
B. Because individual-level theories did not account for influences at higher levels of theoretical aggregation or abstraction such as those factors at the interpersonal (social network) and community level affecting health behavior, to name a few
C. There was no paradigm shift in the 1970s; behavior change theories have continued to focus on individual-level theory throughout the last four decades and do so currently
D. Individual-level models of health behavior tend to explain most all of the variation in a population's health behaviors

54. As with all public health disciplines, health education and health behavior rely on evidence-based theory development, translational research, and professional practice. How are the latter three activities related?

A. Theory development primarily informs professional practice but less so for translational research.
B. Translational research informs theory and not professional practice.

C. Translational research and professional practice inform theory development.
D. Theory development, translational research, and professional practice inform one another.

55. Theoretical frameworks can reflect patterns in social phenomena with respect to healthcare and health behavior on the basis of

A. Systematic inquiry and observations about how aspects of a social phenomena interrelate
B. Nonsystematic inquiry and observations
C. Theory does not reflect patterns and interrelationships in social phenomena
D. Ideological bias of academic researchers and theoreticians

56. Numerous theories, strategies, and models have been developed to inform health promotion and disease prevention practices. As a public health professional, what factor is most important in selecting a particular theoretical framework to understand health behavior?

A. The level of disaggregation of the health behavior problem
B. The scale or unit of analysis of the individual
C. The temporal nature of the behavioral challenge, whether it is a discrete one-time event (e.g., getting a mammogram) or a behavior that requires longer term change over time (e.g., smoking)
D. Whether or not to deconstruct a theoretical framework

57. The Health Belief Model (HBM) posits that individual beliefs about health conditions predict individual health behaviors. Critics claim that HBM cannot explain variation in health behavior across ethnic and racial populations that share beliefs. What is the evidence for this criticism?

A. Research shows that such populations hold the same beliefs about their own susceptibility to a health problem.
B. Research shows that such populations hold differing perceptions of benefits and perceived barriers to taking health actions.
C. Research suggests that the HBM adequately explains ethnic, racial, and cultural variation in health behavior.
D. The HBM is unassailable because it is one of the most relevant and long-standing theories explaining health behavior across racial and ethnic populations.

58. The theory of reasoned action and the closely related theory of planned behavior both suggest that a person's health behavior is determined by his or her intention to perform a behavior. What is the relationship between these theories and the Expectancy-Value Theory?

A. The major constructs (behavioral, normative, and control beliefs) are each further refined into one expectancy construct and one value-based construct.
B. The major constructs (behavioral, normative, and control beliefs) are not further refined into one expectancy construct and one value-based construct.
C. The major constructs (behavioral, normative, and health beliefs) are each further refined into one expectancy construct and one value-based construct.

D. The major constructs (behavioral, normative, and health beliefs) are not further refined into one expectancy construct and one value-based construct.

59. The theory of planned behavior suggests that a person's health behavior is determined by his or her intention to perform a behavior. Which of the following perceptions or attitudes does not comprise behavioral intentions?

A. Attitude toward engaging in a behavior
B. Perceptions of subjective norms regarding engaging in a behavior
C. Perceived behavioral control
D. Perceived mind control

60. The theory of reasoned action and the theory of planned behavior suggest that an individual's health behavior is determined by specific thought processes. According to these theories, which thought process is the strongest predictor of whether a person engages in a health behavior?

A. Perceptions of subjective norms regarding a behavior
B. Perceived behavioral control
C. Behavioral intention
D. Behavioral beliefs

61. Behavior change is any transformation or modification of human behavior, or in reference to public health, a wide range of activities and approaches that focus on the individual, community, and environmental influences on human health behavior. Which of the following theories explicitly assumes that behavior change occurs gradually over time rather than at one discrete point in time?

A. Theory of Planned Behavior/Reasoned Action
B. Health Belief Model
C. Stages of Change/Transtheoretical Model
D. Locus of Control Theory

62. Which one of the following theories or models assumes that populations at risk within the social determinants of health are not prepared for behavior change and will therefore not be well-served by traditional "action-oriented" prevention programs?

A. Social Cognitive Theory
B. Theories of Social Network
C. Health Belief Model
D. Stages of Change/Transtheoretical Model

63. The Transtheoretical Model (TTM) explains an individual's readiness to change his or her behavior. It describes the process of behavior change as occurring in stages. Studies applying TTM to understand tobacco use in the United States discovered that

A. Less than 20% were in the preparation stage, 40% in contemplation
B. Less than 10% were in the preparation stage, 40% in contemplation
C. Less than 5% were in the preparation stage, 30% in contemplation
D. Less than 20% were in the preparation stage, 10% in contemplation

64. Urie Bronfenbrenner is one of the founders and refiners of the Social-Ecological Model, which conceptualizes health broadly and focuses on multiple and layered factors that might affect health. Within this framework, interpersonal models of health behavior theory do not assume that

   A. Health behavior is solely a function of individual attributes.
   B. Health behavior is affected by the social networks people maintain.
   C. Health behavior is affected by the social influences exerted by people in our social networks.
   D. Health behavior is affected by the social support given to and received from people in our social networks.

65. Albert Bandura is one of the founders and refiners of Social Cognitive Theory (SCT), which provides opportunities for social support through instilling expectations, self-efficacy, and using observational learning and other reinforcements to achieve behavior change. SCT approaches health behavior as

   A. A result of a dynamic *interaction* between individuals, their environments, and human capacities for learning and adaptation
   B. A result of individual-level influences only
   C. A result of environmental influences only
   D. Unfolding gradually over time in stages

66. Social Cognitive Theory (SCT), based on Albert Bandura's Social Learning Theory, describes the influence of individual experiences, the actions of others, and environmental factors on individual health behaviors. Which of the following is the most well-known construct in SCT?

   A. Self-efficacy
   B. Reciprocal determinism
   C. Collective efficacy
   D. Reinforcement

67. The ecological model of public health posits that the relationship between health status and social support systems is

   A. Dependent on the type of support and the number of supportive others in one's social network
   B. Consistent across health outcomes
   C. Constant regardless of the type of support or number of supportive others in individuals' social networks
   D. Primarily dependent on the type of support given and received

68. The ecological model of health promotion posits that social support is important for behavior change. Which of the following is NOT an important element of social support systems?

   A. Enhancing existing social network ties in a community or other social collective or group
   B. Developing new social network ties for people in a target population
   C. Enhancing the power of an individual's social network ties by identifying and then utilizing the resources inherent to him or her
   D. Enhancing peer-pressure influence on individuals

69. Gay and bisexual men are the population most affected by HIV in the United States. In 2016, gay and bisexual men accounted for 67% of the 40,324 new HIV diagnoses. Approximately 492,000 sexually active gay and bisexual men are at high risk for HIV. Imagine that you are a health scientist at the Centers for Disease Control and Prevention (CDC) and one of your numerous projects is to create health behavior change interventions around HIV/AIDS among men who have sex with men. Which theoretical approach might you be most likely to employ to help you understand how the spread of the virus goes from a primarily homosexual population into a primarily heterosexual population?

A. Social Cognitive Theory
B. Theories relating to social networks
C. Attribution Theory
D. Social Regulation Theory

70. Approximately 610,000 people die of heart disease in the United States every year, or one in every four deaths. Heart disease is the leading cause of death for both men and women. More than half of the deaths due to heart disease in 2009 were in men. Men aged 35 to 49 years have a twofold greater incidence of coronary heart disease (CHD) than 35- to 49-year-old females. Yet, the prevalence of CHD is comparable in the two genders. What could account for the discrepancy?

A. Risk factors for disease are more common in males.
B. Duration of disease is shorter in females.
C. Case fatality rate for disease is greater in males.
D. Case fatality rate for disease is greater in females.

■ ANSWERS

1. **D.** More than 600,000 people die of heart disease in the United States annually (about 25% of all deaths). Heart disease is the leading cause of death for both men and women. Coronary heart disease is the most common type of heart disease, killing more than 400,000 people annually. About 8.5% of all White men, 7.9% of Black men, and 6.3% of Mexican American men have coronary heart disease. Between 70% and 89% of sudden cardiac events occur in men. Half of the men who die suddenly of coronary heart disease have no previous symptoms. Even if you have no symptoms, you may still be at risk for heart disease.

Incidence rate (or person-time rate) is the number of new cases of disease during a specified time interval.

Point prevalence is the number of current cases (new and preexisting) at a specified point in time, whereas period prevalence is the number of current cases (new and preexisting) over a specified period of time.

Case fatality rate (or case fatality ratio) is the proportion of people who die from a disease among all individuals diagnosed with the disease over a certain period of time.

Men and women have similar risk factors for CHD.

Diabetes

Being overweight or obese

Eating an unhealthy diet

Physical inactivity

Drinking too much alcohol

The most likely way for the prevalence to be similar but incidence to be much higher in men is that the case fatality rate is higher for men. The health-scape of heart disease is changing, along with the metrics.

See: https://www.cdc.gov/heartdisease/facts.htm

  https://www.cdc.gov/csels/dsepd/ss1978/index.html

  https://www.cdc.gov/csels/dsepd/ss1978/lesson3/section2.html

  https://academic.oup.com/eurheartj/article/38/3/181/2967565

2. **C.** A cohort study is similar in concept to the experimental study. In a cohort study, the epidemiologist records whether each study participant is exposed or not, and then tracks the participants to see whether they develop the disease of interest. Note that this differs from an experimental study because, in a cohort study, the investigator observes rather than determines the participants' exposure status. After a period of time, the investigator compares the disease rate in the exposed group with the disease rate in the unexposed group. The unexposed group serves as the comparison group, providing an estimate of the baseline or expected amount of disease occurrence in the community. If the disease rate is substantively different in the exposed group compared to the unexposed group, the exposure is said to be associated with illness.

An alternative type of cohort study is a retrospective cohort study. In this type of study, both the exposure and the outcomes have already occurred. Just as in a prospective cohort study, the investigator calculates and compares rates of disease in the exposed and unexposed groups. Retrospective cohort studies are commonly used in investigations of disease in groups of easily identified people such as workers at a particular factory or attendees at a wedding, or people who ate at a restaurant over a specific period of time. For example, a retrospective cohort study was used to determine the source of infection of cyclosporiasis, a parasitic disease that caused an outbreak among members of a residential facility in Pennsylvania in 2004. The investigation indicated that consumption of snow peas was implicated as the vehicle of the cyclosporiasis outbreak.

See: https://www.cdc.gov/csels/dsepd/ss1978/lesson1/section7.html

3. **D.** Ecological study designs are those in which disease rates are linked to the level of exposure to some risk factor for the target population as a whole. Ecological studies are subject to inference fallacy, whereby inferences about disease status are made about a specific individual in a population of exposed individuals where exposure data are aggregated. Ecological studies are useful for generating hypotheses that can be tested with existing data for large populations and the large number of risk-modifying behaviors that may be investigated.

See: https://www.cdc.gov/csels/dsepd/ss1978/index.html

Grant, W. B. (2014). A multi-country ecological study of cancer incidence rates in 2008 with respect to various risk-modifying factors. *Nutrients, 6*(1), 163–189. doi:10.3390/nu6010163

4. **C.** Disease screening is the process of identifying those individuals who are at sufficiently high risk of a specific disorder to warrant further investigation or direct action. Diagnostic screening tests are used in public health to identify individuals who may have disease, carry vectors of disease, or have acquired immune response to the disease. The sensitivity of a diagnostic test is the ability of the test to detect the health problem that it is intended to detect. Surveillance for the majority of health problems might detect a relatively limited proportion of those that actually occur. The critical question is whether surveillance is sufficiently sensitive to be useful in preventing or controlling the health problem. The specificity of a screening test is the proportion of people who do not have the disorder who test negative on the screening test. In using a diagnostic test, the positive predictive value is the proportion of reported or identified cases that truly are cases, or the proportion of reported or identified epidemics that were actual epidemics. Conducting surveillance that has poor positive predictive value is wasteful, because the unsubstantiated or false-positive reports result in unnecessary investigations, wasteful allocation of resources, and, especially for false reports of epidemics, unwarranted public anxiety.

A sequential screening is a series of two or more tests to double-check or cross-check for disease status. For example, diagnosis of diabetes may depend on measurements of fasting blood sugar concentrations and the concentration of hemoglobin A1C. Prostate cancer screening among men may depend on the outcomes of digital rectal examination and concentration of prostate-specific antigen (PSA). Conducting two tests can increase the positive predictive value of screening tests. If the net sensitivity of two tests is equal to the sensitivity of the first test, then the sensitivity of the first test must be 100%, meaning that all those who tested positive for the first test also tested positive for the second test.

See: https://www.cdc.gov/csels/dsepd/ss1978/lesson5/section7.html

https://www.who.int/diabetes/publications/en/screening_mnc03.pdf

Kramer, B. S., Brown, M. L., Prorok, P. C., Potosky, A. L., & Gohagan, J. K. (1993). Prostate cancer screening: What we know and what we need to know. *Annals of Internal Medicine, 119*, 914–923. doi:10.7326/0003-4819-119-9-119311010-00009

Maxim, L. D., Niebo, R., & Utell, M. J. (2014). Screening tests: A review with examples. *Inhalation Toxicology, 26*(13), 811–828. doi:10.3109/08958378.2014.955932

5. **D.** The attack rate is commonly used in disease outbreak investigations and is a key factor in the formulation of hypotheses. It is calculated as the number of cases in the population at risk divided by the number of people in the population at risk. Sometimes it may be impossible to calculate rates because the population at risk is not known. In such situations, the distribution of cases themselves may help in formulating hypotheses.

The disease status of the chef is irrelevant to the calculation of attack rate.

See: https://www.who.int/foodsafety/publications/foodborne_disease/Section_4.pdf

https://www.cdc.gov/csels/dsepd/ss1978/lesson3/quiz.html

6. **C.** Bias is defined as a systematic deviation of results or inferences from the truth or processes leading to such systematic deviation; any systematic tendency in the collection, analysis, interpretation, publication, or review of data that can lead to conclusions that are systematically different from the truth. In epidemiology, it does not imply intentional deviation.

Information bias is the systematic difference in the collection of data regarding the participants in a study (e.g., about exposures in a case–control study or about health outcomes in a cohort study) that leads to an incorrect result (e.g., risk ratio or odds ratio) or inference. Lead time bias is a kind of information bias associated with systematic error of apparent increased survival based on early detection of disease in an early stage. Length bias is also a kind of information bias associated with the systematic error from detecting disease with a long latency or preclinical period. Referral or volunteer bias is a form of selection bias associated with the systematic error that occurs from detecting disease in persons who are inclined to seek healthcare (regular or wellness checkups). Detection bias is associated with the detection of insignificant disease. Selection bias is the systematic difference in the enrollment of participants in a study that leads to an incorrect result (e.g., risk ratio or odds ratio) or inference.

See: https://www.cdc.gov/csels/dsepd/ss1978/glossary.html

7. **D.** A convenience sample consists of persons whose probability of selection is unknown. It is not possible to know how representative the sample is of the population from which it is selected. In contrast, probability samples have a known probability of their selection, and inferences can be drawn from the sample to the population from which it is selected. The probability sample is representative of the population from which it is drawn. Where populations are hidden because of stigma, discrimination, criminalized behaviors, or where sampling frames do not exist, nonprobability samples are often a necessity. Examples of nonprobability sampling methods include convenience, quota, and snowball (a type of chain-referral) sampling. The U.S. Census Bureau releases interim population projections of the resident population of the United States based on Census 2010 counts. The projections are produced with the general assumption that recent national trends in fertility, mortality, domestic migration, and international migration will continue.

See: https://wonder.cdc.gov/population.html

   https://www.census.gov/data.html

   https://www.cdc.gov/nchs/data/series/sr_02/sr02_113.pdf

   https://www.cdc.gov/nceh/hsb/disaster/casper/sampling.htm

8. **A.** In using a diagnostic test, the positive predictive value is the proportion of reported or identified cases that truly are cases, or the proportion of reported or identified epidemics that were actual epidemics. Conducting surveillance that has poor positive predictive value is wasteful, because the unsubstantiated or false-positive reports result in unnecessary investigations, wasteful allocation of resources, and, especially for false reports of epidemics, unwarranted public anxiety. When considering predictive values of diagnostic or screening tests, it is important to consider the influence of disease prevalence. As disease prevalence increases, the positive predictive value also increases but the negative predictive value decreases.

See: https://www.cdc.gov/csels/dsepd/ss1978/lesson5/appendixa.html

   https://www.cdc.gov/mmwr/preview/mmwrhtml/rr5013a1.htm

9. **B.** Herd immunity or community immunity refers to a situation in which a sufficient proportion of a population is immune to an infectious disease (through vaccination and/or prior illness) to make its spread from person to person unlikely. Even individuals not vaccinated (such as newborns and those with chronic illnesses) are offered some protection because the disease has little opportunity to spread within the community.

See: https://www.cdc.gov/vaccines/terms/glossary.html#commimmunity

10. **B.** Randomized clinical trials or randomized allocation refer to a type of allocation strategy in which participants are assigned to the arms of a clinical trial by chance. External validity refers to whether a program, practice, or policy can demonstrate preventive effects among a wide range of populations and contexts. For example, a parenting skills training program designed to prevent child maltreatment that demonstrated preventive effects in both urban and rural areas with different populations of parents would have high external validity.

The Best Available Research Evidence (BARE) enables researchers, practitioners, and policy makers to determine whether or not a prevention program, practice, or policy is actually achieving the outcomes it aims to and in the way it intends. The more rigorous a study's research design (e.g., randomized control trials, quasi-experimental designs), the more compelling the research evidence.

See: https://clinicaltrials.gov/ct2/about-studies/glossary

https://www.cdc.gov/violenceprevention/pdf/understanding_evidence-a.pdf

Zhang, X., Wu, Y., Ren, P., Liu, X., & Kang, D. (2015). The relationship between external and internal validity of randomized controlled trials: A sample of hypertension trials from China. *Contemporary Clinical Trials Communications, 1*, 32–38. doi:10.1016/j.conctc.2015.10.004

11. **C.** Incidence is a measure of the frequency with which new cases of illness, injury, or other health conditions occur among a population during a specified period.

Incidence proportion, the fraction of persons with new cases of illness, injury, or other health conditions during a specified period, is calculated as the number of new cases divided by the size of the population at the start of the study period.

Incidence rate (density), a measure of the frequency with which new cases of illness, injury, or other health conditions occur, is expressed explicitly per a time frame. Incidence rate is calculated as the number of new cases over a specified period divided by either the average population (usually mid-period) or the cumulative person-time the population was at risk.

See: https://www.cdc.gov/csels/dsepd/ss1978/glossary.html

12. **C.** In a case–control study, investigators start by enrolling a group of people with a certain disease. (At the Centers for Disease Control and Prevention [CDC], such persons are called case-patients rather than cases, because case refers to occurrence of disease, not a person.) As a comparison group, the investigator then enrolls a group of people without the disease (controls). Investigators then compare previous exposures between the two groups. The control group provides an estimate of the baseline or expected amount of exposure in that population. If the amount of exposure among the case group is substantially higher than the amount you would expect based on the control group, then illness is said to be associated with that exposure. The study of hepatitis A traced to green onions, described earlier, is an example of a case–control study. The key in a case–control study is to identify an appropriate control group, comparable to the case group in most respects, in order to provide a reasonable estimate of the baseline or expected exposure.

In a prospective cohort study, the epidemiologist records whether each study participant is exposed or not, and then tracks the participants to see whether they develop the disease of interest. Note that this differs from an experimental study because, in a cohort study, the investigator observes rather than determines the participants' exposure status. After a period of time, the investigator compares the disease rate in the exposed group with the disease rate in the unexposed group. The unexposed group serves as the comparison group, providing an estimate of the baseline or expected amount of disease occurrence in the community. If the disease rate is substantively different in the exposed group compared to the unexposed group, the exposure is said to be associated with illness.

The advantages of case–control studies include being efficient for rare diseases or diseases with a long latency period between exposure and disease manifestation, and it usually costs less and can be completed in a reasonable period of time, particularly when it is difficult to gather exposure data, for example, in a population that is highly mobile. However, case–control studies can be affected by selection or observation bias, and they are not efficient for rare exposures. The estimation of incidence is not possible through case–control study design.

See: https://www.cdc.gov/csels/dsepd/ss1978/lesson1/section7.html

13. **B.** Several models of disease causation have been proposed, including the epidemiologic triad or triangle, the traditional model for infectious disease. The triad consists of an external agent (e.g., infectious pathogen), a susceptible host, and an environment that brings the host and agent together. In this model, disease results from the interaction between the agent and the susceptible host in an environment that supports transmission of the agent from a source to that host. Agent, host, and environmental factors interrelate in a variety of complex ways to produce disease. Different diseases require different balances and interactions of these three components. Development of appropriate, practical, and effective public health measures to control or prevent disease usually requires assessment of all three components and their interactions.

The agent–host–environment model does not work well for many noninfectious diseases. Therefore, several other models that attempt to account for the multifactorial nature of causation have been proposed, including the Rothman Causal Pies model. An individual factor that contributes to cause disease is shown as a piece of a pie. After all the pieces of a pie fall into place, the pie is complete—and disease occurs. The individual factors are called component causes. The complete pie, which might be considered a causal pathway, is called a sufficient cause. A disease may have more than one sufficient cause, with each sufficient cause being composed of several component causes that may or may not overlap. A component that appears in every pie or pathway is called a necessary cause, because without it, disease does not occur. The component causes may include intrinsic host factors as well as the agent and the environmental factors of the agent–host–environment triad. A single component cause is rarely a sufficient cause by itself. For example, even exposure to a highly infectious agent such as measles virus does not invariably result in measles disease. Host susceptibility and other host factors also may play a role.

See: https://www.cdc.gov/csels/dsepd/ss1978/lesson1/section8.html

Rothman, K. J. (1976). Causes. *American Journal of Epidemiology, 104*, 587–592. doi:10.1093/oxfordjournals.aje.a112335

14. **A.** The cause-specific mortality rate is the mortality rate from a specified cause (disease or injury) for a population. The numerator is the number of deaths attributed to a specific cause. The denominator remains the size of the

population at the midpoint of the time period. The fraction is usually expressed per 100,000 population. For example, in the United States, in 2003, a total of 108,256 deaths were attributed to accidents (unintentional injuries), yielding a cause-specific mortality rate of 37.2 per 100,000 population. In this case, the cause-specific mortality rate and incidence rate coincide because of the high case-fatality rate.

See: https://www.cdc.gov/csels/dsepd/ss1978/lesson3/section3.html

15. **A.** The use of multiple tests to screen for disease can be desirable where multiple risk factors or biomarkers are associated with disease symptoms. Multiple tests may be conducted simultaneously or sequentially. In sequential screening, following the initial test, those who tested positive are subjected to a second test to reduce false positives. Thus, sequential screening can increase specificity.

See: https://www.cdc.gov/genomics/gtesting/file/print/FBR/CFClilUti
.pdf

https://www.cdc.gov/tb/publications/ltbi/pdf/USPSTF_Recommen
dation_Statement_Screening_For_Latent_TB_Infection_in_Adults.pdf

16. **B.** The best diagnostic tests are accurate and reproducible. The reproducibility of a test implies getting the same results on the same samples when tested by different individuals or different laboratories. This is the definition of test reliability. Test reliability can be measured by the use of the kappa coefficient, which adjusts the observed agreement for expected chance agreement. Therefore, reliability increases with a higher proportion of concordant observations.

See: https://www.cdc.gov/csels/dsepd/ss1978/lesson5/index.html

Gjørup, T. (1997). Reliability of diagnostic tests. *Acta Obstetricia et Gynecologica Scandinavica. 166*(Suppl.), 9–14.

17. **A.** SMR is the ratio of the observed number of deaths in a study population and the number of deaths that would be expected, based on the age- and sex-specific rates in a standard population and the population size of the study population by the same age/sex groups. Standardization is done to eliminate the distortion caused by different underlying age distributions in different populations. Statistical techniques are used to adjust or standardize the rates among the populations to be compared. These techniques take a weighted average of the age-specific mortality rates and eliminate the effect of different age distributions among the different populations. Mortality rates computed with these techniques are age-adjusted or age-standardized mortality rates. When SMR is higher than 1.0, the number of observed cases is higher than expected.

See: https://www.cdc.gov/csels/dsepd/ss1978/lesson3/section3.html

18. **B.** Infectious disease outbreaks are categorized by the way that the pathogen is spread within the population to infect new susceptible people. The source of the outbreak is the place or object of infection. Common source outbreaks refer to an outbreak where all cases are infected by the same source. Point source outbreaks refer to common source outbreaks where the source has infected cases at one particular geographical location, during a short period of time.

In such situations, the source is said to be located at a single point in time and place. These outbreaks have a typical bell-shaped epidemic curve that increases sharply, peaks, and then declines sharply, which reflects the normal distribution of the incubation period of the causative agent in humans. Therefore, the epidemic curve of a point source outbreak can help identify the moment of transmission. Continuing common source outbreaks refer to cases that have been infected by the same source over a prolonged period of time. For example, during the summer season a recreational lake can be the source of amoeba infections. The shape of the epidemic curve of such outbreaks does not increase sharply and does not peak; instead, it reaches a time-sustained plateau until the source is contained. Propagated outbreaks refer to a situation described by person-to-person transmission and cannot just be a point source outbreak. The shape of the epidemic curve in propagated outbreaks can vary and depends on the contact pattern and the proportion of susceptible individuals. When a transmissible pathogen is introduced into a fully susceptible population (e.g., flu), the epidemic curve increases sharply with incremental jumps, reflecting the generations of cases in the population.

See: https://www.cdc.gov/training/QuickLearns/exposure/pso.html

https://wiki.ecdc.europa.eu/fem/w/wiki/types-of-outbreak

19. **A.** An age-specific mortality rate is a mortality rate limited to a particular age group. The numerator is the number of deaths in that age group; the denominator is the number of persons in that age group in the population. In the United States, in 2003, a total of 130,761 deaths occurred among persons aged 25 to 44 years, or an age-specific mortality rate of 153.0 per 100,000 25- to 44-year olds. Age-adjusted mortality rates can be computed by the direct method. First, the annual age-specific rates for the population of interest are calculated. The product of the age-specific rates and the number in the comparable age-specific group in the standard population equals the expected number of deaths per million population for each age group. The total expected numbers of deaths are then obtained by summing over all age groups. The total expected number of deaths is divided by the sum of the standard population and the resulting quotient is multiplied by 1,000,000 to produce the age-adjusted rate (per million). Indirect age-adjustment involves applying a common set of age-specific rates to the populations whose rates are to be standardized.

See: https://www.cdc.gov/csels/dsepd/ss1978/lesson3/section3.html

Naing, N. N. (2000). Easy way to learn standardization: Direct and indirect methods. *The Malaysian Journal of Medical Sciences: MJMS, 7*(1), 10–15. Retrieved from https://www.ncbi.nlm.nih.gov/pmc/articles/PMC3406211

20. **C.** In a case–control study, investigators start by enrolling a group of people with disease. As a comparison group, the investigator then enrolls a group of people without disease (controls). Investigators then compare previous exposures between the two groups. The control group provides an estimate of the baseline or expected amount of exposure in that population. If the amount of exposure among the case group is substantially higher than the amount you would expect based on the control group, then illness is said to be associated with that exposure. The study of hepatitis A traced to green onions, described earlier, is an example of a case–control study. The key in a case–control study

is to identify an appropriate control group, comparable to the case group in most respects, in order to provide a reasonable estimate of the baseline or expected exposure. Recall bias is more likely to affect results because data is collected retrospectively.

See: https://www.cdc.gov/csels/dsepd/ss1978/lesson1/section7.html

21. **D.** Ecological study designs are those in which disease rates are linked to the level of exposure to some risk factor for the target population as a whole. Ecological studies are subject to inference fallacy, whereby inferences about disease status are made about a specific individual in a population of exposed individuals where exposure data are aggregated. Ecological studies are useful for generating hypotheses that can be tested with existing data for large populations and the large number of risk-modifying behaviors that may be investigated.

    Much epidemiologic research is devoted to searching for causal factors that influence one's risk of disease. Ideally, the goal is to identify a cause so that appropriate public health action might be taken. One can argue that epidemiology can never prove a causal relationship between an exposure and a disease, since much of epidemiology is based on ecologic reasoning. Nevertheless, epidemiology often provides enough information to support effective action. Examples of ecological studies date from the removal of the handle from the Broad St. pump following John Snow's investigation of cholera in the Golden Square area of London in 1854 to the withdrawal of a vaccine against rotavirus in 1999 after epidemiologists found that it increased the risk of intussusception, a potentially life-threatening condition.

    See: https://www.cdc.gov/csels/dsepd/ss1978/lesson1/section7.html

    https://www.cdc.gov/csels/dsepd/ss1978/index.html

    Grant, W. B. (2014). A multi-country ecological study of cancer incidence rates in 2008 with respect to various risk-modifying factors. *Nutrients, 6*(1), 163–189. doi:10.3390/nu6010163

22. **C.** In a case–control study, investigators start by enrolling a group of people with a disease. As a comparison group, the investigator then enrolls a group of people without the disease (controls). Investigators then compare previous exposures between the two groups. The control group provides an estimate of the baseline or expected amount of exposure in that population. If the amount of exposure among the case group is substantially higher than the amount you would expect based on the control group, then illness is said to be associated with that exposure. The study of hepatitis A traced to green onions, described earlier, is an example of a case–control study. The key in a case–control study is to identify an appropriate control group, comparable to the case group in most respects, in order to provide a reasonable estimate of the baseline or expected exposure. Ideally, the control group in a case–control study should be selected from the same population in which cases were selected.

    See: https://www.cdc.gov/csels/dsepd/ss1978/lesson1/section7.html

23. **A.** The matched pair case–control study calculates the statistical relationship between exposures and the likelihood of becoming ill in a given patient population. This study is used to investigate a cause of an illness by selecting a non-ill person as the control and matching the control to a case. The control

can be matched to one or more criteria, and ideally they should be matched on confounding variables of interest to the study hypothesis.

See: https://www.cdc.gov/epiinfo/user-guide/statcalc/matchedpaircase control.html

24. **C.** A systematic difference between cases and controls that results in a mistaken estimate of the association between exposure and disease is referred to as bias. A systematic deviation of results or inferences from the truth or processes leading to such systematic deviation; or any systematic tendency in the collection, analysis, interpretation, publication, or review of data can lead to conclusions that are systematically different from the truth. This does not imply intentional deviation. Information bias is a type of systematic error in the difference in the collection of data regarding the participants in a study (e.g., about exposures in a case–control study, or about health outcomes in a cohort study) that leads to an incorrect result (e.g., risk ratio or odds ratio) or inference. Selection bias is a systematic difference in the enrollment of participants in a study that leads to an incorrect result (e.g., risk ratio or odds ratio) or inference. Bias tends to over- or underestimate the true effect.

See: https://www.cdc.gov/csels/dsepd/ss1978/glossary.html

25. **A.** Surveillance bias, also known as detection bias, can arise in a prospective cohort study when human participants in one exposure group are subjected to increased surveillance, screening, or testing for the outcome, and, as such, have a higher probability of having the study outcome (disease) detected. For example, postmenopausal exposure to estrogen is associated with an increased risk of bleeding that can trigger screening for endometrial cancers, leading to a higher probability of early stage endometrial cancers being detected. Any association between estrogen exposure and endometrial cancer potentially overestimates risk, because unexposed patients with subclinical cancers would have a lower probability of their cancer being diagnosed or recorded. This nonrandom type of misclassification bias can be reduced by selecting an unexposed comparator group with a similar likelihood of screening or testing, selecting outcomes that are likely to be diagnosed equally in both exposure groups, or by adjusting for the surveillance rate in the analysis.

See: http://www.encepp.eu/standards_and_guidances/methodological Guide4_2_2_5.shtml

Haut, E. R. (2011). Surveillance bias in outcomes reporting. *Journal of the American Medical Association, 305*(23), 2462–2463. doi:10.1001/jama.2011.822

Horwitz, R. I., & Feinstein, A. R. (1978). Alternative analytic methods for case-control studies of estrogens and endometrial cancer. *New England Journal of Medicine, 299*(20), 1089–1094. doi:10.1056/NEJM197811162992001

26. **C.** Case–crossover design is a special type of intervention cohort study where the same individuals are exposed to two different interventions over two separate time periods. This can be done if the outcome of the first intervention can be recording in a reasonable period of time so as not to affect the follow-up intervention. Thus, the individuals serve as their own controls.

See Field Epidemiology Manual—A set of training materials for professionals working in intervention epidemiology, public health microbiology, and infection control and hospital hygiene. https://wiki.ecdc.europa.eu/fem/w/wiki/case-cross-over-studies

See: https://www.cdc.gov/niosh/nioshtic-2/20029392.html

27. **D.** The AF (attributable risk percent) is a measure of the public health impact of a causative risk factor (e.g., tobacco smoking). The calculation of AF assumes that the occurrence of disease in the unexposed group represents the baseline or expected risk for that disease (e.g., lung cancer). It further assumes that if the risk of disease in the exposed group is higher than the risk in the unexposed group, the difference can be attributed to the exposure. Thus, the AF is the amount of disease in the exposed group attributable to the exposure. It represents the expected reduction in disease if the exposure (smoking) could be removed (or never existed). Appropriate use of attributable proportion depends on a single risk factor being responsible for a condition. When multiple risk factors may interact (e.g., physical activity and age or health status), this measure may not be appropriate. For example, lung cancer cases may be associated with tobacco smoke, radon, asbestos, and other risk factors. The assumption is that there is no interaction among these risk factors.

See: https://www.cdc.gov/csels/dsepd/ss1978/lesson3/section6.html

28. **A.** Sir Austin Bradford Hill's classic guidelines detailed the association and causation in the relationship between risk factors and diseases. The guidelines were meant to prevent spurious associations that can occur by chance, result from systematic error, or lead to limitations of a study design.

See: https://www.who.int/bulletin/volumes/83/10/792.pdf

https://www.cdc.gov/mmwr/preview/mmwrhtml/00001797.htm

https://www.cdc.gov/csels/dsepd/ss1978/lesson1/section8.html

Cox, L. A., Jr. (2018, November 15). Modernizing the Bradford Hill criteria for assessing causal relationships in observational data. *Critical Review in Toxicology, 48*(8), 682–712. doi:10.1080/10408444.2018.1518404

Rothman, K. J. (1976). Causes. *American Journal of Epidemiology, 104,* 587–592. doi:10.1093/oxfordjournals.aje.a112335

29. **A.** Random or nondifferential misclassification occurs when classifications of disease status or exposure occur equally in all study groups being compared (cases and controls). This means that the probability of exposure being misclassified is independent of disease status and the probability of disease status being misclassified is independent of exposure status. Nondifferential misclassification increases the similarity between the exposed and nonexposed groups and may result in an underestimate (dilution) of the true strength of an association between exposure and disease.

Nonrandom or differential misclassification occurs when the proportions of subjects misclassified differ between the study groups (cases and controls). This means that the probability of exposure being misclassified is dependent on disease status, or the probability of disease status being misclassified is dependent on exposure status. Differential misclassification is considered a more serious problem because the effect is that the observed estimate is either an overestimate or underestimate of the true association.

See: https://www.cdc.gov/niosh/nioshtic-2/00200889.html

https://www.healthknowledge.org.uk/e-learning/epidemiology/
practitioners/errors-epidemiological-measurements

30. **A.** The nature–nurture debate is enduring in disease causation. Increased understanding of gene–environment interactions has revealed insights suggesting that rather than a discrete solution, most disease symptoms are on a continuum where environmental factors influence the genetic predisposition. Study designs where adopted children (siblings) develop with different parents or in different environments can reveal the conservative roles of genetics and the influence of environment on the phenotypes.

See: https://www.sciencedirect.com/topics/medicine-and-dentistry/
adoption-studies

31. **D.** The probability of finding an association as strong as (or stronger than) observable by chance if the null hypothesis (no association) were really true is determined through the statistical significance test. This probability is called a p value. A very small p value means that it is unlikely to observe such an association if the null hypothesis were true. A small p value indicates that the null hypothesis is implausible given the data. If this p value is smaller than some predetermined cutoff (usually 0.05 or 5%), the null hypothesis can be rejected, and the alternative hypothesis that exposure and disease are associated is accepted. The association is then said to be "statistically significant."

See: https://www.cdc.gov/globalhealth/healthprotection/fetp/training_
modules/11/large-data-sets_pw_final_09252013.pdf

https://www.cdc.gov/training/SIC_CaseStudy/Interpreting_Odds_
ptversion.pdf

32. **B.** Statistical power is the likelihood that a study will detect an effect when there is a true effect. If statistical power is high, the probability of making a Type II error decreases (wrongly failing to reject the null hypothesis), as well as concluding there is no effect when, in fact, there is one.

See: https://www.statisticsdonewrong.com/power.html

http://powerandsamplesize.com

33. **A.** There are two types of errors in hypothesis testing. Type I error is rejecting the null when it is true, and Type II error is failing to reject the null when it is false. The probability of a Type I error in hypothesis testing is predetermined by the significance level. The probability of a Type II error depends on the true population mean which is unknown, but can be computed if we know the μ, σ^2, and n. The statistical power of a hypothesis test is 1 minus the probability of a Type II error.

34. **A.** The binomial distribution states the probability that a number of positive outcomes occurs given the expected percentage of positive outcomes and the total number of observations taken.

The Poisson distribution is used to describe the distribution of rare events in a large population or discrete quantitative data such as disease cases in a large population; for example, the number of deaths in a town from a particular disease per day or the number of admissions to a particular hospital.

The normal or Gaussian distribution represents real-valued random variables whose distributions are not known. Normal distribution is defined by a mathematical equation where the mean, median, and mode coincide at the central peak, but the area under the curve helps determine measures of spread such as the standard deviation and confidence interval.

The lognormal distribution is a continuous probability distribution of a random variable whose logarithm is normally distributed.

See: https://www.cdc.gov/csels/dsepd/ss1978/lesson2/section4.html

https://www.pnas.org/content/108/Supplement_3/15549

https://www.cdc.gov/cancer/uscs/technical_notes/stat_methods/confidence.htm

35. C. Population parameters may be estimated as a single value, for example, the mean, or as an interval estimate that specifies a range within which the parameter (mean) is estimated to lie. Confidence intervals show the reliability of the point estimates. Typically, a sufficiently large probability sample will have point estimates that are approximately normally distributed. The end points of the confidence interval, then, are a function of the estimate, its standard error, and a percentile of the normal distribution with zero mean and unit variance, referred to as the standard normal deviate (z score).

Method for calculating a 95% confidence interval for a mean

Step 1. Calculate the mean and its standard error.

Step 2. Multiply the standard error by 1.96.

Step 3. Lower limit of the 95% confidence interval = mean minus 1.96 × standard error.

Upper limit of the 95% confidence interval = mean plus 1.96 × standard error.

For 95%, the z score is **1.960.**

Confidence interval is calculated by

$X \pm zs\sqrt{n}$

where

- X is the mean.
- z is the chosen z score.
- s is the standard deviation.
- n is the number of observations.

The narrower the confidence interval, the more precise the estimate; the range of values in the interval is the range of population values most consistent with the data from the study.

See: https://www.cdc.gov/csels/dsepd/ss1978/lesson2/section7.html

https://www.cdc.gov/cancer/uscs/technical_notes/stat_methods/confidence.htm

https://www.cdc.gov/nchs/tutorials/NHANES/NHANESAnalyses/HypothesisTesting/Info2.htm

https://www.mathsisfun.com/data/confidence-interval.html

36. **C.** The advertised claim that "80% of our customers quit smoking for at least one year" after starting the program is not demonstrably false, but fewer participants successfully quit smoking than expected, but not so few that the advertised claim can be discredited based on the intervals.

37. **B.** The normal or Gaussian distribution represents real-valued random variables whose distributions are not known. Normal distribution is defined by a mathematical equation where the mean, median, and mode coincide at the central peak, but the area under the curve helps determine measures of spread such as the standard deviation and confidence interval.

    See: https://www.cdc.gov/csels/dsepd/ss1978/lesson2/section4.html

38. **B.** The standardized morbidity ratio (SMR) is the ratio of observed to expected number of cases in the study population under the assumption that the morbidity rates for the study population are the same as those for the general population. For nonfatal conditions, the standardized mortality ratio is sometimes known as the SMR.

    The observed number of cases in Woburn is 12. The expected number of cases is 6. SMR = 12/6 = 2.

    p value = 0.014

    Chi-square = 6

    Mid-p exact confidence interval = 1.08, 3.40

    Fisher's exact confidence interval = 1.03, 3.49

    See: http://web1.sph.emory.edu/users/cdckms/exact-midP-SMR.html

    https://www.openepi.com/SMR/SMR.htm

    https://www.openepi.com/PDFDocs/SMRDoc.pdf

39. **C.** To increase statistical power, the following approaches are recommended:

    Increase alpha

    Conduct a one-tailed test

    Increase the effect size

    Decrease random error

    Increase sample size

    Hansen, W. B., & Collins, L. M. (1994). Seven ways to increase power without increasing N. *NIDA Research Monograph, 142,* 184–195. Retrieved from https://www.ncbi.nlm.nih.gov/pubmed/9243537

40. **B.** Measures of central location are single values that represent the center of the observed distribution of values. The different measures of central location represent the center in different ways. The arithmetic mean represents the balance point for all the data. The median represents the middle of the data, with half the observed values below the median and half the observed values above it. The mode represents the peak or most prevalent value. The geometric mean is comparable to the arithmetic mean on a logarithmic scale.

    The median is the number that is halfway in a set of data arranged in order from least to greatest. If there is an even number of items in the dataset, then the median is found by taking the mean (average) of the two middlemost numbers.

See: https://www.cdc.gov/csels/dsepd/ss1978/lesson2/summary.html

41. C.

Total numbers (N): 10

Sum of numbers: 234.0

Mean (average) value: 23.4

Population standard deviation (σ): 3.69

Population variance (σ^2): 13.64

Sample standard deviation (s): 3.89

Sample variance (s2): 15.16

$\mu = M \pm Z(s_M)$

where

M = sample mean

Z = Z statistic determined by confidence level

s_M = standard error = $\sqrt{(s^2/n)}$

$M = 23.4$

$Z = 1.96$

$s_M = \sqrt{(3.69^2/10)} = 1.17$

$\mu = M \pm Z(s_M)$

$\mu = 23.4 \pm 1.96 \times 1.17$

$\mu = 23.4 \pm 2.287$

See: https://www.socscistatistics.com/confidenceinterval/default3.aspx

42. A.

Mean (average) value: 23.4

Sample variance (s^2): 15.16

Sample standard deviation (s): 3.89

Population variance (σ^2): 13.64

Obese BMI = 30

Area under normal distribution curve

$Z = X - u/\sigma$

$30 - 23.4 / 3.89 = 1.69$

Area under curve (z score) = 0.045 or 4.5%

See: http://onlinestatbook.com/2/calculators/normal_dist.html

http://www.z-table.com

43. C. Sensitivity is the ability of a surveillance test to detect the health problem that it is intended to detect (true positives).

Specificity is the ability of a surveillance test to correctly identify a negative result for those who do not have the condition (true negatives).

$$\text{True negatives}/(\text{false positives} + \text{true negatives})$$

Seven students reported BMI <25. 30% of these are false negatives

See: https://www.cdc.gov/csels/dsepd/ss1978/lesson5/appendixa.html

44. B. Tests with low sensitivity are not very useful as screening tests to exclude the presence of a disease in a population. Test sensitivity is independent of disease prevalence; however, the confidence level of a test's sensitivity depends on the sample size. Tests performed on small sample sizes have wide confidence intervals, implying imprecision. The inaccuracy introduced by the false self-reports means that the confidence interval should be higher than originally calculated.

45. C. Positive predictive value is the proportion of reported or identified cases that truly are cases, or the proportion of reported or identified epidemics that were actual epidemics. Conducting surveillance that has poor positive predictive value is wasteful, because the unsubstantiated or false-positive reports result in unnecessary investigations, wasteful allocation of resources, and, especially for false reports of epidemics, unwarranted public anxiety.

Calculation of Positive Predictive Value, Sensitivity, and Specificity for Surveillance				
		True case or outbreak		
		Yes	No	Total
Detected by surveillance?	Yes	True positive (A)	False positive (B)	Total detected by surveillance (A + B)
	No	False negative (C)	True negative (D)	Total missed by surveillance (C + D)
	Total	Total true cases or outbreaks (A + C)	Total non-cases or nonoutbreaks (B + D)	Total (A + B + C + D)

Positive predictive value = A/(A + B)
Sensitivity = A/(A + C)
Specificity = D/(B + D)

See: https://www.cdc.gov/csels/dsepd/ss1978/lesson5/appendixa.html

46. B. The true mean of measurements of a large population is often unknown, so we need confidence intervals for measurements on a sample for which we can be certain of the mean.

Total numbers (N): 50

Mean (average) value after 1 month: 100 mg/dL

Sample variance (s2): 40 mg^2/dL^2

Standard deviation is the square root of the sample variance = 6.32.

$M = 100$

$Z = 1.96$

$s_M = \sqrt{(6.32^2/50)} = 0.89$

$\mu = M \pm Z(s_M)$

$\mu = 100 \pm 1.96 \times 0.89$

$\mu = 100 \pm 1.75$

See: https://www.socscistatistics.com/confidenceinterval/default3.aspx

47. D. The information provided does not include information on the distribution of decreases in fasting blood glucose during the intervention, so we cannot determine the confidence interval for the average decrease.

48. D. The chi-square test is used to test the independence of two variables cross-classified in a two-way table. (A chi-square statistic with n degrees of freedom is based on a statistic equal to the sum of the squares of n independent normally distributed random variables with mean = 0 and unit variance.)

The binomial distribution states the probability that a number of positive outcomes occur given the expected percentage of positive outcomes and the total number of observations taken.

To analyze the Poisson distribution, enter the expected number of positive outcomes in the expected number of events and the value of positive outcomes you would like to determine the probability of the observed number of events.

See: https://www.cdc.gov/epiinfo/user-guide/statcalc/poisson.html

49. A. In a population defined by normal distribution, a two-tailed test is used in null hypothesis testing and testing for statistical significance to examine whether a sample is greater than or less than a certain range of values. The alternative hypothesis is accepted instead of the null hypothesis if the sample being tested falls into either of the critical areas.

Effect size measured by Cohen's d indicates the standardized difference between two means.

The larger the sample variance (σ^2), the lower the statistical power:

$Z = M$(difference) / sigma/square root of N

Increasing σ^2 lowers z and power.

Cohen's $d = (M_2 - M_1)/SD_{pooled}$

$SD_{pooled} = \sqrt{((SD_1^2 + SD_2^2)/2)}$

50. B. Relative Risk (RR) compares the risk of a health event (disease, injury, risk factor, or death) among one group with the risk among another group. It does so by dividing the risk (incidence proportion, attack rate) in group 1 by the risk (incidence proportion, attack rate) in group 2. The two groups are typically differentiated by such demographic factors as sex (e.g., males versus females) or by exposure to a suspected risk factor (e.g., smoking versus nonsmoking). Often, the group of primary interest is labeled the exposed group, and the comparison group is labeled the unexposed group.

Relative risk is a ratio that expresses how many times more probable the outcome is in the exposed group, so, it is best to interpret the results as multiples of risk, for example, "so many times the risk" or "so many times as high as." Hence, smokers had 15 times the risk compared to nonsmokers.

See: https://www.cdc.gov/csels/dsepd/ss1978/lesson3/section5.html

51. **A.** Theories and models used to understand behavioral change include the following:

Learning theories

Health Belief Model

Transtheoretical Model

Relapse Prevention Model

Theory of reasoned action and theory of planned behavior

Social Learning/Social Cognitive Theory

Social support

Ecological approaches

The Social-Ecological Model includes specific reference to the individual

See https://www.cdc.gov/nccdphp/sgr/pdf/chap6.pdf

https://www.cdc.gov/nccdphp/sgr/chap6.htm

https://www.cdc.gov/violenceprevention/publichealthissue/social-ecologicalmodel.html

52. **D.** The human biome project does not exist.

See https://www.healthypeople.gov

https://www.who.int/social_determinants/tools/multimedia/alma_ata/en

Lalonde, M. (1974). *A new perspective on the health of Canadians. A working document.* Ottawa: Government of Canada.

53. **B.** In the Transtheoretical Model, behavior change is conceptualized as a five-stage process or continuum related to an individual's readiness to change: precontemplation, contemplation, preparation, action, and maintenance. A criticism of most theories and models of behavior change is that they emphasize individual behavior change processes and pay little attention to sociocultural and physical environmental influences on behavior, hence, the emergence of socio-ecological models.

See https://www.cdc.gov/nccdphp/sgr/pdf/chap6.pdf

https://wwwn.cdc.gov/CHIdatabase/items/individually-adapted-health-behavior-change

54. **D.** Increasing emphasis has been placed on the importance of evidence-informed prevention strategies and evidence-based decision-making. Definitions of what constitutes "evidence" have been debated but most agree that evidence is extremely important for researchers, practitioners, and

policy makers charged with the task of making decisions around the funding and implementation of disease prevention strategies. Thus, theory, research, and practice should inform one another. This is the foundation of the translational sciences.

See https://www.cdc.gov/violenceprevention/pdf/understanding_evidence-a.pdf

55. **A.** Social phenomena are the individual, external, and social constructions that influence people's lives and development, and are constantly evolving throughout the life course. The health promotion agenda is influenced by Social-Ecological Theory, a systematic approach to understanding the interrelations across the individual-relationship-community-society domains.

See https://www.atsdr.cdc.gov/communityengagement/pce_models.html

56. **C.** The Social-Ecological Model conceptualizes health broadly and focuses on multiple factors that might affect health. This broad approach to thinking of health, advanced in the 1947 Constitution of the World Health Organization, includes physical, mental, and social well-being. The Social-Ecological Model understands health to be affected by the interaction between the individual, the group/community, and the physical, social, and political environments. There is a temporal dimension to health behavior change.

See https://www.atsdr.cdc.gov/communityengagement/pce_models.html

57. **C.** The Health Belief Model provides a theoretical framework to help explain and predict the uptake of disease prevention behaviors. The model posits that persons will engage in a health-protective action if they:

- Believe that a negative health condition can be avoided
- Believe that, by taking a recommended action, they will avoid a negative health condition
- Believe that they can successfully take a recommended health action

According to the model, a person's likelihood of engaging in health-promoting behavior is determined by four main antecedents:

- Perceived susceptibility to a certain health condition
- Perceived severity of the health condition and its consequences
- Perceived barriers to engaging in the advised action
- Perceived benefits to taking health action

These perceptions vary according to various populations and sociocultural attributes, which make generalizability difficult or impossible.

See: https://wwwnc.cdc.gov/eid/article/25/1/18-0824-techapp1.pdf

58. **A.** The theory of reasoned action states that the individual performance of a given behavior is primarily determined by a person's intention to perform that behavior. This intention is determined by two major factors: the person's attitude toward the behavior (i.e., beliefs about the outcomes of the behavior and the value of these outcomes) and the influence of the person's social environment or subjective norm (i.e., beliefs about what other people think the person should do, as well as the person's motivation to comply with the opinions of others). The theory of planned behavior adds to the theory of reasoned action the concept of perceived control over the opportunities, resources, and skills necessary to perform a behavior.

The Expectancy-Value Theory posits that people's achievement-related choices are most proximally determined by expectancies for success and subjective task values. Expectancies refer to how confident an individual is in his or her ability to succeed in a task, whereas task values refer to how important, useful, or enjoyable the individual perceives the task.

See: https://www.cdc.gov/nccdphp/sgr/pdf/chap6.pdf

Ajzen, I. (1988). *Attitudes, personality, and behavior* (U.S. ed.). Chicago, IL: Dorsey Press.

59. **A.** There is no "perceived mind control."

The theory of planned behavior adds to the theory of reasoned action the concept of perceived control over the opportunities, resources, and skills necessary to perform a behavior.

See: https://www.cdc.gov/nccdphp/sgr/pdf/chap6.pdf

60. **C.** Behavioral intention is defined as a person's perceived likelihood or subjective probability that he or she will engage in a particular behavior. Intention is behavior-specific and operationalized by direct questions such as "I intend to do_____," with Likert scale response choices to measure relative strength of intention. Intention reflects how hard a person is willing to try, and how motivated the person is, to perform the behavior. The theory of reasoned action states that individual performance of a given behavior is primarily determined by a person's intention to perform that behavior. This intention is determined by two major factors: the person's attitude toward the behavior (i.e., beliefs about the outcomes of the behavior and the value of these outcomes) and the influence of the person's social environment or subjective norm (i.e., beliefs about what other people think the person should do, as well as the person's motivation to comply with the opinions of others).

See: https://chirr.nlm.nih.gov/behavioral-intention.php

https://www.cdc.gov/nccdphp/sgr/pdf/chap6.pdf

61. **C.** In the Transtheoretical Model, behavior change is conceptualized as a five-stage process or continuum related to an individual's readiness to change: precontemplation, contemplation, preparation, action, and maintenance. A criticism of most theories and models of behavior change is that they emphasize individual behavior change processes and pay little attention to sociocultural and physical environmental influences on behavior; hence, the emergence of socio-ecological models.

See: https://www.cdc.gov/nccdphp/sgr/pdf/chap6.pdf

https://wwwn.cdc.gov/CHIdatabase/items/individually-adapted -health-behavior-change

62. **D.** In the Transtheoretical Model, behavior change is conceptualized as a five-stage process or continuum related to an individual's readiness to change: precontemplation, contemplation, preparation, action, and maintenance. A criticism of most theories and models of behavior change is that they emphasize individual behavior change processes and pay little attention to sociocultural and physical environmental influences on behavior, hence, the emergence of socio-ecological models.

See: https://www.cdc.gov/nccdphp/sgr/pdf/chap6.pdf

https://wwwn.cdc.gov/CHIdatabase/items/individually-adapted
-health-behavior-change

63. A. In the TTM, behavior change is conceptualized as a five-stage process or continuum related to an individual's readiness to change: precontemplation, contemplation, preparation, action, and maintenance. A criticism of most theories and models of behavior change is that they emphasize individual behavior change processes and pay little attention to sociocultural and physical environmental influences on behavior, hence, the emergence of socio-ecological models.

See: https://mdquit.org/health-behavior-models/transtheoretical-model
-ttm

Campbell, S., Bohanna, I., Swinbourne, A., Cadet-James, Y., McKeown, D., & McDermott, R. (2013). Stages of change, smoking behaviour and readiness to quit in a large sample of indigenous Australians living in eight remote north Queensland communities. *International Journal of Environmental Research and Public Health, 10*(4), 1562–1571. doi:10.3390/ijerph10041562

Prochaska, J. O., Redding, C. A., & Evers, K. E. (2015). The Transtheoretical Model and stages of change (Chapter 7). In K. Glanz, B. K. Rimer, & K. Viswanath (eds.), *Health Behavior: Theory, Research, and Practice* (5th ed). pp. 125–148.

Spencer, L., Pagell, F., Hallion, M. E., & Adams, T. B. (2002). Applying the Transtheoretical Model to tobacco cessation and prevention: A review of literature. *American Journal of Health Promotion, 17*(1), 7–71. doi:10.4278/0890-1171-17.1.7

64. A. The Social-Ecological Model conceptualizes health broadly and focuses on multiple factors that might affect health. This broad approach to thinking of health, advanced in the 1947 Constitution of the World Health Organization, includes physical, mental, and social well-being. The Social-Ecological Model understands health to be affected by the interaction between the individual, the group/community, and the physical, social, and political environments.

Both the community engagement approach and the Social-Ecological Model recognize the complex role played by context in the development of health problems as well as in the success or failure of attempts to address these problems. Health professionals, researchers, and community leaders can use this model to identify factors at different levels (the individual, the interpersonal level, the community, society) that contribute to poor health and to develop approaches to disease prevention and health promotion that include action at those levels. This approach focuses on integrating approaches to change the physical and social environments rather than modifying only individual health behaviors.

Four core principles that underlie the ways the Social-Ecological Model can contribute to efforts to engage communities:

- Health status, emotional well-being, and social cohesion are influenced by the physical, social, and cultural dimensions of the individual's or community's environment and personal attributes (e.g., behavior patterns, psychology, and genetics).

- The same environment may have different effects on an individual's health depending on a variety of factors, including perceptions of ability to control the environment and financial resources.
- Individuals and groups operate in multiple environments (e.g., workplace, neighborhood, larger geographic communities) that "spill over" and influence each other.
- There are personal and environmental "leverage points," such as the physical environment, available resources, and social norms, that exert vital influences on health and well-being.

See: https://www.atsdr.cdc.gov/communityengagement/pce_models.html

65. **A.** Social Cognitive Theory proposes that behavior change is affected by environmental influences, personal factors, and attributes of the behavior itself. Each may affect or be affected by either of the other two. A central tenet of Social Cognitive Theory is the concept of self-efficacy. A person must believe in his or her capability to perform the behavior (i.e., the person must possess self-efficacy) and must perceive an incentive to do so (i.e., the person's positive expectations from performing the behavior must outweigh the negative expectations). Additionally, a person must value the outcomes or consequences that he or she believes will occur as a result of performing a specific behavior or action. Outcomes may be classified as having immediate benefits (e.g., feeling energized following physical activity) or long-term benefits (e.g., experiencing improvements in cardiovascular health as a result of physical activity).

See https://www.cdc.gov/nccdphp/sgr/pdf/chap6.pdf

66. **A.** Social Cognitive Theory proposes that behavior change is affected by environmental influences, personal factors, and attributes of the behavior itself. Each may affect or be affected by either of the other two. A central tenet of Social Cognitive Theory is the concept of self-efficacy. A person must believe in his or her capability to perform the behavior (i.e., the person must possess self-efficacy) and must perceive an incentive to do so (i.e., the person's positive expectations from performing the behavior must outweigh the negative expectations). Additionally, a person must value the outcomes or consequences that he or she believes will occur as a result of performing a specific behavior or action. Outcomes may be classified as having immediate benefits (e.g., feeling energized following physical activity) or long-term benefits (e.g., experiencing improvements in cardiovascular health as a result of physical activity).

See: https://www.cdc.gov/nccdphp/sgr/pdf/chap6.pdf

67. **A.** Community-based social support interventions focus on changing physical activity behavior through building, strengthening, and maintaining social networks that provide supportive relationships for behavior change (e.g., setting up a buddy system or a walking group to provide friendship and support).

The Social-Ecological Model conceptualizes health broadly and focuses on multiple factors that might affect health. This broad approach to thinking of health, advanced in the 1947 Constitution of the World Health Organization, includes physical, mental, and social well-being. The Social-Ecological Model understands health to be affected by the interaction between the individual, the group/community, and the physical, social, and political environments.

See: https://www.cdc.gov/mmwr/preview/mmwrhtml/mm5417a4.htm

https://wwwn.cdc.gov/CHIdatabase/items/social-support-in -community-settings

68. **D.** Peer pressure is not an agreeable form of social support.

Community-based social support interventions focus on changing physical activity behavior through building, strengthening, and maintaining social networks that provide supportive relationships for behavior change (e.g., setting up a buddy system or a walking group to provide friendship and support).

The Social-Ecological Model conceptualizes health broadly and focuses on multiple factors that might affect health. This broad approach to thinking of health, advanced in the 1947 Constitution of the World Health Organization, includes physical, mental, and social well-being. The Social-Ecological Model understands health to be affected by the interaction between the individual, the group/community, and the physical, social, and political environments.

See: https://www.cdc.gov/ncbddd/childdevelopment/positiveparenting/ adolescence.html

https://www.cdc.gov/mmwr/preview/mmwrhtml/mm5417a4.htm

https://wwwn.cdc.gov/CHIdatabase/items/social-support-in -community-settings

69. **B.** Social networks can be a key factor in determining how healthy a community is. For one thing, they can create social supports that provide a buffer against the stressors that damage health. Social networks may also have negative effects on health. "Clusters" of obesity within a network of people were studied over time. Their longitudinal analysis suggested that these clusters were not merely the result of like-minded or similarly situated people forming ties with one another, but rather reflected the "spread" of obesity among people who were connected to each other. Although not everyone agrees on how social networks affect health, they seem to play a role, together with culture, economics, and other factors, that is important for both individuals and communities.

See: https://www.atsdr.cdc.gov/communityengagement/pce_social_ health.html

70. **D.** It is illegal to conduct research with children without informed consent through parental approval, although there are variations on the policy.

National Institutes of Health (NIH) policy (NOT-OD-18-116) requires individuals of all ages, including children, to be included in NIH-supported research unless there is a scientific or ethical reason not to include them. There are also specific requirements that apply to research involving children in 45 Code of Federal Regulations (CFR) 46 Subpart D. NIH defines a child as an individual under the age of 18. Note that "children" is defined in 45 CFR 46 Link to Non-U.S. Government Site—Click for Disclaimer as "persons who have not attained the legal age for consent to treatments or procedures involved in the research, under the applicable law of the jurisdiction in which the research will be conducted." Important points from 45 CFR 46 regarding research with children:

Exemption 2 does not apply to research with children except for research involving observations of public behavior when the investigator(s) do not participate in the activities being observed.

Research with children may require assent from the child in addition to permission from a parent(s).

Research involving greater than minimal risk is permitted with children only under specific conditions, and requirements depend on the prospect or absence of direct benefit to the individual participants.

When children are wards of the State or other agency/institution/entity, an advocate may be required in addition to an individual acting on behalf of the child as a guardian or in loco parentis.

The federal regulations list eight required elements of informed consent. These are the following:

1. Purpose and procedures—You must tell a prospective participant that the study involves research, explain the purpose of the study and the length of time you expect the person to participate, describe the procedures to be followed, and identify any experimental procedures.
2. Risks—You must describe any reasonably foreseeable risks or discomforts to the prospective participant.
3. Benefits—You must describe any benefits to the prospective participant or to others which may reasonably be expected from the research.
4. Alternatives—You must disclose any appropriate alternative procedures or courses of treatment that might benefit the prospective participant.
5. Confidentiality—You must tell prospective participants whether their records will be kept confidential and, if so, explain the level of confidentiality.
6. When there is greater than minimal risk—You must tell prospective participants whether they will receive any compensation and/or medical treatments if injury occurs and, if so, what compensation or treatment will consist of, or where to obtain further information.
7. Persons to Contact—You must tell prospective participants whom to contact if they have questions about the research and their rights as study participants, and whom to contact if they have an injury that may be related to the research.
8. Voluntary participation, refusal, and withdrawal—You must state that participation is voluntary, that refusal to participate involves no penalty or loss of benefits to which the person is otherwise entitled, and that the person may discontinue participation at any time without penalty.

See: https://www.hhs.gov/ohrp/regulations-and-policy/regulations/45
-cfr-46/index.html

2

Communication

INTRODUCTION

Communication is a main pillar of effective public health practice because of the need to reach large populations with timely and effective information about disease prevention. The field of public health has borrowed extensively from other disciplines to develop theoretical frameworks for effective communication. For example, mass communication, advertising, and marketing have long relied on understandings of human behavior and psychology to frame messages that support behavior modification and adoption of best practices. The digital information age is upon us, and public health communication strategies have had to adapt quickly to use new opportunities to message individuals, communities, and globally distributed populations through the use of the Internet, social media networks, and text messaging. Modern competencies in public health communication must reflect mastery of the various dimensions of information, including content, format, media, delivery, and feedback mechanisms, to ensure that communication is effective and responsive to new information and information technologies. Communication competencies are tested with questions designed to examine broad knowledge of principles and strategies of effective public health communication and advocacy. Practicing with these questions should enable you to

- Ensure health literacy concepts are applied in communication efforts

- Identify communication gaps

- Propose recommendations for improving communication processes

- Exercise a variety of communication strategies and methods targeting specific populations and venues to promote policies and programs

- Communicate effectively and convey information in a manner that is easily understood by diverse audiences (e.g., including persons of limited English proficiency, those who have low literacy skills or are not literate, individuals with disabilities, and those who are deaf or hard of hearing)

- Choose communication tools and techniques to facilitate discussions and interactions
- Assess the health literacy of populations served
- Use risk communication approaches to address public health issues and problems
- Set communication goals, objectives, and priorities for a project
- Inform the public about health policies, programs, and resources
- Apply ethical considerations in developing communication plans and promotional initiatives
- Create and disseminate educational information relating to specific emerging health issues and priorities to promote policy development
- Communicate the role of public health within the overall health system (e.g., national, state, county, local government) and its impact on the individual
- Communicate with colleagues, patients, families, or communities about health disparities and healthcare disparities
- Communicate lessons learned to community partners or global constituencies
- Apply facilitation skills in interactions with individuals and groups
- Communicate results of population health needs and asset assessments
- Communicate with other health professionals in a responsive and responsible manner that supports a team approach to maintaining health of individuals and populations
- Provide a rationale for program proposals and evaluations to lay, professional, and policy audiences
- Communicate results of evaluation efforts

■ QUESTIONS

1. Ineffective communication is one of the reasons behind public confusion about research findings that affect compliance with recommendations for disease prevention including vaccination. Which among the following is NOT part of the strategies for effective communication in public health?

   A. Collaborate with communication and informatics specialists in the process of design, implementation, and evaluation of public health programs
   B. Apply legal and ethical principles to the use of information technology and resources in public health settings
   C. Use informatics and communication methods to advocate for community public health programs and policies

D. Rely on information provided by corporations marketing products linked to adverse health outcomes

2. Which of the following is likely to be the single-most effective method for communicating health education to middle-aged women in a Hispanic American community characterized by lower socioeconomic status?

    A. Public service spot on National Public Radio
    B. Community health workers in hairdresser shops, convenience stores, and grocery markets
    C. Reverse 911 (mass telephone broadcasts to dialing area)
    D. Articles in the highest circulating newspaper

3. Which of the following factors is not an essential requirement for effective public health emergency preparedness?

    A. Identifying surge capacity in the public health infrastructure
    B. Developing channels for real-time interagency communication
    C. Training key decision-makers and first responders for coordinated action
    D. Developing an alternative to the color-coded public alert system

4. Communicating the performance of healthcare organizations to patients and the general public is an important function of the government. For example, the California Office of the Patient Advocate rates Health Management Organizations, and the Kaiser Permanente model is often highly rated in healthcare delivery because it

    A. Pays physicians lower salaries than levels set by the federal government
    B. Separates the health insurer and health provider into two distinct organizational units
    C. Does not tailor its insurance policies to young, healthy individuals
    D. Integrates primary, secondary, and tertiary care through effective provider communication to ensure best patient outcomes

5. Which of the following is a compelling reason for using documentary photography and image search in global health?

    A. To communicate complex, large-scale stories
    B. Because pictures of disease and sick people in other countries can be really sickening
    C. To encourage individualized and selective understanding of challenges among politicians, software developers, bankers, and researchers, among others potentially involved in solutions
    D. To compete for an Oscar award

6. The National Cancer Institute recognizes four components of a health communication program cycle. Which of the following is NOT among the components?

    A. Planning and strategy development
    B. Developing and pretesting concepts, messages, and materials
    C. Jettisoning the program
    D. Assessing effectiveness and making refinements

7. Core functions of communication between healthcare provider and patients DO NOT include

   A. Enabling patient self-management
   B. Exchanging information
   C. Managing uncertainty
   D. Ignoring emotions

8. The CDC Clear Communication Index is a research-based tool to plan and assess public communication materials. The index assesses communications materials in seven areas, including all of the following EXCEPT

   A. Language
   B. Standard design
   C. State of the science
   D. Risk

9. The CDC Clear Communication Index was developed to comply with which federal mandate?

   A. Federal Communications Commission Act of 1934
   B. Plain Writing Act of 2010
   C. Patient Protection and Affordable Care Act of 2010
   D. Telecommunications Act of 1996

10. The National Action Plan to Improve Health Literacy is based on which principle(s)?

   A. Some people have the right to health information that helps them make informed decisions.
   B. Health services should be delivered in ways that are easy to understand and that improve health, longevity, and quality of life.
   C. Health information on individuals should be provided only upon request by third parties.
   D. Health information belongs to health insurance agencies.

11. The National Action Plan to Improve Health Literacy contains seven goals that will improve health literacy and strategies for achieving them. The goals DO NOT include

   A. Develop and disseminate health and safety information that is accurate, accessible, and actionable
   B. Promote changes in the healthcare system that improve health information, communication, informed decision-making, and access to health services
   C. Incorporate accurate, standards-based, and developmentally appropriate health and science information and curricula in child care and education through the university level
   D. Adopt a single universal language in which health literature is archived

12. The primary audience in preventive health communication is defined as

   A. A group of influencers such as religious leaders or stars with direct and immediate influence on targeted populations

B. Individuals, including patients or vulnerable people, who are expected to act by changing behavior in response to health communication messages
C. A group with indirect influence on the primary audience
D. A group with tangential interests in the target health behavior

13. Core health communication strategies include the following EXCEPT

A. Engagement
B. Persuasion
C. Policies, laws, and regulations
D. Intimidation

14. The elaboration likelihood model of persuasion (ELM) proposes the following major routes to persuasion:

A. The decision-making route
B. The central route
C. The peripheral route
D. The challenging route

15. The Health Belief Model may be used to identify communication opportunities by identifying barriers to engagement according to modifiable variables that include the following EXCEPT

A. Perceived benefits
B. Self-efficacy
C. Perceived threat
D. Extrasensory perception

16. The use of social marketing in health communication may identify the "product" being marketed as the following EXCEPT

A. A physical material such as condoms
B. Services such as cancer screening
C. Behaviors such as exercising
D. Interactions such as mind control

17. Social marketing strategies can be used to increase the value of a product by modifying the following EXCEPT

A. The price or cost of the product
B. The placement or location of the product
C. The perception of the product
D. False advertisement

18. The Agency for Healthcare Research and Quality (AHRQ) developed the Health Literacy Universal Precautions Toolkit to improve the following EXCEPT

A. Spoken communication
B. Body language
C. Written communication
D. Telepathic communication

19. "Risk communication" in public health defines the terms "risk," "hazard," and "exposure." "Risk" is

   A. The probability of harm
   B. The source of potential harm
   C. The contact with a harmful situation
   D. The cost of potential harm

20. "Risk communication" in public health defines the terms "risk," "hazard," and "exposure." "Hazard" is

   A. The probability of harm
   B. The source of potential harm
   C. The contact with a harmful situation
   D. The cost of potential harm

21. "Risk communication" in public health defines the terms "risk," "hazard," and "exposure." "Exposure" is

   A. The probability of harm
   B. The source of potential harm
   C. The contact with a harmful situation
   D. The cost of potential harm

22. The Centers for Disease Control and Prevention uses a Crisis Emergency Communication Planning Cycle consisting of the following phases EXCEPT

   A. Precrisis actions
   B. Initial communication
   C. Maintaining communication
   D. Postcrisis correction

23. The Centers for Disease Control and Prevention developed the Single Overriding Communications Objective (SOCO) to

   A. Assist scientists in framing the results of their research for public communication
   B. Narrow down the content of press releases to a single point
   C. Establish a hierarchy of communications objectives
   D. Assist scientists in framing the results of their research for peer-reviewed publication

24. "Health numeracy" is

   A. The ability of individuals to understand health information text
   B. The ability of numerous people to interpret textual health information together
   C. The ability of individuals to understand quantitative health information
   D. The ability of numerous people to interpret qualitative health information

25. "Fear appeal" is

    A. A public health communication strategy that aims to modify health behavior by creating anxiety about potential hazard, risk, or exposure in populations receiving a fearful message

    B. The attraction that people have for fearsome situations, for example, the popularity of horror movies

    C. A legal term referring to the appeal of a conviction based on fear of the judiciary

    D. A public health communications strategy for health promotion based on fear of foreigners

26. "Public health advocacy" is

    A. Practiced only by legally qualified advocates and solicitors in legal practice

    B. The communication process of gaining political commitment for a specific public health goal or program

    C. The communication process of forcing opponents of successful public health intervention programs such as vaccination to obey the law

    D. The communication process of forcing adherents of a questionable alternative healthcare practice to cease and desist

27. Public right-to-know laws are embodied in U.S. federal and state laws as

    A. The legal principle that individuals have the right to know the hazardous chemicals to which they may be exposed in their daily living

    B. The legal right of public agencies to know information about the health status of every individual in a population

    C. The legal principle that in a democratic society, populations are always right in their request for information about individual health

    D. The legal principle that in a democratic society, individuals are always right in their request for information about other individuals' health

28. Under U.S. federal law, "informed consent" is associated with public health activities regarding

    A. Human participants in research

    B. The consensual relationship between two adults guided by the exchange of information

    C. Consenting adults informing one another about their health status

    D. Consenting children informing one another about social welfare

29. Ensuring that "informed consent" is an effective communication tool is the responsibility of the following EXCEPT

    A. Institutional review board

    B. The investigator

    C. The sponsor

    D. The patient

30. Informed consent forms originally written in the English language must be translated

    A. If the individual cannot read English but is fluently literate in another language
    B. If the individual can read and understand English only at the sixth-grade level
    C. Under no circumstances; informed consent forms should not be translated into other languages because the intended meaning will be lost in translation
    D. If the first language of the investigator is not English

31. A public health "policy brief" is

    A. A very short policy established by the U.S. House of Representatives on vaccination where the scientific evidence is indisputable
    B. A very short policy established by the U.S. Senate on vaccination where the scientific evidence is indisputable
    C. A brief policy on a public health topic that can withstand presidential veto
    D. A concise summary of information that can help the target audience understand and make decisions about government policies on matters of significance to public health

32. Public health communication should NOT abide by which of the following principles of ethics?

    A. Beneficence
    B. Maleficence
    C. Respect for personal autonomy
    D. Justice

33. In the year 2020, the best media for communicating drug abuse prevention with adolescents and young adults in the United States is

    A. AM radio broadcast
    B. Books available in the library
    C. Digital social media
    D. FM radio

34. Resilient public alert and warning tools are essential to save lives and protect property during times of national, state, regional, and local public health emergencies. In the United States, the Emergency Alert System (EAS) is operated by

    A. The White House
    B. The U.S. Department of State
    C. The U.S. Department of Homeland Security
    D. The U.S. Department of Health and Human Services

35. Which of the following is NOT included in the World Health Organization's six principles for effective communication?

A. Defensible
B. Accessible
C. Understandable
D. Credible

36. The best definition of "health informatics" is

    A. The process of manipulating health information to fit a health belief theory
    B. The process of digitally doctoring health information to fit a health belief theory
    C. The application of information engineering to the field of healthcare
    D. The storage of "big data" in a centralized healthcare system

37. The best definition of "electronic health record" is

    A. A real-time, patient-centered record that makes information available instantly and securely to authorized users
    B. A real-time, patient-centered record that makes information available instantly and securely to any user
    C. A real-time record of how comfortable individuals are in navigating electronic media for health communication
    D. A real-time record of the competency of healthcare providers that can be checked by patients

38. The following are included in the ethical codes of conduct regarding communication of personal health information EXCEPT

    A. Confidentiality
    B. Security
    C. Privacy
    D. Maleficence

39. Peer-reviewed journal articles are best for communicating with the following public health audiences:

    A. Government policy makers
    B. Active researchers
    C. Journalists
    D. Health insurers

40. The application of consumer-oriented marketing techniques in the design, implementation, and evaluation of health promotion is

    A. Consumer health
    B. Health informatics
    C. Health economics
    D. Social marketing

41. Mass immunization campaigns may be necessary when responding to specific public health threats. For example, during the pandemic swine flu outbreak in 2009, California stockpiled vaccine doses, many of which went unused, in part

because of an unsuccessful communications campaign. The following populations are targets for successful communication in immunization campaigns EXCEPT

A. Caregivers
B. Communities that are hard to reach
C. Populations that have long-held mistrust of the health system
D. Those on the waiting list to receive Shingrix

42. Global "public health days" are an opportunity to raise awareness and understanding about critical health issues and mobilize support for action. The World Health Organization marks seven health campaigns annually, including the following EXCEPT

A. World Health Day, 7 April
B. World Malaria Day, 25 April
C. World No Tobacco Day, 31 May
D. World War Day, 28 July

43. The basic model of communication is usually presented as a unidirectional flow of information with three variables: sender, message, and receiver. Two additional variables are included in health promotion to suggest a bidirectional flow of information. One of these variables is

A. Gullibility
B. Resistance
C. Feedback
D. Temperance

44. The content of a public health message may contain both verbal and nonverbal communication. Verbal communication includes

A. Body language
B. Words
C. Proxemics
D. Hand gestures

45. The content of a public health message may contain both verbal and nonverbal communication. Nonverbal communication includes all EXCEPT

A. Paralinguistic features
B. Standing features
C. Kinesic elements
D. Intonational features

46. Prosodic elements in health communication include

A. Intonation
B. Eye contact
C. Gestures
D. Posture

47. The major categories of communication include the following, EXCEPT

    A. Intrapersonal
    B. Interpersonal
    C. Organizational
    D. Global

48. The "Communication–Persuasion Model" (CPM) of health communication is different from other health promotion models because

    A. CPM focuses on mass media
    B. CPM targets only populations at risk
    C. CPM cannot be evaluated for effectiveness
    D. CPM focuses on direct marketing

49. The Information–Communication Matrix (IPM) posits that an individual's choice regarding health can be influenced by the following EXCEPT

    A. External factors, for example, financial price
    B. Internal directive factors, for example, beliefs
    C. Internal dynamic factors, for example, age
    D. Exterior factors such as skin color

50. Health communications strategies can be informed by theoretical models including the following EXCEPT

    A. Theory of planned behavior
    B. Health Belief Model
    C. Transtheoretical model of perceived behavioral control
    D. Communism theory

51. The generally used terminology for the application of digital communication technology in healthcare is

    A. Digital-health
    B. Analog-health
    C. Techno-health
    D. E-health

52. Electronic devices such as mobile phones, messaging technologies, and social networking applications are often used for communication in healthcare, and are collectively referred to as

    A. Short message service
    B. App-Health
    C. Remote sensing
    D. M-Health

53. Health communication strategies include framing messages to influence behavior change. For example, a message framed to emphasize the cost to the

individual for neglecting to take action on a health issue such as preventive check-ups is referred to as

A. Gain-framed messages
B. Loss-framed messages
C. Neutrally framed messages
D. Co-benefit-framed messages

54. The individual capacity to access, understand, appraise, and apply health information toward making beneficial health decisions is referred to as

A. Health literacy
B. Health accessibility
C. Health awareness
D. Health appraisal

55. The structure of the Claude Shannon–Warren Weaver model of communication consists of

A. Precontemplation, contemplation, preparation, action, maintenance
B. Product, price, place, promotion
C. Source, transmitter, channel, receiver, destination
D. Product, precision, perception, particularity

56. Individual-centered health communication ideas include strategies for the following EXCEPT

A. Examining the biological basis of disease
B. Understanding the social determinants of disease
C. Integrating disease prevention approaches
D. Population health management

57. According to the "Prospect Theory" of information framing, most people consider the following in making decisions:

A. Potential gains
B. Past losses
C. Past gains
D. Their budget

58. The behavior change approach to health promotion is based on the assumption that

A. People are irrational decision-makers.
B. People use information about risks and benefits of their behaviors.
C. People rely on their neighbors to make decisions about health behaviors.
D. Shaming pressure works.

59. Evaluation of the once-popular "fear appeal" model of health communication has shown that

A. Fear tactics are the most appropriate strategy to promote healthy behavior.

B. Stimulation of fear is less effective than provision of information that encourages effective behavioral responses.

C. Evidence is inconclusive about the effectiveness of fear appeal.

D. Fearsome messages are cost-effective.

60. Medical communication is defined as the development and production of materials that deal specifically with medicine or healthcare focused mostly on the interaction with patients. The following skills are required for professional medical communicators EXCEPT

A. Communication expertise

B. Awareness of ethical standards

C. Knowledge of healthcare systems

D. Friending physicians

▥ ANSWERS

1. **D.** Health communication is defined as *the study and use of communication strategies to inform and influence individual decisions that enhance health.* Health communication can take many forms: written and verbal, traditional, and new media outlets. All strategic communication planning involve some variation on these steps:

   - Review background information to define the problem (What's out there?)
   - Set communication objectives (What do we want to accomplish?)
   - Analyze and segment target audiences (Who do we want to reach?)
   - Develop and pretest message concepts (What do we want to say?)
   - Select communication channels (Where do we want to say it?)
   - Select, create, and pretest messages and products (How do we want to say it?)
   - Develop promotion plan/production (How do we get it used?)
   - Implement communication strategies and conduct process evaluation (Getting it out there)
   - Conduct outcome and impact evaluation (How well did we do?)

   In general, it is not appropriate to use unverified information from a corporation being regulated in advocating behavior change through health communication.

   See: https://www.cdc.gov/healthcommunication/healthbasics/WhatIsHC .html

   https://npin.cdc.gov/pages/health-communication-strategies

   https://npin.cdc.gov/pages/health-communication-strategies -methods

2. **B.** Effective communication methods should take into consideration sociocultural factors that accommodate the target population's time-activity patterns, preferred authoritative source of credible information, access, and trust factors.

   Knowing the habits and preferences of Hispanics/Latinos can help you tailor compelling health messages for this audience. Consider custom publications because these have proven to be an effective way to communicate with the Hispanic/Latino market. Companies such as Sears and Procter & Gamble have invested millions of dollars to reach (and enhance their relationships with) Hispanic/Latino consumers through custom publications in Spanish that address their lifestyle interests and needs. Consider using bilingual ad messages to appeal to Hispanic/Latino teens—especially from English-language celebrities "who happen to slip in some Spanish." Hispanic/Latino teens respond best to this message type because it mirrors their own usage patterns. Coordinate community outreach activities through established and trusted organizations and people. For example, *promotoras* are trusted community health advisors and can be accessed through Community Health Centers. They visit homes and individually work with families.

See: https://www.cdc.gov/healthcommunication/pdf/audience/audience
insight_culturalinsights.pdf

3. **D.** Surge capacity assessments, designing and testing effective highly coordinated interagency communication, and coordinated actions are all essential for emergency preparedness. Color-coded public alert systems have been tested (e.g., post 9–11 homeland security systems) and they have variable effectiveness.

In 2011, the Department of Homeland Security (DHS) replaced the color-coded alerts of the Homeland Security Advisory System (HSAS) with the National Terrorism Advisory System (NTAS), designed to more effectively communicate information about terrorist threats by providing timely, detailed information to the American public.

See: https://www.dhs.gov/national-terrorism-advisory-system

4. **D.** The California Office of the Patient Advocate has consistently rated Kaiser Permanente as the highest quality Health Management Organization (HMO) in the state. The ratings are based on criteria that capture Quality of Medical Care (QMC), including a set of national standards for quality of care to ensure that health plans offer good quality preventive care to their members; and Patients Overall Experience (POE), including "Getting Care Easily," "Satisfaction With Plan Services," and "Satisfaction With Plan Doctors." In 2019, Kaiser Permanente scored five stars on QMC and four stars on POE.

There is no evidence that Kaiser Permanente pays physicians at a lower rate than other HMOs. Health insurance is integrated with health provision. There is no discrimination according to age in access to healthcare.

See: http://reportcard.opa.ca.gov/rc/HMO_PPOCombined.aspx

https://about.kaiserpermanente.org/our-story/news/accolades-and
-awards/kaiser-permanentes-overall-quality-of-medical-care-earns
-highest

5. **A.** Much of the information critical to the communication of public health messages is pictorial rather than text-based. Centers for Disease Control and Prevention's (CDC) Public Health Image Library (PHIL) was created as an organized, universal electronic gateway to CDC's pictures. CDC welcomes public health professionals, the media, laboratory scientists, educators, students, and the worldwide public to use this material for reference, teaching, presentation, and public health messages.

See: https://phil.cdc.gov

http://www.resource-media.org/free-image-libraries-global-health
-womens-storytelling

Houts, P. S., Doak, C. C., Doak, L. G., & Loscalzo, M. (2006, May). The role of pictures in improving health communication: A review of research on attention, comprehension, recall, and adherence. *Patient Education and Counseling, 61*(2), 173–190. doi:10.1016/j.pec.2005.05.004

6. **C.** Understanding what health communication can and cannot do is critical to communicating successfully. Health communication is one tool for promoting or improving health. Changes in healthcare services, technology, regulations, and policy are often also necessary to completely address a health problem.

Communication alone can

- Increase the intended audience's knowledge and awareness of a health issue, problem, or solution
- Influence perceptions, beliefs, and attitudes that may change social norms
- Prompt action
- Demonstrate or illustrate healthy skills
- Reinforce knowledge, attitudes, or behavior
- Show the benefit of behavior change
- Advocate a position on a health issue or policy
- Increase demand or support for health services
- Refute myths and misconceptions
- Strengthen organizational relationships

See: https://www.cancer.gov/publications/health-communication/pink -book.pdf

7. **D.** Good medical care depends upon effective communication between patients and healthcare providers. Ineffective communication can lead to improper diagnosis and delayed or improper medical treatment. If patients have limited English proficiency or are deaf or hard-of-hearing, they may require interpreters or other services to help communicate effectively with healthcare providers. Many hospitals are actively taking steps to improve effective communication. However, hospitals face increasing challenges to meet the communication needs of an increasingly diverse population. Ideas about health and behaviors are shaped by the communication, information, and technology that people interact with every day. Health communication and health information technology are central to healthcare, public health, and the way our society views health. These processes make up the ways and the context in which professionals and the public search for, understand, and use health information, significantly impacting their health decisions and actions.

See: https://www.healthypeople.gov/2020/topics-objectives/topic/health -communication-and-health-information-technology

https://www.hhs.gov/civil-rights/for-individuals/special-topics/ hospitals-effective-communication/index.html

8. **B.** The CDC Clear Communication Index (Index) is a research-based tool to help you develop and assess public communication materials. The Index has four introductory questions and 20 scored items drawn from scientific literature in communication and related disciplines. The items represent the most important characteristics that enhance and aid people's understanding of information.

See: https://www.cdc.gov/ccindex/index.html

9. **B.** The Clear Communication Index (Index) provides a set of research-based criteria to develop and assess public communication products. The Index supports the efforts of the Centers for Disease Control and Prevention (CDC) to comply with the Plain Writing Act of 2010 and achieve goals set forth in the National Action Plan to Improve Health Literacy and the CDC Action Plan to Improve Health Literacy.

The 20 items in the Index build on and expand plain language techniques described in the Federal Plain Language Guidelines.

See: https://www.cdc.gov/healthliteracy/pdf/clear-communication-user
-guide.pdf

10. **B.** The National Action Plan to Improve Health Literacy seeks to engage organizations, professionals, policy makers, communities, individuals, and families in a linked, multi-sector effort to improve health literacy. The Action Plan is based on two core principles:

1. All people have the right to health information that helps them make informed decisions.
2. Health services should be delivered in ways that are easy to understand and that improve health, longevity, and quality of life.

See: https://health.gov/communication/initiatives/health-literacy-action
-plan.asp

11. **D.** The Action Plan to Improve Health Literacy contains seven goals that will improve health literacy and strategies for achieving them:

- Develop and disseminate health and safety information that is accurate, accessible, and actionable
- Promote changes in the healthcare system that improve health information, communication, informed decision-making, and access to health services
- Incorporate accurate, standards-based, and developmentally appropriate health and science information and curricula in child care and education through the university level
- Support and expand local efforts to provide adult education, English language instruction, and culturally and linguistically appropriate health information services in the community
- Build partnerships, develop guidance, and change policies
- Increase basic research and the development, implementation, and evaluation of practices and interventions to improve health literacy
- Increase the dissemination and use of evidence-based health literacy practices and interventions

See: https://health.gov/communication/initiatives/health-literacy-action
-plan.asp

12. **A.** One of the key steps in the health communication and social marketing process is identifying the population segments that can benefit from a specific health behavior. The more that is known about the primary segment, the better we can reach them with messages, activities, and policies. The upfront research includes understanding the needs and wants of the primary target audience on a more personal level, and their motivations and lifestyles so we can truly engage with them. This effort will pay dividends later when we begin preparing your campaign activities, health messages, channels, and campaign materials.

See: https://www.cdc.gov/healthcommunication/audience/index.html

13. **D.** Intimidation is not an effective way to deliver health information; it is more likely to produce the opposite of the desired impact. Health communication can take many forms: written and verbal, traditional, and new media outlets. While you might be excited to get started with your new program, you must first develop a sound strategic plan. All strategic communication planning involves some variation on these steps:

Identify the health problem and determine whether communication should be part of the intervention

Identify the audience for the communication program and determine the best ways to reach them

Develop and test communication concepts, messages, and materials with representatives of the target audiences

Implement the health communication program based on results of the testing

Assess how effectively the messages reached the target audience and modify the communication program if necessary

See: https://www.cdc.gov/healthcommunication/healthbasics/HowToDo .html

https://www.cdc.gov/cancer/dcpc/research/articles/aamm_phm_ 2015.htm

14. **D.** The elaboration likelihood model of persuasion recognizes that at times audiences are active, thinking about messages and the arguments in those messages. At other times target audiences are passive, needing persuasion through a peripheral route. Two conditions determine whether the audience is doing central or peripheral processing: Central processing requires that the audience have both the ability and motivation to think about a message. Factors that influence the audience include involvement, argument quality, argument quantity, credibility.

See: http://www.cios.org/encyclopedia/persuasion/Helaboration_ 7evaluation.htm

https://www.cdc.gov/cancer/dcpc/research/articles/aamm_phm_ 2015.htm

15. **D.** The Health Belief Model has been used extensively in public health, noting that two factors influence the adoption of a health protective behavior: (1) a feeling of being personally threatened by a disease, and (2) a belief that the benefits of adopting the protective health behavior will outweigh the perceived costs of adopting that behavior. The Health Belief Model has been incorporated into several public health communication campaigns. Extrasensory perception or ESP, or "sixth sense," is not a scientifically verifiable communication mode.

See: https://www.cdc.gov/nccdphp/dch/programs/healthycommunities program/tools/pdf/apply_theory.pdf

16. **D.** "Mind control" is not an acceptable form of social marketing. Health communication and social marketing may have some differences, but they share a common goal: creating social change by changing people's attitudes, external structures, and/or modifying or eliminating certain behaviors. Generally, a person in social marketing or health communications will create and use

products, programs, or interventions as a means to the same end: to promote health changes in individuals and communities, using strategies and tactics based on science and consumer research. Sometimes you may hear the term "health marketing." In this context, health marketing is a blending of multiple disciplines: the theoretical underpinnings of social marketing with the outreach communication strategies found in health communications. The Centers for Disease Control and Prevention (CDC) uses both social marketing and health communication practices, which are both overlapping and complementary, in its approach to promoting or "marketing" health to the public.

See: https://www.cdc.gov/healthcommunication/healthbasics/WhatIsHC.html

https://www.cdc.gov/healthcommunication/index.html

17. D. Deception or false advertisement (15 United States Code 54) is illegal and ultimately not an effective way to communicate health information.

Health communication and social marketing may have some differences, but they share a common goal: creating social change by changing people's attitudes, external structures, and/or modifying or eliminating certain behaviors. Generally, a person in social marketing or health communications will create and use products, programs, or interventions as a means to the same end: to promote health changes in individuals and communities, using strategies and tactics based on science and consumer research. Sometimes you may hear the term "health marketing." In this context, health marketing is a blending of multiple disciplines: the theoretical underpinnings of social marketing with the outreach communication strategies found in health communications. The Centers for Disease Control and Prevention (CDC) uses both social marketing and health communication practices, which are both overlapping and complementary, in its approach to promoting or "marketing" health to the public.

See: https://www.govinfo.gov/app/details/USCODE-2011-title15/USCODE-2011-title15-chap2-subchapI-sec54

https://www.cdc.gov/healthcommunication/healthbasics/WhatIsHC.html

https://www.cdc.gov/healthcommunication/index.html

18. D. There is no credible scientific evidence in support of telepathic communication.

The Agency for Healthcare Research and Quality (AHRQ) Health Literacy Universal Precautions Toolkit, Second Edition, can help primary care practices reduce the complexity of healthcare, increase patient understanding of health information, and enhance support for patients of all health literacy levels. Health literacy universal precautions are the steps that practices take when they assume that all patients may have difficulty comprehending health information and accessing health services. Health literacy universal precautions are aimed at

- Simplifying communication with and confirming comprehension for all patients, so that the risk of miscommunication is minimized
- Making the office environment and healthcare system easier to navigate
- Supporting patients' efforts to improve their health

See: https://www.ahrq.gov/professionals/quality-patient-safety/quality
-resources/tools/literacy-toolkit/index.html

19. **A.** Risk is defined as the probability that an event will occur. It can also be defined as the probability that a health effect will occur after an individual has been exposed to a specified amount of a hazard. Risk assessment is the process of gathering all available information on the toxic effects of a chemical and evaluating it to determine the possible risks associated with exposure. The process of gathering and evaluating the information can be divided into the following:

- Hazard identification
- Hazard evaluation or dose-response assessment
- Exposure assessment
- Risk characterization

Virtually every day, crisis and emergency risk communication are needed somewhere in public health. Whenever a crisis occurs, communicators must be ready to provide information to help people make the best possible decisions for their health and well-being. This must be done in rapid time frames and without knowing everything about the crisis. Yet often the types of disasters that public health must address can be anticipated. The Centers for Disease Control and Prevention (CDC) has developed a process for planning and conducting crisis and emergency risk communication. On this page you will find this process and a wealth of information to help you prepare if an emergency occurs and you are part of the response team.

The right message at the right time from the right person can save lives. The CDC's Crisis and Emergency Risk Communication (CERC) draws from lessons learned during past public health emergencies and research in the fields of public health, psychology, and emergency risk communication. The CDC's CERC program provides training, tools, and resources to help health communicators, emergency responders, and leaders of organizations communicate effectively during emergencies.

See: https://www.atsdr.cdc.gov/training/toxmanual/pdf/module-3.pdf

　　https://www.atsdr.cdc.gov/publications_risk_comm.html

　　https://www.cdc.gov/csels/dsepd/ss1978/lesson3/section5.html

20. **B.** Hazard identification—This first step in risk assessment consists of collecting data from different sources to determine whether a risk factor (e.g., a chemical substance) is dangerous (toxic or carcinogenic). It involves gathering and examining data from toxicological and epidemiological studies.

Epidemiology is the study of the causative factors that are associated with the occurrence and number of cases of disease and illness in a specific population. Information from these studies should answer these questions:

Does exposure to the substance produce any adverse effects?

If yes, what are the circumstances associated with the exposure?

See: https://www.atsdr.cdc.gov/training/toxmanual/pdf/module-3.pdf

21. **C.** Exposure is defined as the contact with a risk factor by swallowing, breathing, or touching the skin or eyes. Exposure may be short-term (acute exposure), of intermediate duration, or long-term (chronic exposure). Related phrases are

    Exposure assessment: The process of finding out how people come into contact with a hazardous substance, how often and for how long they are in contact with the substance, and how much of the substance they are in contact with.

    Exposure-dose reconstruction: A method of estimating the amount of people's past exposure to hazardous substances. Computer and approximation methods are used when past information is limited, not available, or missing.

    Exposure investigation: The collection and analysis of site-specific information and biologic tests (when appropriate) to determine whether people have been exposed to hazardous substances.

    Exposure pathway: The route a substance takes from its source (where it began) to its end point (where it ends), and how people can come into contact with (or get exposed to) it. An exposure pathway has five parts: a source of contamination (such as an abandoned business); an environmental media and transport mechanism (such as movement through groundwater); a point of exposure (such as a private well); a route of exposure (eating, drinking, breathing, or touching); and a receptor population (people potentially or actually exposed). When all five parts are present, the exposure pathway is termed a completed exposure pathway.

    Exposure registry: A system of ongoing follow-up of people who have had documented environmental exposures.

    See: https://www.atsdr.cdc.gov/glossary.html

22. **D.** Every emergency evolves. For communicators, it's important to understand that crises happen in phases; and understanding the pattern of a disaster can help communicators anticipate problems and appropriately respond. The CDC's Crisis and Emergency Risk Communication (CERC) Communication Lifecycle identifies the types of information that need to be delivered during different phases of an emergency. The stages are

    Precrisis

    Initial

    Maintenance

    Resolution

    Evaluation

    The precrisis phase, which occurs before the onset of the emergency, is the best time for a communicator to prepare by creating a crisis communication plan, drafting messages, identifying possible audiences, and predicting communication needs. When a new disaster happens, these ready resources can help communicators respond rapidly. Strong communication using CERC principles is vital in the initial phase of a response, when there is the greatest confusion and least amount of available information. It's important to remember that as the emergency response progresses, available information and audience needs will change. Communication resources and strategies must adapt to meet these evolving needs.

All crises will go through all five stages, although the length of time for each stage will vary for each crisis, and even for different stakeholders who are affected. For example, as Zika virus disease (Zika) continues to initially affect new areas, some have been maintaining their outbreak response for a while. Others are in the precrisis phase, preparing for the eventuality that they too may have to deal with Zika soon. Even in the same location, pregnant women may experience a higher level of initial anxiety, while the larger populations quickly move on to the maintenance phase. Organizations addressing Zika are faced with the challenge of simultaneously communicating to diverse audiences experiencing different phases of the outbreak.

See: https://emergency.cdc.gov/cerc/cerccorner/article_051316.asp

23. **A.** The Single Overriding Communications Objective (SOCO) is the outcome or change desired as a result of health communication. The SOCO is not the message. Advisories need a clear, consistent message. The SOCO Worksheet is a tool to create a specific message. Use the message developed in the SOCO Worksheet for all communication with the public and partners, including briefings and press releases. The point of contact information identifies the communication contact for the advisory. The SOCO approach applies to any water system communication.

See: https://www.who.int/risk-communication/training/Module-D1.pdf?ua=1

24. **C.** Literacy, numeracy, and technology skills are increasingly important in today's information-rich environments. What people know and what they do with what they know have a major impact on their life chances. For example, people with lower literacy proficiency are more likely than those with better literacy skills to report poor health. Numeracy is the ability to access, use, interpret, and communicate mathematical information and ideas, and to engage in and manage mathematical demands of a range of situations in adult life.

See: https://www.cdc.gov/healthliteracy/learn/UnderstandingLiteracy.html

25. **A.** A "fear appeal" is defined as a message that attempts to provoke fear in order to divert behavior through the threat of impending danger or harm to health. It presents a risk, presents the vulnerability to the risk, and then may, or may not, suggest a form of protective action; for example, placing pictures of lung cancer patients or symptoms on cigarette cartons.

See: https://www.cdc.gov/healthcommunication/pdf/thisjustin/tji_17_200912.pdf

https://onlinelibrary.wiley.com/doi/full/10.1002/ijop.12042

26. **B.** Advocacy is a key health promotion activity for overcoming major barriers to public health and occupational health. The barriers addressed by advocacy are poor living and working conditions, rather than individual or behavioral barriers. The modern use of the term advocacy gained momentum from the

Ottawa Charter on Health Promotion (a landmark definition of health promotion): "Political, economic, social, cultural, environmental, behavioral, and biological factors can all favor health or be harmful to good health. Health promotion aims at making these conditions favorable through advocacy for health."

See: https://www.who.int/occupational_health/topics/workplace/en/index2.html

https://npin.cdc.gov/subjects/advocacy

https://www.cdc.gov/publichealthgateway/policy/national-organiza tions.html

https://phadvocates.org/who-we-are

27. **A.** In the practice of environmental health, public right-to-know laws take two forms: community right to know and workplace right to know, particularly regarding potential exposure to hazardous chemicals and agents. Broadly, the Freedom of Information Act, known as the FOIA, is a law that gives any person the right to request federal agency records. Like all federal agencies, the CDC is required to disclose records requested in writing by individuals (regardless of citizenship), partnerships, corporations, and organizations unless the records (or a part of the records) are protected from disclosure by any of the nine exemptions contained in the law. The FOIA also requires federal agencies to make certain types of information available to the public without the need to submit a request. As the U.S. leading public health agency, the CDC is dedicated to saving lives and protecting the health of Americans. CDC ensures its science and research activities, as well as employees, comply with various federal laws, regulations, and policies in order to exercise the highest level of scientific integrity. At the core of this mission is information sharing—not just health information and disease study results, but information the CDC gathers as part of a continuous process of putting information into action. As a science-based agency funded by U.S. taxpayers, CDC is committed to openness and accountability.

See: https://www.cdc.gov/od/foia/resources/infographics/foia-at-cdc .htm

https://www.nih.gov/institutes-nih/nih-office-director/office-commu nications-public-liaison/freedom-information-act-office/freedom-infor mation-act-5-usc-552

28. **A.** Informed consent is a process in which patients or human participants in research are given important information, including possible risks and benefits, about a medical procedure or treatment, genetic testing, or a clinical trial. This is to help them decide whether they want to be treated, tested, or take part in the trial. Patients are also given any new information that might affect their decision to continue. Also called consent process.

The HHS regulations at 45 CFR part 46 for the protection of human subjects in research require that an investigator obtain the legally effective informed consent of the subject or the subject's legally authorized representative, unless (1) the research is exempt under 45 CFR 46.101(b); (2) the IRB finds and documents that informed consent can be waived (45 CFR 46.116(c) or (d)); or (3) the IRB finds and documents that the research meets the requirements of the HHS Secretarial waiver under 45 CFR 46.101(i) that permits a waiver of the general requirements for obtaining informed consent in a limited class of research in emergency settings. When informed consent is required, it must be sought prospectively, and documented to the extent required under HHS regulations at 45 CFR 46.117. (Food and Drug Administration [FDA] regulations at 21 CFR part 50 may also apply if the research involves a clinical investigation regulated by FDA.)

Code of Federal Regulations (Title 21, Volume 1) Revised as of April 1, 2018 (CITE: 21CFR50):

Sec. 50.20 General requirements for informed consent.

Except as provided in 50.23 and 50.24, no investigator may involve a human being as a subject in research covered by these regulations unless the investigator has obtained the legally effective informed consent of the subject or the subject's legally authorized representative. An investigator shall seek such consent only under circumstances that provide the prospective subject or the representative sufficient opportunity to consider whether or not to participate and that minimize the possibility of coercion or undue influence. The information that is given to the subject or the representative shall be in language understandable to the subject or the representative. No informed consent, whether oral or written, may include any exculpatory language through which the subject or the representative is made to waive or appear to waive any of the subject's legal rights, or releases or appears to release the investigator, the sponsor, the institution, or its agents from liability for negligence.

[46 FR 8951, Jan. 27, 1981, as amended at 64 FR 10942, Mar. 8, 1999]

See: https://www.hhs.gov/ohrp/regulations-and-policy/guidance/faq/informed-consent/index.html

https://www.cancer.gov/publications/dictionaries/cancer-terms/def/informed-consent

https://www.accessdata.fda.gov/scripts/cdrh/cfdocs/cfcfr/CFRSearch.cfm?CFRPart=50&showFR=1&subpartNode=21:1.0.1.1.20.2

29. B. It is the responsibility of the investigator, project sponsor, and review boards to obtain informed consent from patients or study participants. The obtaining of informed consent shall be deemed feasible unless, before use of the test article (except as provided in paragraph (b) of this section), both the investigator and a physician who is not otherwise participating in the clinical investigation certify in writing all of the following:

1. The human subject is confronted by a life-threatening situation necessitating the use of the test article.
2. Informed consent cannot be obtained from the subject because of an inability to communicate with, or obtain legally effective consent from, the subject.
3. Time is not sufficient to obtain consent from the subject's legal representative.
4. There is no available alternative method of approved or generally recognized therapy that provides an equal or greater likelihood of saving the life of the subject.

See: https://www.hhs.gov/ohrp/regulations-and-policy/guidance/faq/informed-consent/index.html

30. A. Informed consent is a process, not just a form. Information must be presented to enable persons to voluntarily decide whether or not to participate as a research subject. It is a fundamental mechanism to ensure respect for persons through provision of thoughtful consent for a voluntary act. The procedures used in obtaining informed consent should be designed to educate the subject population in terms that they can understand. Therefore, informed consent language and its documentation (especially explanation of the study's purpose, duration, experimental procedures, alternatives, risks, and benefits) must be written in "lay language" (i.e., understandable to the people being asked to participate). The written presentation of information is used to document the basis for consent and for the subjects' future reference. The consent document should be revised when deficiencies are noted or when additional information will improve the consent process.

See: https://www.hhs.gov/ohrp/regulations-and-policy/guidance/informed-consent-tips/index.html

31. D. Policy is an important tool for improving population health. Decision-makers often look to public health professionals for surveillance data, research findings, and evidence-based interventions and guidelines to help inform policy decisions. The Centers for Disease Control and Prevention (CDC) has identified four types of briefing documents that can be used to clearly communicate public health evidence. Public health professionals can use the following resources to develop briefs that succinctly inform decision-makers and stakeholders of the best available evidence on a public health problem, policy, method, or approach.

Policy briefs provide a summary of evidence-based best practices or policy options for a public health issue. They also include information on the background and significance of the issue as well as current status and potential next steps.

See: https://www.cdc.gov/policy/polaris/training/policy-resources-writing-briefs.html

https://www.cdc.gov/ruralhealth/diabetes/policybrief.html

32. D. Maleficence is the act of committing harm or evil.

Public health ethics involves a systematic process to clarify, prioritize, and justify possible courses of public health action based on ethical principles, values, and beliefs of stakeholders, as well as scientific and other information.

Beneficence means that persons are treated in an ethical manner not only by respecting their decisions and protecting them from harm, but also by making efforts to secure their well-being. Such treatment falls under the principle of beneficence. The term "beneficence" is often understood to cover acts of kindness or charity that go beyond strict obligation. In this document, beneficence is understood in a stronger sense, as an obligation. Two general rules have been formulated as complementary expressions of beneficent actions in this sense: (1) do not harm and (2) maximize possible benefits and minimize possible harms.

See: https://www.cdc.gov/od/science/integrity/phethics/index.htm

https://www.apha.org/-/media/files/pdf/membergroups/ethics/ethics_brochure.ashx

33. **C.** As a health communicator, you craft health and safety messages that can have a profound impact on the public. Using social media, these messages can reach more audiences and have an even greater impact on the public. This guide aims to assist you in translating your messages so they resonate and are relevant to social media audiences, and encourage action, engagement, and interaction. It is largely tactical, giving you specific ways to write for social media channels. Although a wide variety of social media tools exist, this guide will focus on three specific channels: Facebook, Twitter, and text messages (short message service or SMS). The Centers for Disease Control and Prevention (CDC) uses social media to provide users with access to credible, science-based health information when, where, and how you want it. A variety of social media tools are used to reinforce and personalize messages, reach new audiences, and build a communication infrastructure based on open information exchange.

See: https://www.cdc.gov/socialmedia/tools/guidelines/guideforwriting
.html

https://www.cdc.gov/socialmedia/tools/index.html

34. **C.** Resilient public alert and warning tools are essential to save lives and protect property during times of national, state, regional, and local emergencies. The Emergency Alert System (EAS) is used by alerting authorities to send warnings via broadcast, cable, satellite, and wireline communications pathways. EAS participants, which consist of broadcast, cable, satellite, and wireless providers, are the stewards of this important public service in close partnership with alerting officials at all levels of government. The EAS is also used when all other means of alerting the public are unavailable, providing an added layer of resiliency to the suite of available emergency communication tools.

Federal Emergency Management Agency constantly works to improve the EAS to better ensure seamless integration of CAP-based and emerging technologies. The U.S. EAS is a national public warning system that requires TV and radio broadcasters, cable television systems, wireless cable systems, satellite digital audio radio service providers, direct broadcast satellite service providers, and wireline video service providers to offer to the president the communications capability to address the American public during a national emergency. The system also may be used by state and local authorities to deliver important emergency information such as AMBER (missing children) alerts and emergency weather information targeted to a specific area.

See: https://www.fema.gov/emergency-alert-system

https://www.fcc.gov/consumers/guides/emergency-alert-system-eas

35. **A.** WHO principles for effective communications framework support the broad range of communication activities occurring across all parts and levels of WHO, including the following principles:

- Accessible to decision-makers
- Actionable by decision-makers
- Credible and trusted as perceived by decision-makers
- Relevant to decision-makers

- Timely to enable decision-making
- Understandable to decision-makers

See: https://www.who.int/communicating-for-health/principles/en/

36. C. Public health informatics is the systematic application of information, computer science, and technology to public health practice, research, and learning.

See: https://www.cdc.gov/publichealth101/informatics.html

https://www.cdc.gov/phifp/overview/index.html

37. A. Electronic health records (EHRs) allow for the systematic collection and management of patient health information in a form that can be shared across multiple healthcare settings. By providing easier access to patients' medical records, EHRs can help improve healthcare quality, efficiency, and safety. These systems can also promote use of preventive services, improve public health surveillance, and support research to improve population health. But despite these advantages, the expense of system implementation has slowed EHR adoption rates. With U.S. healthcare expenditures exceeding $2.5 trillion yearly (17% of our GDP), such investments must provide cost-effective support for better health at the individual and population levels.

EHRs are replacing paper medical records in most medical environments, but EHRs typically do not contain information about patient work. When it is available, healthcare providers can use information about their patients' work to provide the most appropriate care. In addition, healthcare organizations can use work information to identify groups of patients who may be at risk for harmful exposures or health problems, or who may benefit from specific interventions. Patient work information in EHRs and other health information systems also can be used to support public health activities, such as case reporting and disease registries.

See: https://www.cdc.gov/grand-rounds/pp/2011/20110721-electronic -records.html

https://www.cdc.gov/niosh/topics/ehr/default.html

https://www.cdc.gov/nchs/fastats/electronic-medical-records.htm

38. D. Maleficence is the act of committing harm or evil.

Federal law, good statistical practice, and our ethical obligations to the American people all require that any personal information collected by the National Center for Health Statistics (NCHS) be treated with the utmost concern for the privacy of those who provide it.

The NCHS collects detailed and often highly personal information from its respondents. Since this information is used for a variety of important purposes, it is critical that it be accurate. Respondents must be able to trust that information they provide to NCHS will be treated with respect, and that the answers they provide will not put them at risk. For that reason, NCHS takes all steps possible to protect the confidentiality of individually identifiable information.

Legally, NCHS is not permitted to release personal information to anyone—except for those persons or organizations we have clearly mentioned to the respondent before we ask them any questions. All of our respondents have the chance to make up their minds—without any pressure from us—as to (a) whether they want to participate in our surveys and (b) whether they agree with how we would use their information and who we would share it with. When they choose to provide us information, we rigorously observe the restrictions imposed by what we have promised them.

Federal law, upheld by the Fifth Circuit Court of Appeals, prohibits NCHS from releasing personal information to anyone without consent—no matter who the person is and no matter how carefully the person says he or she will take care of the information.

See: https://www.cdc.gov/nchs/about/policy/confidentiality.htm

39. **B.** Peer review is the process by which research is assessed for quality, relevancy, and accuracy by the active peers of the producer of the research. The National Library of Medicine (NLM) plays a pivotal role in translating biomedical research into practice. As the world's largest biomedical library, NLM creates and hosts major resources, tools, and services for literature, data, standards, and more, sending more than 100 terabytes of data to nearly five million users and receiving more than 10 terabytes of data from more than 3,000 users every weekday.

Scientists, health professionals, and the public in the United States and around the world search the Library's online information resources billions of times each year. In addition, NLM leads research and research training in biomedical informatics, information science, and data science. It conducts intramural research and training in its own laboratories and supports extramural research and training in institutions across the United States.

NLM is part of the National Institutes of Health (NIH), U.S. Department of Health and Human Services, in Bethesda, Maryland, tracing its roots to the founding of the library of the U.S. Army Surgeon General in 1836.

See: https://www.nih.gov/about-nih/what-we-do/nih-almanac/national -library-medicine-nlm

40. **D.** Social marketing is the use of marketing theory, skills, and practice to achieve social change, promote the general health, raise awareness, and induce changes in behavior. Community mobilization models for HIV prevention include social marketing campaigns.

See: https://effectiveinterventions.cdc.gov/en/community-and-structural -level/group-3/social-marketing

41. **D.** Immunization is one of the most successful and cost-effective health interventions and prevents between two and three million deaths every year. Immunization protects against diseases such as diphtheria, measles, pertussis (whooping cough), pneumonia, polio, rotavirus diarrhea, rubella, and tetanus. The benefits of immunization are increasingly being extended from children to adolescents and adults, providing protection against life-threatening diseases such as influenza, meningitis, and cancers (cervical and liver cancers).

However, even now, around 22 million infants are not fully immunized with routine vaccines and more than 1.5 million children under 5 die from diseases that could be prevented by existing vaccines. A mass vaccination campaign is a particular challenge to Adverse Events Following Immunization surveillance. It involves administration of vaccine doses to a large population over a short period of time. As a result, adverse events may be more noticeable to staff and to the public.

Two vaccines are licensed and recommended to prevent shingles in the United States. Zoster vaccine live (ZVL, Zostavax) has been in use since 2006. Recombinant zoster vaccine (RZV, Shingrix) has been in use since 2017 and is recommended by ACIP as the preferred shingles vaccine.

See: https://www.who.int/campaigns/immunization-week/2013/campaign_essentials/en/

https://www.cdc.gov/about/24-7/savinglives/diphtheria/campaign.html

https://vaccine-safety-training.org/mass-vaccination-campaigns.html

https://www.cdc.gov/vaccines/vpd/shingles/public/shingrix/index.html

42. **D.** There is no world war day.

Global public health days offer great potential to raise awareness and understanding about health issues and mobilize support for action, from the local community to the international stage. There are many world days observed throughout the year related to specific health issues or conditions—from Alzheimer's to zoonoses.

However, WHO focuses particular attention on the 7 separate days and one whole week that WHO Member States have mandated as "official" global public health days. These are

World Tuberculosis Day, 24 March

World Health Day, 7 April

World Malaria Day, 25 April

World No Tobacco Day, 31 May

World Immunization Week, 24 to 30 April

World Blood Donor Day, 14 June

World Hepatitis Day, 28 July

World Antibiotics Awareness Week, 12 to 18 November

World AIDS Day, 1 December

See: https://www.who.int/campaigns

43. **B.** There are numerous definitions of health communication. The National Cancer Institute and the Centers for Disease Control and Prevention use the following: The study and use of communication strategies to inform and influence individual and community decisions that enhance health. The Shannon and Weaver's linear model of communication was expanded in 1960 by David Berlo who created the Sender-Message-Channel-Receiver (SMCR) Model of Communication, which separated the model into clear components. Recognition of receiver resistance is another dimension that may be used to refine effectiveness of communication and promotion strategies.

See: https://health.gov/communication/literacy/quickguide/quickguide.pdf

https://www.cancer.gov/publications/health-communication/pink-book.pdf

44. **B.** Health communication can take many forms: written and verbal (words), traditional, and new media outlets. Proxemics is the branch of knowledge that deals with the amount of space that people feel is necessary to set between themselves and others.

See: https://npin.cdc.gov/pages/health-communication-strategies

45. **D.** Intonational refers to the "tone" of verbal communication. The pattern or melody of pitch changes in connected speech, especially the pitch pattern of a sentence, which distinguishes kinds of sentences or speakers of different language cultures. Kinesics is the interpretation of body motion communication such as facial expressions and gestures, as well as nonverbal behavior related to movement of any part of the body or the body as a whole.

See: https://npin.cdc.gov/pages/health-communication-strategies

46. **A.** Intonational refers to the "tone" of verbal communication. the pattern or melody of pitch changes in connected speech, especially the pitch pattern of a sentence, which distinguishes kinds of sentences or speakers of different language cultures.

See: https://npin.cdc.gov/pages/health-communication-strategies

47. **D.** Traditional interventions are no longer seen as enough to effectively prevent and control major health threats such as antimicrobial resistance, measles, and HIV. Research shows that properly designed behavior-based health communication activities can have a significant positive impact on health-related attitudes, beliefs, and behaviors. The complexity of communication variables makes it difficult if not impossible to create a single model for global health communication. The World Health Organization recognizes that effective, integrated and coordinated communication is integral to carrying out WHO's goal to build a better, healthier future for people all over the world. The purpose of this Framework is to describe a strategic approach for effectively communicating WHO information, advice, and guidance across a broad range of health issues: from chronic health issues to emerging and novel risks. Although techniques, audiences, and channels for WHO's communication products and activities differ, they all have the same goal:

To provide information, advice, and guidance to decision-makers (key audiences) to prompt action that will protect the health of individuals, families, communities, and nations.

See: https://www.who.int/mediacentre/communication-framework.pdf

https://www.cdc.gov/healthcommunication/healthbasics/WhatIsHC.html

https://ecdc.europa.eu/en/health-communication/facts

48. **A.** The communication–persuasion matrix was developed by William J. McGuire, and focuses on mass media strategies, which are used in campaigns such as anti-smoking advertisements.

See: https://www.bartleby.com/essay/Evaluating-Health-Campaigns-with
-the-Communication-Persuasion-PKZCK2JDB6A

http://agris.fao.org/agris-search/search.do?recordID=US20130
1443767

http://dahl.at/wordpress/2012/02/27/mcguire-communication
-persuasion-matrix

49. D. Effective communication is a key component of successful project management and delivery. It is often estimated that 80% of a project manager's job revolves around communication with the project team, client, and executive management. Without effective communication, vital information may not be exchanged effectively. A lack of communication may even delay or prohibit the execution or completion of scheduled tasks. Project success increases exponentially by avoiding communication issues.

The Communication Matrix should describe the communications approach for each communication vehicle and include information on target audience, distribution/purpose, and frequency, owner, and distribution vehicle; whether the communication should remain internal or is allowed externally; and any additional comments. Include items such as project meetings, project reporting, product documentation, test results, and metrics.

Consideration for exterior factors such as skin color is inappropriate.

See: https://www2.cdc.gov/cdcup/library/practices_guides/CDC_UP_
Communication_Management_Practices_Guide.pdf

50. D. Communism is defined as a political theory advocating class war, leading to a society in which all property is publicly owned and each person works and is paid according to his or her abilities and needs. This has nothing to do with health communication. Effective communication is a key component of successful project management and delivery. It is often estimated that 80% of a project manager's job revolves around communication with the project team, client, and executive management. Without effective communication, vital information may not be exchanged effectively. A lack of communication may even delay or prohibit the execution or completion of scheduled tasks. Project success increases exponentially by avoiding communication issues. The Communication Matrix should describe the communications approach for each communication vehicle and include information on target audience, distribution/purpose, and frequency, owner, and distribution vehicle; whether the communication should remain internal or is allowed externally; and any additional comments. Include items such as project meetings, project reporting, product documentation, test results, and metrics.

Consideration for exterior factors such as skin color is inappropriate.

See: https://www2.cdc.gov/cdcup/library/practices_guides/CDC_UP_
Communication_Management_Practices_Guide.pdf

51. D. E-Health is the use of information and communication technologies to improve people's health and healthcare.

Although the terms "telemedicine" and "telehealth" are often used to describe similar types of technologies, the term "telemedicine" has historically been used to refer specifically to bilateral, interactive health communications with clinicians on both "ends" of the exchange (e.g., videoconferenced grand rounds, x-rays transmitted between radiologists or consultations where a remote practitioner presents a patient to a specialist), whereas the term "telehealth" incorporates not only technologies that fall under "telemedicine," but also direct, electronic patient-to-provider interactions and the use of medical devices (e.g., smartphone applications ["apps"], activity trackers, automated reminders, blood glucose monitors) to collect and transmit health information, often with the intent to monitor or manage chronic conditions. Currently, there are four basic modalities, or methods, of telehealth.

The term "E-Health" is generally used to describe an even broader array of digital information tools, including electronic health records (EHRs), which facilitate the exchange of patient data between healthcare professionals. E-Health may include computerized physician order entry mechanisms, e- prescribing, and clinical decision support tools, which provide information electronically to providers about protocols and standards for use in diagnosing and treating patients.

See: https://aspe.hhs.gov/system/files/pdf/206751/TelemedicineE-HealthReport.pdf

https://health.gov/communication/ehealth/default.htm

52. D. Mobile health (mHealth) is the use of smartphone apps designed to foster health and well-being. These apps range from programs that send targeted text messages aimed at encouraging healthy behaviors to alerts about disease outbreaks to programs or apps that help patients with reminders to adhere to specific care regimens. Increasingly, smartphones may use cameras, microphones, or other sensors or transducers to capture vital signs for input to apps and bridging into RPM.

See: https://aspe.hhs.gov/system/files/pdf/206751/TelemedicineE-HealthReport.pdf

53. B. A loss-framed message presents negative outcomes, or the absence of positive outcomes associated with not performing a particular health-promoting behavior, whereas a gain-framed message presents beneficial outcomes or the absence of negative outcomes related to performing the behavior.

See: https://fns-prod.azureedge.net/sites/default/files/LitReview_Framing.pdf

54. A. Health literacy is the degree to which individuals have the capacity to obtain, process, and understand basic health information and services needed to make appropriate health decisions.

Health literacy is dependent on individual and systemic factors:

- Communication skills of lay persons and professionals
- Lay and professional knowledge of health topics
- Culture
- Demands of the healthcare and public health systems
- Demands of the situation/context

Health literacy affects people's ability to

- Navigate the healthcare system, including filling out complex forms and locating providers and services
- Share personal information, such as health history, with providers
- Engage in self-care and chronic-disease management
- Understand mathematical concepts such as probability and risk

See: https://health.gov/communication/literacy/quickguide/factsbasic.htm

55. **C.** The Shannon–Weaver model of communication refers to an integrated concept of information source, message, transmitter, signal, channel, noise, receiver, and information destination. Other components include the probability of error, encoding, decoding, information rate, and channel capacity. The model has been used in structuring health communication strategies.

Shannon, C. E., & Weaver, W. (1963). *The mathematical theory of communication.* Urbana, IL: University of Illinois Press. ISBN 978-0-252-72548-7

56. **D.** The Centers for Disease Control and Prevention (CDC) views population health as an interdisciplinary, customizable approach that allows health departments to connect practice to policy for change to happen locally. This approach utilizes nontraditional partnerships among different sectors of the community—public health, industry, academia, healthcare, local government entities, and so on—to achieve positive health outcomes. Population health brings significant health concerns into focus and addresses ways that resources can be allocated to overcome the problems that drive poor health conditions in the population. Public health works to protect and improve the health of communities through policy recommendations, health education, and outreach, and research for disease detection and injury prevention. It can be defined as what "we as a society do collectively to assure the conditions in which people can be healthy." On the other hand, population health provides "an opportunity for healthcare systems, agencies, and organizations to work together in order to improve the health outcomes of the communities they serve."

See: https://www.cdc.gov/pophealthtraining/whatis.html

https://www.cdc.gov/diabetes/ndep/pdfs/population_health_management_-webinar_slides.pdf

57. **A.** Prospect theory was developed by Daniel Kahneman and Amos Tversky as a psychologically more accurate description of decision-making. The theory describes the way that individuals make decisions based on the potential value of losses and gains rather than the final outcome. The theory has been applied to refine health communication strategies.

Harrington, N. G., & Kerr, A. M. (2017). Rethinking risk: Prospect theory application in health message framing research. *Health Communication, 32*(2), 131–141. doi:10.1080/10410236.2015.1110004

Kahneman, D., & Tversky, A. (1979). Prospect theory: An analysis of decision under risk. *Econometrica, 47*(2), 263–291. doi:10.2307/1914185

58. **B.** In the transtheoretical model (stages of change model), behavior change has been conceptualized as a five-stage process or continuum related to a person's readiness to change precontemplation, contemplation, preparation, action, and maintenance. Individuals use continuous assessment of risks and benefits of behavior to proceed through the stages of change.

See: https://www.cdc.gov/nccdphp/sgr/chap6.htm

https://www.ruralhealthinfo.org/toolkits/health-promotion/2/theories-and-models/stages-of-change

59. **B.** The use of fear appeals in health promotion is controversial. Proponents are confident in their efficacy, whereas opponents are confident that fear appeals backfire. A meta-analysis of 248 studies concluded that fear appeals are effective at positively influencing attitude, intentions, and behaviors; there are very few circumstances under which they are not effective; and there are no identified circumstances under which they backfire and lead to undesirable outcomes. Another study concluded that "In spite of the evidence against its use, it seems likely that appeal to fear will continue to be used in conjunction with other public awareness initiatives to modify recognized detrimental behaviors such as smoking and drunk driving as well as silent killers such as hypertension. However, when used to promote a treatment that has no evidentiary basis such as subluxation-based practice in chiropractic the appeal to fear is a fallacy and must be stopped."

Simpson, J. K. (2017). Appeal to fear in health care: Appropriate or inappropriate? *Chiropractic & Manual Therapies, 25,* 27. doi:10.1186/s12998-017-0157-8

Tannenbaum, M. B., Hepler, J., Zimmerman, R. S., Saul, L., Jacobs, S., Wilson, K., & Albarracín, D. (2015). Appealing to fear: A meta-analysis of fear appeal effectiveness and theories. *Psychological Bulletin, 141*(6), 1178–1204. doi:10.1037/a0039729

60. **D.** The American Medical Writers Association provides guidelines on essential skill sets for medical communication, which include expertise in written and verbal communication, commitment to the principles of ethics, and knowledge of healthcare systems.

Befriending a physician is not a required skill of AMWA members.

See: https://www.amwa.org/page/Med_Communication

3

Leadership

■ INTRODUCTION

In the book *Milestones in Public Health* published in 2006 by Pfizer Global Pharmaceuticals, nine major accomplishments and challenges reveal the role of leaders in advancing the agenda of strategies to improve the health of populations. Leaders are "made not born"! Although certain individual personalities may be conducive to leading organizations and teams to accomplish their goals, there is evidence that leadership skills can be acquired through training and practice. It is difficult to learn everything that one needs to lead a public health agency only through pedagogy because on-the-job experience contributes a lot to learning how to navigate the variety of stakeholders and personalities that must collaborate to achieve successful implementation of strategies to prevent disease in populations. Studying and analyzing the questions in this section will enrich competencies in the following topic areas:

- Utilize critical analysis to prioritize and justify actions and allocation of resources

- Apply team-building skills

- Apply organizational change management concepts and skills

- Apply conflict management skills

- Implement strategies to support and improve team performance

- Apply negotiation skills

- Establish and model standards of performance and accountability

- Guide organizational decision-making and planning based on internal and external assessments

- Prepare professional development plans for self or others

- Develop strategies to motivate others for collaborative problem-solving, decision-making, and evaluation

- Develop capacity-building strategies at the individual, organizational, or community level
- Communicate an organization's mission, goals, values, and shared vision to stakeholders
- Create teams for implementing health initiatives
- Develop a mission, goals, values, and shared vision for an organization or the community in conjunction with key stakeholders
- Implement a continuous quality improvement plan
- Develop a continuous quality improvement plan
- Evaluate organizational performance in relation to strategic and defined goals
- Implement organizational strategic planning processes
- Assess organizational policies and procedures regarding working across multiple organizations
- Align organizational policies and procedures with regulatory and statutory requirements
- Maximize efficiency of programs
- Ensure that informatics principles and methods are used in the design and implementation of data systems

■ QUESTIONS

1. Practicing public health with the utmost attention to professionalism encourages trust in the public of recommendations to improve collective health. The following are among the tenets of public health professionalism, EXCEPT

   A. Promoting variable standards of personal and organizational integrity, compassion, honesty, and respect for all people
   B. Analyzing determinants of health and disease using an ecological framework
   C. Analyzing the potential impacts of legal and regulatory environments on the conduct of ethical public health research and practice
   D. Distinguishing between population and individual ethical considerations in relation to the benefits, costs, and burdens of public health programs

2. Bisphenol-A is a high-volume production chemical used in the manufacture of plastics. There is controversy regarding population exposure and potential health effects. As research is ongoing to collect more data, some jurisdictions are taking action to ban the chemical from potential routes of exposure, including food cans and drinking bottles. At the same time, lobbying by plastics manufacturers have intensified the claim that bisphenol-A is harmless. As a leader of a public health agency weighing your options on whether to propose a ban

on bisphenol-A in your community, your leadership should draw upon the following guidelines, EXCEPT

A. Development of strategies to motivate others for collaborative problem-solving, decision-making, and evaluation
B. Demonstrate transparency, integrity, and honesty in all actions
C. Describe alternative strategies for collaboration and partnership among organizations, focused on public health goals
D. Demonstrate conniving skills to counteract lobbying strategies

3. On February 9, 2010, First Lady Michelle Obama announced a "very ambitious" program to end the American plague of childhood obesity in a single generation. This is an example of public health leadership, defined as "the ability to create and communicate a shared vision for a changing future; champion solutions to organizational and community challenges; and energize commitment to goals." To be successful, however, the announcement must be followed with specific actions associated with leadership skills in public health. These may include the following:

A. Withholding state funds from counties that do not abide by Obama's strategy to combat obesity
B. Encouraging legal action against parents whose children are obese
C. Applying social justice and human rights principles when addressing community needs to address the obesity epidemic
D. Requiring routine periodical reporting of caloric intake by all American children

4. Imagine that you are the head of the unit of the County Healthcare Agency during a resurgence of the H1N1 pandemic. Which of the following does NOT represent attributes of leadership in public health that ensure effective discharge of your responsibilities?

A. Apply social justice and human rights principles when addressing community needs
B. Develop strategies to motivate others for collaborative problem-solving, decision-making, and evaluation
C. Engage in dialogue and learning from others to advance public health goals to contain the pandemic
D. Apply clandestine strategies to discharge your responsibilities and achieve your goals

5. Which of the following leadership strategies is likely to be the most effective for the project director of a university research team in designing and implementing an evaluation study of the long-term effects of an intervention to prevent drug abuse in a lower socioeconomic status community?

A. Co-opt one of the community leaders by promising special treatment for his family in the course of the study
B. Clearly demonstrate academic credentials and track record to convince community representatives of the team's leadership expertise, skills, and knowledge of the problem

C. Convey an attitude of solicitous, maternal concern, assuring community leaders that whatever the team does will benefit the community
D. Invite community leaders to work collaboratively to plan, develop, and implement the research study and intervention program

6. It is typical that many programs and initiatives compete for financial resources in a public health agency responsible for protecting population health through implementation of activities to prevent disease. Which of the following are processes for prioritizing funding?

A. A formulaic strategic plan
B. A S.P.O.T. (Strengths, Problems, Opportunities and Threats) Analysis
C. A detailed budget plan
D. A preemptive strategic plan

7. The distinctive feature of the "situational theory of leadership" (also known as Hersey–Blanchard Situational Leadership Theory) is that

A. Personality traits of the leader dictate the leadership approach
B. Events happening dictate the leadership approach
C. Subordinate consensus dictates the leadership approach
D. The financial profit margin dictates the leadership approach

8. The best definition of an "organization" with respect to public health is

A. A group of individuals working in the same region affected by a disease burden
B. The physical location where people work on public health issues
C. A group of people focused on making profit by selling vaccines
D. A deliberate arrangement of people to accomplish a specific purpose

9. According to the Mintzberg theory of management, the 10 major management roles can be grouped into which of the following categories?

A. Leadership, resource allocation, and planning roles
B. Decision-making, leadership, and planning roles
C. Informational, interpersonal, and decisional roles
D. Networking, controlling, and communication roles

10. According to the Mintzberg theory of management, the interpersonal category of management roles includes

A. Leadership, monitor, and spokesperson roles
B. Leadership, disseminator, and liaison roles
C. Leadership, figurehead, and monitor roles
D. Leadership, figurehead, and liaison roles

11. According to the Mintzberg theory of management, the informational category of management roles includes

A. Spokesperson, monitor, and disseminator roles
B. Liaison, leadership, and spokesperson roles

C. Disseminator, leadership, and liaison roles

D. Spokesperson, leadership, and entrepreneur roles

12. According to the Mintzberg theory of management, the decisional category of management roles includes

A. Disturbance handler, resource allocator, and spokesperson

B. Negotiator, entrepreneur, and resource allocator

C. Disseminator, monitor, and spokesperson

D. Entrepreneur, leadership, and figurehead

13. According to Robert L. Katz's theory, the three categories of management skills are

A. Negotiating, organizational, and analytical skills

B. Negotiating, conceptual, and analytical skills

C. Negotiating, human, and analytical skills

D. Technical, human, and conceptual skills

14. The formal framework for dividing, grouping, and coordinating jobs and responsibilities in a public health agency is captured in the

A. Policies and procedures

B. Vision statement

C. Mission statement

D. Organizational structure

15. Public health leaders often have to make decisions based on incomplete information. The type of decision-making in which the solution is considered "good-enough" is

A. Satisficing

B. Intuitive

C. Programmed

D. Rational

16. Public health advocates often demand that the very best decisions are made to protect every individual in a population that may be vulnerable to a risk factor. This type of decision-making is

A. Satisficing

B. Programmed

C. Maximizing

D. Rational

17. The main difference between "rational" and "intuitive" decision-making is

A. There is no real difference between them; the outcome is often the same.

B. Rational decision-making takes more time.

C. Intuitive decision-making takes more time.

D. Rational decision-making relies on conscious, not subconscious reasoning.

18. Different types of decision-making strategies may be required in public health emergency preparedness compared with emergency response. These are described as combinatorial or positional decision-making. The main difference between these two strategies is

    A. Combinatorial decision-making takes steps toward a predetermined final outcome, whereas positional decision-making responds to emerging events.
    B. Combinatorial decision-making requires more time.
    C. Positional decision-making requires more time.
    D. Combinatorial decision-making requires teamwork.

19. Public health leaders and managers may use computerized decision-support systems for all of the following EXCEPT

    A. Declaration of disease outbreak
    B. Declaration of a pandemic
    C. Assuming the position of stakeholders
    D. Resource allocation

20. In a public health agency, the continuous line of authority that clarifies who reports to who throughout the agency is referred to as

    A. Supply chain
    B. The matrix
    C. Chain of command
    D. Bottom-up approach

21. The obligation of employees in a public health agency to perform their assigned activities is referred to as

    A. United front
    B. Unity of command
    C. Chain of command
    D. Responsibility

22. Public health leaders should be skilled in managing change. To minimize resistance to change, leaders should do the following:

    A. Avoid conflict
    B. Communicate information about the change honestly, thoroughly, and openly
    C. Implement the change rapidly with minimal consultation
    D. Implement the change abruptly

23. The organizational culture or organizational climate of a public health agency can be defined as

    A. The set of values and norms shared by employees of the agency
    B. The carbon footprint of the agency
    C. The number of cultures acceptable to the agency leadership
    D. The latitudinal location of the agency

24. Most public health projects require the contribution of experts in various disciplines. Which leadership or management style is most likely to be effective for such projects?

A. Middle management
B. Authority management
C. Team management
D. Top management

25. Public health agencies are often required to optimize efficiency of operations to

A. Minimize employee time-off due to labor union contracts
B. Maximize outputs and minimize inputs
C. Avoid taxation
D. Avoid laying off good employees

26. To promote change in procedures or practices, leaders target those who are recognized as opinion leaders and role models with information about the change. These targeted individuals are

A. Early adopters
B. Early majority
C. Innovators
D. Risk takers

27. The focus of data analysis is to

A. Collect data from various sources
B. Organize data for efficient retrieval
C. Identify data sources for research funding
D. Transform data into a form that reveals structure, trend, or other useful information

28. System analysis is typically conducted to

A. Review a proposal for feasibility
B. Explore potential vendor solutions
C. Identify management needs
D. Investigate users' needs to design functional requirements of a system of operation

29. Organization theory is relevant to the implementation of health information technology because

A. All theories are relevant.
B. Organization theory helps to identify concepts that are relevant for informatics practice.
C. Organization theory is not relevant to health informatics.
D. Organization theory informs the organization as a whole.

30. A public health leader must understand the process through which innovative approaches to disease prevention diffuse through agencies and populations. Everett Rogers' theory on the Diffusion of Innovation is relevant to the understanding because it identifies which four elements?

A. The creative class, the neighborhood, the cost, and advertisement
B. The Internet presence, social network, communication savvy, and business strategy
C. The innovation, communication channels, time, and social system
D. The advertisement options, early adopters, economic costs, and disease burden

31. The five stages in Everett Rogers' theory of innovation-decision process are

A. Early adopters, later adopters, early majority, late majority, and laggards
B. Innovation, communication, time, social network, and economy
C. Innovation, communication, evaluation, analysis, and decision
D. Knowledge, persuasion, decision, implementation, and confirmation

32. To launch a new public health technology system (e.g., the 2013 launching of Internet-based enrollment in the provisions of the Patient Protection and Affordable Care Act), it is preferably to avoid publicizing a "go live" date because

A. Going "live" makes people think about mortality.
B. Implementing technology occurs over time and "go live" implies it is a single point in time.
C. "Go live" might be misunderstood as going to a specific place in person.
D. "Go live" might be misunderstood as a medical theater procedure.

33. The mobilization of healthcare information electronically across public health agencies within a regional healthcare system is referred to as

A. Health information exchange
B. Health informatics
C. Health information management
D. Health information technology

34. Interactive computer programs designed to assist health professionals with decision-making tasks are referred to as

A. Telemedicine
B. E-Health
C. m-Health
D. Health decision-support systems

35. The health information organization that connects healthcare stakeholders under a governing structure for health information exchange is called

A. Regional Health Information Organization (RHIO)
B. Health Information Exchange (HIE)

C. Health and Human Services (HHS)

D. Health Management Organization (HMO)

36. The detailed and overarching organizational work plan for the healthcare organization's quality improvement activities is referred to as the

A. Organizational structure

B. Organizational work plan

C. Quality improvement plan

D. Organizational activity plan

37. A public health agency's plan for improving quality should include the following characteristics EXCEPT

A. Siloed processes with expert leaders collaborating every 2 weeks on time-sensitive resources

B. Use of data and measurable outcomes to determine progress toward relevant, evidence-based benchmarks

C. Focus on linkages, efficiencies, and provider and client expectations in addressing outcome improvement

D. Continuous process that is adaptive to change and that fits within the framework of other programmatic quality assurance and quality improvement activities

38. The organizational structure for implementing a quality improvement plan should have the following key components EXCEPT

A. Clearly visible leadership

B. Board of directors

C. Information management technology

D. No leadership input from outside the agency

39. A public health agency plans to reduce the proportion of diabetes patients whose HbA1c levels are less than 9%. What information is needed to develop a quality improvement project based on this quality improvement plan?

A. Baseline data on HbA1c levels in the population

B. A control population where the placebo intervention is provided

C. Information on diabetes prevalence in the control population

D. Genetic profile of insulin gene polymorphism

40. The following dimensions are essential in developing a quality improvement plan for a healthcare agency EXCEPT

A. Safety

B. Timeliness

C. Frequency

D. Efficiency

41. Successful implementation of quality improvement in a public health agency requires the following EXCEPT

    A. A process for identifying organizational problems
    B. A process for solving organizational problems
    C. A process for providing ongoing education and training for all staff of the organization in principles, tools, and techniques of continuous improvement
    D. A process for undermining organizational competitors

42. To be effective, leaders of public health agencies must acquire and implement team-building skills. The principles of team-building DO NOT include

    A. Articulation of clear goals
    B. Division of labor
    C. Constructive conflict resolution
    D. Individualized and individual performance-oriented reward systems

43. The five stages of team development are

    A. Forming, storming, norming, performing, and adjourning
    B. Planning, forming, performing, evaluating, and adjourning
    C. Planning, forming, norming, evaluating, and adjourning
    D. Forming, norming, performing, evaluating, and adjourning

44. In an interprofessional healthcare team, each member should

    A. Assume a leadership stance
    B. Assume that the leader is the physician
    C. Assume that the leader is the public health professional
    D. Assume the leader with the most interdisciplinary training is the leader

45. Sustaining essential public health practice competencies requires

    A. College-level continuing education
    B. Specialty-based case studies
    C. Mentorship leadership training
    D. Multidisciplinary instruction

46. A possible strategy for dealing with difficult interprofessional situations is

    A. Using an influential leader to address misunderstandings and conflicts
    B. Reporting conflicts to higher organizational levels
    C. Encouraging the participation of team members in managing differences and conflict resolution
    D. Addressing individuals who express disparate opinions

47. Successful interprofessional teamwork needs

    A. Respect for hierarchy
    B. Challenging practical information
    C. Challenging role development
    D. Respecting ethical values

48. An important responsibility of an influential public health team leader is

    A. The ability to delegate team activities
    B. Providing a safe environment for participation
    C. Keeping clear, professional boundaries
    D. Proposing divisions of labor

49. The management style recommended for providing team-based healthcare is

    A. Authoritative
    B. Task-oriented
    C. Participatory
    D. Transformational

50. An effective skill in managing interprofessional conflict that may arise in public health practice is

    A. Offering feedback
    B. Suggesting solutions
    C. Challenging evidence
    D. Promoting debate

51. An essential skill for providing team-based public health services is

    A. Creative teaching
    B. Challenging leadership
    C. Critical thinking
    D. Commitment to change

52. Effective interprofessional teams in public health practice result from the following EXCEPT

    A. Defining clear purpose and roles for members and the team
    B. Friendships
    C. Communication
    D. Personal and team accountability

53. What is the first step in the process of capacity building?

    A. Assess capacity needs
    B. Assess capacity assets
    C. Engage stakeholders in capacity development
    D. Develop a capacity development response

54. Building capacity for public health agencies requires a clear method of communication flow, as well as mutual understanding of roles and responsibility. This method is defined as the

    A. Vision and scope
    B. Conceptual approach
    C. Organizational structure
    D. Organizational approach

55. Developing capacity for a public health agency requires an articulation of what the agency seeks to accomplish and the program the agency wishes to follow. These requirements are codified in the

    A. Organizational structure
    B. Vision and strategy
    C. Conceptual framework
    D. Organizational approach

56. Building capacity of a public health agency requires information about the agency's understanding of the world. This information is usually articulated in the company's

    A. Conceptual framework
    B. Vision and strategy
    C. Organizational attitude
    D. Organizational structure

57. A public health agency's general expression of its overall purpose is its

    A. Mission
    B. Vision
    C. Goals
    D. Strategy

58. Implementing the strategic plan of a public health agency involves

    A. Senior managers and board members only
    B. Senior and middle managers only
    C. Managers at all levels
    D. Senior managers only

59. In public health, scenario planning is useful to

    A. Consider alternate futures no matter how implausible they are
    B. Ensure that managers implement scenarios they know can work in practice
    C. Develop contingency plans for each scenario
    D. Build only short-term plans

60. Which terminology is used for a public health agency's capacity to renew and recreate its strategic capabilities to meet the needs of a changing environment?

    A. Core competence
    B. Competence replacement
    C. Renewable resources
    D. Dynamic capabilities

■ ANSWERS

1. **A.** Promotion of unequal (variable) standards in desirable attributes is inappropriate and inconsistent with the tenets of public health professionalism. Professional development is a systematic process that strengthens how professionals obtain and retain knowledge, skills, and attitudes. Professionalism isn't one thing; it's a combination of qualities.

   See: https://www.cdc.gov/healthyschools/trainingtools.htm

   https://www.dol.gov/odep/topics/youth/softskills/Professionalism .pdf

2. **D.** "Conniving," or the tendency to do something immoral, illegal, or harmful, is the opposite of what is expected from good leaders. Instead, advocacy and coalition building are essential skills. Training and professional development strengthen the public health workforce by helping professionals learn new skills and advance their careers to become leaders in their agencies.

   See: https://www.cdc.gov/publichealthgateway/nlaph/index.html

3. **C.** Withholding funds from evidence-based public health intervention is not consistent with leadership.

   Threatening litigation (fear appeal) is controversial, and not likely to be effective in this case.

   Monitoring caloric intake for all American children is not logistically possible, will be too expensive to attempt, and may be counterproductive.

   The application of social justice and human rights principles is a leadership quality.

   > "Often, when we talk about this issue, we begin by citing sobering statistics like the ones you've heard today – that over the past three decades, childhood obesity rates in America have tripled; that nearly one third of children in America are now overweight or obese – one in three. But these numbers don't paint the full picture. These words – "overweight" and "obese" – they don't tell the full story. This isn't just about inches and pounds or how our kids look. It's about how our kids feel, and how they feel about themselves. It's about the impact we're seeing on every aspect of their lives."
   >
   > — First Lady Michelle Obama (2010)

   See: https://obamawhitehouse.archives.gov/realitycheck/the-press-office/ remarks-first-lady-michelle-obama

   https://www.cdc.gov/nccdphp/dch/programs/healthycommunities program/tools/pdf/SDOH-workbook.pdf

   https://www.hhrjournal.org/2019/06/health-is-a-human-right-at -cdc/

4. **D.** "Clandestine" implies something or some action that is kept secret or done secretively, especially because it is illegal. This is not consistent with public health leadership. Training and professional development strengthen the public health workforce by helping professionals learn new skills and advance their careers to become leaders in their agencies.

See: https://www.cdc.gov/publichealthgateway/nlaph/index.html

5. **D.** Co-opting, credential bragging, and solicitous behaviors are not consistent with effective leadership in community engagement. Community engagement is the process of working collaboratively with and through groups of people affiliated by geographic proximity, special interest, or similar situations to address issues affecting the well-being of those people. It is a powerful vehicle for bringing about environmental and behavioral changes that will improve the health of the community and its members. It often involves partnerships and coalitions that help mobilize resources and influence systems, change relationships among partners, and serve as catalysts for changing policies, programs, and practices.

See: https://www.atsdr.cdc.gov/communityengagement/pce_what.html

6. **B.** A formulaic plan is generally not strategic because it is predictable and produced according to a slavishly followed rule or style; therefore, it is unresponsive to program needs.

The budget plan comes after the prioritization of objectives.

A preemptive strategic plan implies an attempt to forestall something, rather than being proactive.

Analysis of strengths, problems, opportunities, and threats is a reliable planning scheme.

See: https://communityconnections.unl.edu/40aabb4b-98ec-4eb1-b7da
    -d695febffdfa.pdf

7. **B.** The situational theory of leadership takes the approach that no single leadership style is consistently applicable in all situations. Instead, the situation dictates the type of leadership and strategies that are best for particular tasks. The most effective leaders are adaptable and can quickly identify type of task, nature of the team, and other environmental or situational factors that are likely to be effective. The theory is also known as the Hersey–Blanchard Situational Leadership Theory.

See: https://www.verywellmind.com/what-is-the-situational-theory-of
    -leadership-2795321

Rabarison, K., Ingram, R. C., & Holsinger, J. W., Jr. (2013). Application of situational leadership to the national voluntary public health accreditation process. *Frontiers in Public Health, 1*, 26. doi:10.3389/fpubh.2013.00026

8. **D.** A public health organization is a systematic arrangement of people with a specific purpose and with expertise to create conditions that keep people healthy.

See: https://www.cdc.gov/about/organization/cio.htm

9. **C.** The Mintzberg theory posits that managerial skills are learned through experience and not simply by pedagogy. According to this theory, there are three major managerial categories: informational, interpersonal, and decisional roles, under which there are 10 roles or functions.

Planning roles and networking are important, but not major categories.

Glouberman, S., & Mintzberg, H. (2001, January 1). Managing the care of health and the cure of disease—Part I: Differentiation. *Health Care Management Review, 26* (1), 56–69.

> http://www.mintzberg.org/blog/hospital-management

Mintzberg, H. (1989). *Mintzberg on management: Inside our strange world of organizations.* New York, NY: Simon and Schuster; 418 pages; ISBN 0029213711, 9780029213711.

Mintzberg, H. (2012). Managing the myths of health care. *World Hospitals and Health Services, 48*(3), 4–7.

10. **D.** The *interpersonal* category of skills essential for managerial leaders includes the following three roles: ceremonial *figurehead,* inspirational *leader,* and networking *liaison.* Monitoring, spokesperson, and disseminator skills are included in the *informational* category of management.

See: https://www.business.com/articles/management-theory-of-henry -mintzberg-basics/

Mintzberg, H. (1975). The manager's job: Folklore and fact. *Harvard Business Review, 53*(4), 49–61. (https://uci.primo.exlibrisgroup.com/permalink/ 01CDL_IRV_INST/m9vhfd/proquest1296458764)

11. **A.** The *informational* category of management roles includes interior *monitor* of information, interior *disseminator* of information, and external communication *spokesperson.* Liaison, leadership, and entrepreneurial skills are not included in the informational category.

See: https://www.business.com/articles/management-theory-of-henry -mintzberg-basics/

Mintzberg, H. (1975). The manager's job: Folklore and fact. *Harvard Business Review, 53*(4), 49–61.

12. **B.** The *decisional* category of management skills includes innovation-inclined *entrepreneur, resource-allocator,* and an interior *negotiator.* Dissemination and monitoring are included in the informational category, and disturbance handling is not part of the decisional category of skills.

See: https://www.business.com/articles/management-theory-of-henry -mintzberg-basics/

Mintzberg, H. (1975). The manager's job: Folklore and fact. *Harvard Business Review, 53*(4), 49–61.

13. **D.** Robert L. Katz's theory posits that managers need three essential skills that can be developed and cultivated. *Technical skills* are the specific knowledge and techniques needed to perform specific tasks proficiently. *Human skills* involve the ability to work well with other people both individually and in a group. *Conceptual skills* are the skills that managers use to think and to conceptualize about abstract and complex situations.

Harvard Business Review. (1974). Skills of an effective administrator. https://hbr.org/1974/09/skills-of-an-effective-administrator

Peterson, T. O., & Van Fleet, D. D. (2004). The ongoing legacy of RL Katz: An updated typology of management skills. *Management Decision, 42* (10), 1297–1308.

14. **D.** An organizational structure is a system that defines how activities are coordinated to achieve the goals of an organization such as a public health agency.

See: https://www.cdc.gov/about/organization/orgchart.htm

Jacobides, M. G. (2007). The inherent limits of organizational structure and the unfulfilled role of hierarchy: Lessons from a near-war. *Organization Science, 18*(3), 455–477.

15. **A.** Satisficing is the "strategy" of accepting the status quo as satisfactory. According to David Nelson, "People are exposed to hundreds of media messages each day, mostly in the form of advertising. The human brain is remarkably adept at blocking information a person does not consider relevant. A person can hone-in quickly on information that is salient, which explains the tendency of people to rapidly scan Web sites. Information seekers tend to work no harder than they need to in order to find relevant information (i.e., they are cognitive misers). Once they determine that what they have is good enough, they rarely search further. This tendency, first described in the 1950s, is referred to as satisficing and is especially common among people who are time-pressured, such as journalists and health care providers. People exposed to excessive information tend to rely on simple rules such as selecting the first item from a lengthy list."

See: https://www.cdc.gov/pcd/issues/2007/jan/06_0119.htm

16. **C.** Traditionally, public health emergency response has focused on maximizing population health, for example, through saving the most lives. However, some have challenged this assumption and have suggested that fairness considerations be more explicitly included in policy decisions, even if doing so does not maximize population health. Conflict between providing "fair chances" and maximizing "best outcomes" arises when there are relatively small differences in expected benefits that may be gained by people in different prioritization groups.

See: https://www.cdc.gov/about/pdf/advisory/ventdocument_release .pdf

17. **A.** Rational decision-making involves taking sequential steps designed to approach and secure a desired goal. Intuitive decision-making involves instinctive, subjective, and subconscious steps in the path toward the desired goal.

See: https://journals.sagepub.com/doi/pdf/10.1177/0170840616655483

https://the-happy-manager.com/articles/intuition-and-decision -making/

https://www.cdc.gov/niosh/mining/UserFiles/works/pdfs/jadmus .pdf

18. **A.** Combinatorial decision-making involves having a clearly defined outcome and taking a series of steps that link the initial position with the final outcome in a secure narrowly defined path. Numerous alternative paths are quickly rejected based on predetermined criteria (hence the term combinatorial). Positional decision-making involves a more flexible approach that bases decisions on consideration of each new opportunity created by responding to prevailing situations.

See: https://courses.lumenlearning.com/wm-principlesofmanagement/chapter/styles-of-decision-making/

https://www.cdc.gov/features/understandingevidence/index.html

19. **C.** Computers are (not yet) able to replace human thought processes in stakeholder consultation. Stakeholders are people or organizations invested in the program, interested in the results of the evaluation, and/or with a stake in what will be done with the results of the evaluation. Representing their needs and interests throughout the process is fundamental to good program evaluation.

See: https://www.cdc.gov/eval/guide/step1/index.htm

20. **C.** Chain of command is the procedural order in which authority and power in an agency is held and/or delegated from top management to every employee at every level of the agency. In general, instructions flow downward along the chain of command and accountability flows upward.

See: https://wwwnc.cdc.gov/eid/article/16/6/10-0345_article

21. **D.** Responsibility is defined as the state or fact of having a duty to deal with something or of having control over someone. For example, the Centers for Disease Control and Prevention (CDC) as an organization is responsible for controlling the introduction and spread of infectious diseases, and provides consultation and assistance to other nations and international agencies to assist in improving their disease prevention and control, environmental health, and health promotion activities. Individuals within CDC are charged with specific responsibilities.

See: https://www.cdc.gov/maso/pdf/cdcmiss.pdf

22. **B.** The primary purpose of a change management system is to provide a standard process for submitting, documenting, and reviewing changes in preparation for prioritizing those corrections/enhancements. It identifies what changes to make, the authority for approving changes, the support for implementing changes, and the process for formal deviations and waivers from the original agreed upon requirements. The change management process establishes an orderly and effective procedure for tracking the submission, coordination, review, evaluation, categorization, and approval for release of all changes to the project's baselines. The change management system defines the guidelines for the management of project change and describes in detail how changes will be documented, organized, and managed.

Each change request is unique and the proper evaluation of each change request is a vital management practice. The way that change requests are evaluated depends on their importance and urgency with the objective of

- Understanding the impact of the changes on all affected parties
- Ensuring that all eventualities are considered
- Consolidating all the individual impact analyses for the purpose of making an informed management decision
- Ensuring that due diligence has been exercised in the evaluation of the change request
- Ensuring that all affected parties have been consulted
- Evaluating the impact of the change being considered and weigh the cost against the benefits of the original change request

See: https://www2.cdc.gov/cdcup/library/practices_guides/CDC_UP_ Change_Management_Practices_Guide.pdf

23. **A.** Organizational culture includes an organization's expectations, experiences, and philosophy, as well as the values that guide member behavior, and is expressed in member self-image, inner workings, interactions with the outside world, and future expectations. Culture is based on shared attitudes, beliefs, customs, and written and unwritten rules that have been developed over time and are considered valid.

Creating a working environment where employee health and safety is valued, supported, and promoted through workplace health programs, policies, benefits, and environmental changes is an important part of organizational change. Organizational and culture change involves all levels of the organization and establishes the workplace health program as a routine part of business operations aligned with overall business goals. The results of this organizational and culture change include engaged and empowered employees, an impact on healthcare costs, and improved worker productivity.

See: https://gothamculture.com/what-is-organizational-culture -definition/

https://www.cdc.gov/niosh/twh/essentials.html

https://www.cdc.gov/workplacehealthpromotion/model/ evaluation/organizational.html

https://www.cdc.gov/workplacehealthpromotion/tools-resources/ pdfs/NHWP-WH101-Leadership-07172012.pdf

24. **C.** The aim of good team management is to provide well-coordinated services to the community in an appropriate, efficient, equitable, and sustainable manner. This can only be achieved if key resources for service provision, including human resources, finances, hardware, and process aspects of care delivery, are brought together at the point of service delivery and are carefully synchronized.

See: https://www.who.int/management/en/

25. **B.** Measurable productivity and efficiency are important attributes of well-functioning public health agencies. Improved productivity can come at the expense of efficiency, and improved efficiency can reduce productivity. Productivity is the quantity of work produced by a team, whereas efficiency refers to the resources used to produce that work; hence, maximizing outputs and minimizing inputs is a potential way to accomplish high productivity efficiently.

See: https://www.cdc.gov/workplacehealthpromotion/model/
evaluation/productivity.html

26. **C.** Innovation diffusion theory addresses how new ideas are spread among groups of people. Innovations are not accepted or adopted simultaneously by everyone in a society. The following are the five established adopter categories distributed in a normal curve:

- *Innovators* are people who want to be the first to try the innovation. They have a sense and aptitude for adventure. These people are willing to take risks. Not much cajoling or "selling" of new ideas or behaviors needs to be done for this group.
- *Early adopters* are thought leaders. They thrive in leadership roles and embrace change opportunities. They do not need repeated information to convince them to change.
- *Early majority* are rarely leaders, but they do adopt new ideas before the average person. Their adoption of innovation awaits testimonials.
- *Late majority* are skeptical of innovation, and will only proceed to adopt after it has been tried by the majority.
- *Laggards* are conservative, and not likely to adopt innovative ideas or practices without a campaign based on fear appeals or peer pressure.

Dearing, J. W. (2009). Applying diffusion of innovation theory to intervention development. *Research on Social Work Practice, 19*(5), 503–518. doi:10.1177/1049731509335569

27. **D.** Evidence-based public health practice requires the collection of large amounts of data. Data analysis is the process of evaluating collected data with data processing tools (increasingly computer-driven analytical and statistical software) to reveal information about the disease burden or effectiveness of interventions and policy decision-making.

See: https://www.cdc.gov/brfss/data_tools.htm

https://www.cdc.gov/datastatistics/index.html

28. **D.** Systems represent a set of items working together as parts of a mechanism or an interconnecting network. Systems analysis is the process of collecting and interpreting data about a system, troubleshooting problems, and solving problems that arise within the system, or as a result of external factors impinging on the system.

Public health grapples with many problems that are challenging and difficult to resolve. The Centers for Disease Control and Prevention's (CDC) Thinking in Systems (TiS) can help public health professionals think more effectively, and systemically, about the issues they face. This can lead to identifying possible policy solutions that may not have been readily apparent, which can be helpful in the realm of using policy to improve the health and well-being of populations.

See: https://www.cdc.gov/policy/polaris/tis/index.html

29. **B.** Organizational theory addresses the structure and function of organizations, which are defined as units of interacting individuals or groups that are structured and managed to meet a specific need or purpose. The Organizational Theory in Health Care Association (OTHC) is the only U.S. association that is dedicated exclusively to research on healthcare organization and management.

Aarts, J., Peel, V., & Wright, G. (1998). Organizational issues in health informatics: A model approach. *International Journal of Medical Informatics, 52*, 235–242. doi:10.1016/S1386-5056(98)00142-7

   http://www.ot-hc.org

30. **C.** Diffusion of innovation theory presents the following four main interacting elements:

The innovation, communicated through certain channels, over a time period, and among members of a social system

Innovation: It is an idea, practice, or object.

Communication: The process by which participants create and share information to one another in order to reach a mutual understanding

Time: Time involved in the innovation–decision process, the time taken to adopt an innovation by the adopter, and the adoption rate across the social system

Social system: These are a set of interrelated social units.

Dearing, J. W. (2009). Applying diffusion of innovation theory to intervention development. *Research on Social Work Practice, 19*(5), 503–518. doi:10.1177/1049731509335569

31. **D.** Diffusion of innovation theory proposed a five-step process through which new ideas are passed across certain channels over time in society:

- Knowledge—target individuals become aware of an innovation with some knowledge of functions
- Persuasion—target individuals form a favorable or unfavorable attitude toward the innovation
- Decision—target individuals engage in activities that lead to adoption or rejection of the innovation
- Implementation—target individuals use the innovation
- Confirmation—target individuals evaluate the outcome of decision about an innovation

Dearing, J. W. (2009). Applying diffusion of innovation theory to intervention development. *Research on Social Work Practice, 19*(5), 503–518. doi:10.1177/1049731509335569

32. B. "Go live date" is a phrase used in announcing the start-date of an operation, especially digital communication including website access. The potential problems associated with unforeseen glitches have led to modification of the go live date to "rollout day" or beta-testing period.

See: https://digital.hbs.edu/platform-rctom/submission/the-failed-launch -of-www-healthcare-gov/

http://cshca-wpengine.netdna-ssl.com/wp-content/uploads/2011/06 /9-Go-Live-Planning-Tips-for-Success.pdf

https://www.forbes.com/sites/lorenthompson/2013/12/03/healthca re-gov-diagnosis-the-government-broke-every-rule-of-project-manage ment/#11d8e5406b7f

33. A. Almost 85% of all health data is now electronic. With the proliferation of disease outbreaks and the need for fast access to patient healthcare data, bridging the electronic exchange of information between public health and healthcare is essential for timely, accurate, and accessible disease surveillance.

See: https://www.cdc.gov/surveillance/innovation/sharing-data-digitally. html?CDC_AA_refVal=https%3A%2F%2Fwww.cdc.gov%2Fsurveilla nce%2Fbridging-public-health-and-health-care-better-exchange-better -data.html

https://www.himss.org/news/cdc-and-health-information-exchanges

34. D. Telemedicine or telehealth, E-Health, and m-Health are typically about data collection. The Centers for Disease Control and Prevention's (CDC) National Center for Chronic Disease Prevention and Health Promotion uses several approaches to help improve the health of rural residents. One approach is telehealth, which is the delivery of healthcare through technology such as mobile phones or computers. It can help reduce barriers to care for people who live far away from specialists or who have transportation or mobility issues. The use of mobile and wireless technologies to support the achievement of health objectives (m-Health) has the potential to transform the face of health service delivery across the globe.

Clinical decision support (CDS) is computer-aided provision to clinicians, staff, patients, or other individuals with knowledge and person-specific information, intelligently filtered or presented at appropriate times, to enhance health and healthcare. CDS encompasses a variety of tools to enhance decision-making in the clinical workflow. These tools include computerized alerts and reminders to care providers and patients; clinical guidelines; condition-specific order sets; focused patient data reports and summaries; documentation templates; diagnostic support; and contextually relevant reference information, among other tools.

See: https://www.cdc.gov/chronicdisease/resources/publications/factshe ets/telehealth-in-rural-communities.htm

https://www.who.int/goe/publications/goe_mhealth_web.pdf

https://www.healthit.gov/topic/safety/clinical-decision-support

https://blogs.cdc.gov/publichealthmatters/2018/03/tackling-ehealth
-literacy/

35. **A.** Regional Health Information Organization (RHIO)—An organization that brings together healthcare stakeholders within a defined geographic area and governs health information exchange (HIE) among them for the purpose of improving health and care in that community. RHIOs are a component of the structure intended to implement the Nationwide Health Information Network (NwHIN). RHIOs facilitate electronic medical records and electronic health records or healthcare professionals; personal health records for individuals; and support electronic communications across these domains.

   See: https://www.cdc.gov/cliac/docs/addenda/cliac0811/O_addendum_
   EHR_Related_Acronyms_and_Terms.pdf

36. **C.** Quality improvement in public health is the use of a deliberate and defined improvement process, such as Plan-Do-Check-Act, which is focused on activities that are responsive to community needs and improving population health. It refers to a continuous and ongoing effort to achieve measurable improvements in the efficiency, effectiveness, performance, accountability, outcomes, and other indicators of quality in services or processes which achieve equity and improve the health of the community

   See: https://www.cdc.gov/publichealthgateway/performance/definitions
   .html

   https://www.cdc.gov/publichealthgateway/performance/index.html

   https://www.cdc.gov/publichealthgateway/performance/resources
   .html

   https://www.phaboard.org/wp-content/uploads/2018/11/FINAL_
   PHAB-Acronyms-and-Glossary-of-Terms-Version-1.5.pdf

   Riley, W. J., Moran, J. W., Corso, L. C., Beitsch, L. M., Bialek, R., & Cofsky, A. (2010). Defining quality improvement in public health. *Journal of Public Health Management and Practice*, 2010, *16*(1), pp.5–7.

37. **A.** Public health practice demands the contributions of many different sectors working together as a system. Siloed processes are counterproductive. For example, the CDC policy process includes five domains that often overlap or occur in a different order. However, in an ideal scenario, a problem is defined; potential policy solutions are identified, analyzed, and prioritized; and the best solution is adopted and evaluated.

   See: https://www.cdc.gov/nphpsp/Improvement/Performance%20Impro
   vement-Post%20Assessment%20Reports/Post%20Assessment%20Repo
   rt1.pdf

   https://www.cdc.gov/policy/polaris/training/policy-cdc-policy
   -process.html

38. **D.** External advisory boards are essential for public health agencies, and members are typically leaders in their respective disciplines to enrich the quality improvement plan of an agency such as the Centers for Disease Control and

Prevention, where the Advisory Committee to the Director, CDC, was established under Section 222 of the Public Health Service Act (42 U.S.C. § 217a), as amended. The committee is governed by the provisions of the Federal Advisory Committee Act, as amended, 5 U.S.C. App., which sets forth standards for the formation and use of advisory committees.

Purpose

The Secretary, Department of Health and Human Services (HHS); the Assistant Secretary for Health; and, by delegation, the Director, Centers for Disease Control and Prevention (CDC), are authorized under Section 301 [42 U.S.C. Section 241] and Section 311 [42 U.S.C. Section 243] of the Public Health Service Act, as amended, to: (1) conduct, encourage, cooperate with, and assist other appropriate public authorities, scientific institutions, and scientists in the conduct of research, investigations, experiments, demonstrations, and studies relating to the causes, diagnosis, treatment, control, and prevention of physical and mental diseases, and other impairments; (2) assist States and their political subdivisions in the prevention of infectious diseases and other preventable conditions, and in the promotion of health and well-being; and (3) train State and local personnel in health work.

Function

The Advisory Committee to the Director, CDC, shall advise the Secretary, HHS, and the Director, CDC, on policy and broad strategies that will enable the CDC to fulfill its mission of protecting health through health promotion, prevention, and preparedness. The committee recommends ways to prioritize the CDC's activities, improve results, and address health disparities. It also provides guidance to help the CDC work more effectively with its various private and public sector constituents to make health protection a practical reality.

See: https://www.cdc.gov/about/advisory/advcharter.htm

39. **A.** The Diabetes HbA1c quality measure is designed to measure the percentage of patients aged 18 through 75 years with type 1 or type 2 diabetes mellitus that had a most recent hemoglobin A1c (HbA1c) greater than 9 percent. Identifying HbA1c values greater than 9 percent among adult patients aged 18–75 years allows an organization the opportunity to focus on those patients who are in poor control and at highest risk. Consider the characteristics of a good performance measure and the IOM framework, Envisioning the National Healthcare Quality Report:

   - Relevance: Does the performance measure relate to a frequently occurring condition or have a great impact on patients at an organization's facility?
   - Measurability: Can the performance measure realistically and efficiently be quantified given the facility's finite resources?
   - Accuracy: Is the performance measure based on accepted guidelines or developed through formal group decision-making methods?
   - Feasibility: Can the performance rate associated with the performance measure realistically be improved given the limitations of the clinical services and patient population?

To ensure that a performance measure has these characteristics, it is often based on, or aligned with, current evidence-based guidelines and proven measures.

The diabetes HbA1c measure aligns with measures endorsed by the National Committee for Quality Assurance (NCQA) and similar performance metrics used by HRSA grantees and programs. The measure also aligns with those adapted by the Office of Regional Operations (ORO) and is similar to the one used by the Bureau of Primary Health Care (BPHC) in the clinical portion of its Uniform Data Systems (UDS) process. Similar measures also exist in the national measure set for Healthy People 2020.

See: https://www.hrsa.gov/sites/default/files/quality/toolbox/508pdfs/ diabetesmodule.pdf

40. **C.** Safety, timeliness, and efficiency are essential best practices for quality improvement. The frequency of conducting improvements is irrelevant. The National Public Health Performance Standards (NPHPS or the Standards) provide a framework to assess capacity and performance of public health systems and public health governing bodies. This framework can help identify areas for system improvement, strengthen state and local partnerships, and ensure that a strong system is in place for providing the 10 essential public health services.

Using the NPHPS assessment can help ensure that health agencies can respond effectively to both day-to-day public health issues and public health emergencies. The Standards can

- Improve organizational and community communication and collaboration
- Educate participants about public health and the interconnectedness of activities
- Strengthen the diverse network of partners within state and local public health systems
- Identify strengths and weaknesses to address in quality improvement efforts
- Provide a benchmark for public health practice improvements

See: https://www.cdc.gov/publichealthgateway/nphps/index.html

https://www.mphiaccredandqi.org/wp-content/uploads/2013/12/ 2012_02_28_Guidebook_web_v2.pdf

41. **D.** Cooperation among public health agencies and organizations is essential for population health, as "disease knows no boundaries." Therefore, undermining competitors is counterproductive.

The U.S. public health system is most effective when the federal government teams up with partner organizations to address emerging outbreaks and other natural or human-made disasters, develop the public health workforce, communicate public health information, translate science to practice, and evaluate effective public health services.

Public health partners have the reach, influence, access, and capabilities to coordinate an effective public health response and to strengthen public health systems and services. A key role for public health partners is to provide capacity-building assistance to ensure a capable and efficient public health system and workforce.

The Center for State, Tribal, Local, and Territorial Support (CSTLTS) coordinates funding opportunities that provide capacity-building assistance to grantees. CSTLTS also administers the Preventive Health and Health Services Block Grant, which provides all 50 states, the District of Columbia, two American Indian tribes, and eight U.S. territories with funding to address their unique public health needs in innovative and locally defined ways.

See: https://www.cdc.gov/publichealthgateway/partnerships/index.html

42. **D.** The four principles of effective team building are defining criteria for goals and success, rewarding success through division of labor, leading by examples, and providing clear guidance on constructive conflict resolution procedures. In public health, good teams have talented individuals willing to collaborate with others. Teamwork and individualism are like opposite attributes of a team, but individualism should be subordinate to the team in terms of reward systems.

See: https://www.apa.org/monitor/2018/09/cover-teams-health-care

43. **A.** "Tuckman's Stages" (named after Bruce Wayne Tuckman with contributions by Mary Ann Jensen) for teams to develop effective functioning are the following:

   – Stage 1: Forming
   – Stage 2: Storming
   – Stage 3: Norming
   – Stage 4: Performing
   – Stage 5: Adjourning

"Evaluating" is not one of the stages.

See: https://www.atsdr.cdc.gov/communityengagement/pce_program_phases.html

   https://www.projectsmart.co.uk/the-five-stages-of-team-development-a-case-study.php

44. **A.** In a team, every member should feel valued and be recognized for the skills that he or she brings to the team. The leadership stance is not a posture, but rather an attitude of collaboration and determination to get the work done.

See: http://app.ihi.org/LMS/Content/21cd2568-2e1e-4c0f-bf23-8c62971b0cb1/Upload/L%20101%20SummaryFINAL.pdf

   https://www.cdc.gov/globalhealth/leadership/default.htm

45. **A.** Public health practice has traditionally been at the graduate level with the Master of Public Health competencies being the entry-level degree. There is a rapid growth in undergraduate public health degree programs, and the graduates are filling needed workforce roles. The college-level continuing education remains the essential level to update competencies.

Allegrante, J. P., Moon, R. W., Auld, M. E., & Gebbie, K. M. (2001). Continuing-education needs of the currently employed public health education workforce. *American Journal of Public Health, 91*(8), 1230–1234. doi:10.2105/ajph.91.8.1230

See: http://www.phf.org/programs/corecompetencies/Pages/Core_Competencies_Domains.aspx

https://www.cdc.gov/publichealthgateway/professional/index.html

46. **C.** Alternative Dispute Resolution (ADR) is a collection of processes used to informally, and confidentially, resolve conflicts or disputes. These processes are called alternative because they are an alternative to grievances and complaints; however, it does not displace those traditional processes. For example, the Centers for Disease Control and Prevention (CDC) and Agency for Toxic Substances Disease Registry teams have access to ADR for the following actions:

- Advice about how to deal directly with a concern
- Uncertainty about taking a problem through other channels
- Uncertainty about who to talk with about a problem or concern
- Informal, nonescalating approach
- Impartial perspective
- Discussion of strategies or possible options for resolving a concern
- Maintenance of the greatest possible flexibility in how to approach a concern
- Sounding board

ADR is generally voluntary. However, CDC and ATSDR managers and supervisors are required to participate in resolution processes when employees choose this mechanism to resolve workplace disputes. ADR empowers and enables the participating parties to develop and seek mutually acceptable solutions, which they choose to meet their needs. Generally, ADR uses a neutral third party to help the parties communicate, develop ideas, and resolve the dispute.

Some reasons for using ADR are the following:

- It is faster, cheaper, easier, less formal, and less confrontational or adversarial.
- It encourages creativity and searching for practical solutions.
- It avoids the unpredictability involved when decisions are rendered as a result of the traditional dispute resolution mechanisms.
- The process usually results in improved communications between disputing parties and is therefore better for ongoing relationships.
- It increases workplace morale and can make you feel better about coming to work.
- Solutions tend to be durable or long lasting since they have the "buy-in" of all parties involved.
- It avoids publicity.
- The parties retain control of the outcome.
- There is no risk since all statutory entitlements remain intact.

47. **D.** An effective team should have a code of ethics regarding appropriate behavior based on the team's values. Every member of the team should respect these ethical values. For example, the Centers for Disease Control and

Prevention (CDC) provides guidance on ethics and compliance activities for all employees and those who conduct transactions with the agency.

See: https://www.cdc.gov/ethics/index.html

48. **B.** To be effective, any public health program needs the meaningful participation of team members. Team members have much to gain from a successful program and the most to lose if the program fails. They also often know the most about potential hazards associated with their jobs. Successful programs tap into this knowledge base. Team member participation means that workers are involved in establishing, operating, evaluating, and improving the safety and health program.

In an effective safety and health program, all team members

- Are encouraged to participate in the program and feel comfortable providing input and reporting safety or health concerns
- Have access to information they need to participate effectively in the program
- Have opportunities to participate in all phases of program design and implementation
- Do not experience retaliation when they raise safety and health concerns; report injuries, illnesses, and hazards; participate in the program; or exercise safety and health rights

See: https://www.osha.gov/shpguidelines/worker-participation.html

49. **C.** Participatory management is particularly suited to building effective public health teams as a system in which members take an active role in the decision-making process as it relates to the way the team operates. Participative or democratic leadership encourages input from the group where each member has some level of influence over the final decision. Such leaders also communicate well what needs to get completed. However, they are less specific in how they expect it to be done. Instead, they opt for providing guidance after consulting with the group. As a result, group members feel more engaged in the decision-making process; team cooperation and motivation is often more positive and effective. Leaders utilizing this style are often viewed more favorably than those using an authoritarian or task-oriented, or transformational, style.

See: https://www2a.cdc.gov/cdcup/library/newsletter/CDC_UP_News letter_v5_i4.htm

50. **A.** The capacity to facilitate the resolution of conflicts within the public health agency, in the community, and with other stakeholder groups. Offering feedback is a way to secure best practices and not have repeated conflicts.

See: https://www.cdc.gov/nceh/ehs/corecomp/corecompetencies.htm

51. **D.** Team-based practice is not new in public health, but its implementation can be challenging. Practice facilitators assist in implementing team-based care through the following actions:

Preparing for the transition to team-based care:

Help identify a change champion for team-based care who can lead the effort

Increase his or her knowledge about care teams and how teamwork differs from traditional approaches by providing training and resources

Provide examples of best practices and set up virtual or in-person site visits

Setting up teams:

Create new workflows of how teams will deliver care

Assign roles and responsibilities that enable working at the level of licensure

Create new ways of communicating that strengthen team approaches to care:

Previsit planning

While patient is in the office

Postvisit

Performance and feedback

Optimizing already existing care teams by helping team members clarify roles, tasks, and expectations; redesign workflow based on these things; and improve communication and problem-solving skills

Set up performance measures to monitor the care team's effectiveness (see Module 7 on performance measurement)

See: https://www.ahrq.gov/professionals/prevention-chronic-care/
improve/system/pfhandbook/mod19.html

52. **B.** Friendship among team members is desirable, but not essential for effective performance. All team members should be aware of the purpose of the teams and their roles.. Effective communication and accountability are essential at all levels. The evidence for implementing team-based care in healthcare systems and practices is very strong. Solid evidence shows that this strategy achieves desired outcomes, with studies demonstrating internal and external validity. This strategy has also been independently replicated, which shows reliability of impact. Several randomized controlled trials, which are often considered the gold standard in research, have been conducted and show positive results from using multidisciplinary teams as a way to improve hypertension control. Various organizations, such as the American Medical Association and the Agency for Healthcare Research and Quality (AHRQ), have developed guidelines to help healthcare systems and practices implement this strategy as part of their policies and protocols.

See: https://www.cdc.gov/dhdsp/pubs/docs/CPA-Team-Based-Care.pdf

https://www.cdc.gov/dhdsp/pubs/guides/best-practices/team
-based-care.htm

53. **B.** Assessing and cataloging the existing capacity of an agency is the first step in capacity building because the catalog can reveal gaps in the coverage of functions, personnel, and resources that are needed to fulfill the objectives that the agency seeks to pursue under a strategic plan. Thus, identifying assets comes before needs assessment, stakeholder engagement, and capacity development response.

See: https://effectiveinterventions.cdc.gov/docs/default-source/general
-docs/Capacity_Building_Eval_Guide_ECB_102010_Final.pdf

http://www.gdrc.org/uem/undp-cb.html

54. C. The organizational structure of a public health agency is a system that outlines how certain activities are directed in order to achieve goals, including rules, roles, responsibilities, and communication pathways for information flow across the structure.

See: https://www.cdc.gov/maso/OfficialMissionStatementsCharts.html

55. B. The vision statement defines the goal of an organization, whereas the strategy is a plan that describes the tactics for how the plan will be executed to achieve the vision.

See: https://www.cdc.gov/eeo/aboutus/mission.htm

56. A. An organization's conceptual framework is the overall picture of the organization's ideas, resources, and goals, including the approach and methodology adopted to proceed. The conceptual framework is a "big picture" testament that captures the organization's understanding of the world (e.g., the role of disease in human welfare, disease eradication, equity, and justice).

See: https://www.cdc.gov/dhdsp/programs/spha/roadmap/docs/
Strategic%20Partnering%20Conceptual%20Framework_ac.pdf

57. A. The mission statement is a formal description of the aims and values of a public health agency. It describes the reason for the organization's existence, and why its goals matter.

For example: The Centers for Disease Control and Prevention (CDC) works 24/7 to protect America from health, safety, and security threats, both foreign and in the United States. Whether diseases start at home or abroad, are chronic or acute, curable or preventable, human error or deliberate attack, the CDC fights disease and supports communities and citizens to do the same.

The CDC increases the health security of our nation. As the nation's health protection agency, the CDC saves lives and protects people from health threats. To accomplish its mission, the CDC conducts critical science work and provides health information that protects the nation against expensive and dangerous health threats, and responds when these arise.

See: https://www.cdc.gov/about/organization/mission.htm

58. C. The implementation of a strategic plan turns promises into actions toward achieving the objectives and goals. All managers should be involved in the implementation.

See: https://www.cdc.gov/about/organization/strategic-framework/
index.html

https://www.cdc.gov/program/performance/fy2000plan/2000ii.htm

59. B. Scenario planning involves brainstorming about possible environmental or social conditions in the future, and how the organization will respond under various combinations of futuristic assumptions. It is not wise to implement actions based on scenarios that are doomed to failure. Scenario planning is often included in long-term strategic plans.

See: https://www.cdc.gov/foodsafety/pdfs/ifsac-strategic-plan-2017-2021
.pdf

60. **D.** Dynamic capabilities refer to an organization's ability to integrate, build, and reconfigure internal and external competencies to address rapidly changing environments. In 2011, the Centers for Disease Control and Prevention (CDC) established 15 capabilities that serve as national standards for public health preparedness planning. Since then, these capability standards have served as a vital framework for state, local, tribal, and territorial preparedness programs as they plan, operationalize, and evaluate their ability to prepare for, respond to, and recover from public health emergencies.

See: https://www.davidjteece.com/dynamic-capabilities

https://www.cdc.gov/cpr/readiness/capabilities.htm

4 Law and Ethics

■ INTRODUCTION

Effective public health practice relies on the conviction that when we have compelling evidence to prevent disease in populations, we must act accordingly. However, it is not always clear that what is in the best .interests of a population is also in the best interest of every individual member of the population. To navigate between public and private interests, and population and individual interests in public health, societies have established codes of ethics and legally binding stipulations to guide public health practice. These codes of ethics and law are constantly being tested, challenged, refined, and reviewed. For example, in April 2019, nearly 1,000 residents of Los Angeles, California, were quarantined because they were exposed to individuals confirmed to have measles virus infection. Quarantine laws are designed to be in the best interest of the population, even though some individuals may feel that the law infringes on their individual rights. The measles outbreak is also associated with different interpretations of the requirement for vaccination against preventable infectious diseases. Some parents chose not to vaccinate their children, thereby weakening the herd immunity that protects the population. Many states are tightening the loopholes through which anti-vaccination options are permissible. Research that is intended to produce generalizable evidence is also subject to strict codes of ethics and law, according to federal mandates. However, research ethics and law can vary across national boundaries, making the work of public health practitioners challenging. The questions on law and ethics are designed to examine broad knowledge of aspirational conduct and codes of conduct for public health research and practice across national and international domains. Practicing with these questions should enable you to

- Identify regulations regarding privacy, security, and confidentiality; for example, personal health information

- Design strategies to ensure implementation of laws and regulations governing the scope of one's legal authority

- Apply basic principles of ethical analysis to issues of public health research, practice, and policy
- Ensure the application of ethical principles in the collection, maintenance, use, and dissemination of data and information
- Manage potential conflicts of interest encountered by practitioners, researchers, and organizations
- Advise on the laws, regulations, policies, and procedures for the ethical conduct of public health research, practice, and policy
- Identify environmental, social justice, and other factors that contribute to health disparities
- Apply social justice and human rights principles when addressing community needs

■ QUESTIONS

1. In 2004, the State of Massachusetts implemented a "smoke-free workplace law" that has been shown by public health researchers to prevent 270 deaths from acute myocardial infarction annually. In contrast, California's proposition 99, passed in 1988, implemented a tax on cigarette packaging, leading, in part, to a 19% decrease in lung cancer rates. Imagine that you are a public health consultant recruited to advise a developing country on the development of appropriate policies to reduce tobacco-related disease burden. Which of the following is NOT included in policy development as a function of public health practice?

   A. Develop policies and plans that support individual and community health efforts
   B. Inform, educate, and empower people about health issues
   C. Research for new insights and innovative solutions to health problems
   D. Mobilize community partnerships to identify and solve health problems

2. In 2010, the U.S. Congress passed a Healthcare Reform Bill, and President Obama signed the legislation into law on March 23, 2010. The bill will make $15 billion available for "disease prevention" strategies, but there is a sharp disagreement between public health officials and nonprofit organizations over how to spend the funds over the next 10 years. Which of the following is definitely NOT an investment in disease prevention?

   A. Stem cell research and development
   B. Anti-malaria drug research and development
   C. Green parks development in urban centers
   D. Missile defense programs

3. What does the word "quarantine" mean in public health practice?

   A. Quarantine is used to separate and restrict the movement of well persons who may have been exposed to a communicable disease to see if they become ill.

B. Quarantine is an experimental design for investigating the influence of a public health intervention program according to four divisions of a population.

C. Quarantine is a term that captures the variations in disease incidence over the four seasons of the year.

D. Quarantine means the administration of four doses of an experimental drug in a clinical trial.

4. The Public Health Code of Ethics is useful for the following, EXCEPT

A. Defining a field of research and practice

B. Making public health agencies accountable

C. Creating an ethical environment

D. Stipulating moral standards of behavior that affect public health in a community

5. The following are aspiration codes of ethics in public health, EXCEPT

A. Public health should address principally the fundamental causes of disease and requirements for health, aiming to prevent adverse health outcomes.

B. Public health should achieve community health in a way that respects the rights of individuals in the community.

C. Public health policies, programs, and priorities should be developed and evaluated through processes that prioritize input from experts.

D. Public health should advocate for, or work for the empowerment of, disenfranchised community members, ensuring that the basic resources and conditions necessary for health are accessible to all people in the community.

6. "Confidentiality" is one of the cornerstone ethical standards in public health practice. The following are key guidelines on confidentiality, EXCEPT

A. Public health institutions should protect the confidentiality of information that can bring harm to a corporation if made public.

B. Public health institutions should protect the confidentiality of information that can bring harm to a community if made public.

C. Exceptions to the confidentiality ethic must be justified on the basis of the high likelihood of significant harm to the individual.

D. Exceptions to the confidentiality ethic must be justified on the basis of the high likelihood of significant harm to others.

7. The Code of Federal Regulations (45 CFR 46) defines research as "A systematic investigation, including research development, testing and evaluation, designed to develop or contribute to generalizable knowledge." Public health practice relies on the results of research, and ethical standards apply to all research conducted to investigate strategies to advance health in communities. Ethical guidelines about public health research DO NOT apply to

A. Research involving humans

B. Research involving inanimate substances such as water and air quality

C. Biological processes not involving humans

D. Research involving plants on their own

8. Identify the most influential event that led to the Health and Human Services (HHS) Policy for Protection of Human Subjects.

   A. Nuremberg trials
   B. Syphilis study at Tuskegee
   C. Jewish chronic disease hospital study
   D. Willowbrook study

9. What are the three ethical principles that constitute the basis for the Health and Human Services (HHS) Human Subjects Regulations (45 CFR 46)?

   A. Honesty, trust, and respect
   B. Informed consent, institutional review board (IRB) review, and research integrity
   C. Respect for persons, beneficence, and justice
   D. Protections for pregnant women, prisoners, and children

10. Which of the following should be eliminated or minimized in public health research designs?

    A. Coercion
    B. Team research
    C. Recruitment of diverse research participants for new protocols
    D. Ecological study design

11. Which of the following is NOT a scenario in human participants research that requires public health investigators to obtain informed consent?

    A. Investigators must obtain informed consent if the study involves interactions with human research participants.
    B. Investigators must obtain informed consent if the study involves interventions with human research participants.
    C. Investigators must obtain informed consent if the study involves collection of private information from or about human research participants.
    D. Investigators must obtain informed consent if the study involves observations of human behavior in a public setting.

12. What is NOT an appropriate method for maintaining confidentiality of private information obtained from human subjects?

    A. Keeping data in a password-protected database
    B. Storing images in a secured cabinet
    C. Coding data or specimens and keeping the key to the code in a separate, locked drawer
    D. Keeping confidential information on your private mobile phone

13. In localities where community consent is the norm

    A. A family member's consent for another individual may be sufficient, as long as community consent is given.
    B. Federal regulations preclude the conduct of U.S. taxpayer-funded research.

C. Community consent to participate in the research study is sufficient and no institutional review board (IRB) approval is required.

D. In addition to the cultural norm, individual informed consent is required.

14. The institutional review board (IRB) is a group of people, often affiliated with a research institution, who review scientific protocols for research involving humans and who decide whether the proposed study design is ethical. The IRB considers proposals to conduct research with human subjects according to the following categories EXCEPT

A. Exempt review
B. Expedited review
C. Full committee review
D. Exceptional review

15. The prevention of human disease is a time-honored and honorable goal of public health practice. Recent developments in the analysis of the human genome have introduced a powerful but controversial tool for diagnosis and prevention. Hence, the field of genetic counseling has gained in importance for public health. From a public health perspective, the ethical issues surrounding genetic counseling include all of the following EXCEPT

A. Autonomy: The right of individuals to act freely with adequate information
B. Beneficence and Justice: Information should be helpful and available to all
C. Confidentiality: All information is private and not to be shared with others
D. Genetic License: Permanent waiver of rights to use of individual genetic information

16. Which entity has regulatory authority for the protection of human subjects for Public Health Service-funded research?

A. Office of Human Research Protections (OHRP)
B. National Institutes of Health (NIH)
C. Department of Health and Human Services (HHS)
D. Centers for Disease Control and Prevention (CDC)

17. All research that involves interaction or intervention with humans or human samples/data, whether they are alive or dead, is human subjects research.

A. True
B. False
C. It depends on the cause of death.
D. Only in the case of samples, not data

18. Who should determine whether proposed studies are exempt from regulatory requirements?

A. The investigator
B. Human participants in the research
C. Institutionally designated authority
D. A focus group of RO1-funded investigators

19. After informed consent for a research study is given, a research participant must complete the study.

   A. True
   B. False
   C. Except if the principal investigator releases the participant
   D. Except if the research participant suffers from unacceptable side effects

20. Potential participants in a public health research study must understand that enrolling in the research is voluntary and that they may withdraw from the study at any time without penalty or loss of benefits.

   A. True
   B. False
   C. Human participants in research may enjoy the benefits of voluntary participation, but they must return all forms of financial compensation to the principal investigator if they chose to withdraw.
   D. Human participants permanently forfeit all rights to their samples and data already collected if they prematurely withdraw from the study.

21. In general, informed consent should be a process rather than a onetime event.

   A. True
   B. False
   C. Informed consent is administered twice, at the beginning and at the end of the study only.
   D. Informed consent is administered three times: at the beginning, the middle, and the end of the study only.

22. In order to participate in research, children must

   A. Provide written informed consent
   B. Provide written permission
   C. Provide assent, unless the institutional review board (IRB) determines that they are too young
   D. Sign, or put an "X" on the assent document

23. For research involving pregnant women, participation requires

   A. That women have completed the first trimester
   B. That the study be conducted first in men
   C. Permission of the father of the fetus
   D. Consideration of risks and potential benefits for the fetus and the pregnant woman

24. Why might an individual have diminished autonomy?

   A. He or she is a young adult.
   B. He or she is incarcerated.
   C. He or she is conscious.
   D. He or she is careless

25. Risks to research participants must be completely eliminated for the study to be considered ethical.

    A. True
    B. False
    C. Only financial risks need to be completely eliminated.
    D. Only health needs need to be completely eliminated.

26. When are researchers specifically required by National Institutes of Health (NIH) policy to describe data and safety monitoring?

    A. For all research involving human subjects
    B. For all research involving children as subjects in research
    C. For all clinical trials
    D. For all research with prisoners

27. There must be equipoise in order to justify conducting a clinical trial.

    A. True
    B. False
    C. Only when the protocol demands it
    D. Except for trials for new pharmaceuticals

28. If a researcher determines that his/her study poses no more than minimal risk as defined in 45 CFR 46, there is no need for the protocol to have institutional review board (IRB) review and approval.

    A. True
    B. False
    C. Except when the risk concerns financial status.
    D. Except when the risk concerns physical health status.

29. For HIV antiretroviral treatment trials conducted in developing countries, the National Institutes of Health (NIH) expects investigators/contractors to address the provision of antiretroviral treatment to trial participants after their completion of participation in the clinical trial.

    A. True
    B. False
    C. Only if the GDP of the developing country is lower than projected after the study
    D. Only if the country does not manufacture its own antiretroviral therapeutics

30. Children must be included in all National Institutes of Health (NIH)-supported human subjects research unless

    A. The researcher is not a pediatrician.
    B. Past experience has shown it is time-consuming and expensive to recruit children.
    C. There are scientific and ethical reasons to exclude them.
    D. The researcher does not possess the pediatric equipment necessary to involve children in the proposed research.

31. Which of the following is TRUE regarding applications for National Institutes of Health (NIH)-funded research overseas?

    A. It is illegal to spend NIH funds in research overseas.
    B. Research conducted overseas is subject to Health and Human Services (HHS) Human Subjects Regulations (45 CFR 46) and local regulations and policies.
    C. Research conducted overseas is only subject to local regulations and policies.
    D. Research conducted overseas need not address human subjects protections.

32. In localities where community consent is the norm

    A. A family member's consent for another individual may be sufficient, as long as community consent is given.
    B. Federal regulations preclude the conduct of PHS-funded research.
    C. Community consent to participate in the research study is sufficient and no institutional review board (IRB) approval is required.
    D. In addition to the cultural norm, individual informed consent is required.

33. The history of ethical regulations in human subjects research began with the

    A. Nuremberg Code
    B. Declaration of Helsinki
    C. Belmont Report
    D. Common Rule

34. A student is conducting a research project that involves using a survey. The survey asks subjects about their highest level of education, political affiliation, and views on various social issues. No identifiable information will be collected. This study would be categorized as which type of review?

    A. Not human subjects
    B. Full board review
    C. Exempt review
    D. Expedited review

35. What is the institutional review board (IRB) charged with?

    A. Conducting inquiries into scientific misconduct
    B. Reviewing manuscripts prior to submission for publication
    C. Protecting the rights and welfare of human subjects
    D. Making sure that human subjects are paid at least minimum wage

36. The Belmont principle of beneficence requires that

    A. Potential benefits justify the risks of harm.
    B. Subjects derive individual benefit from study participation.
    C. The study makes a significant contribution to generalizable knowledge.
    D. Risks are managed so that they are no more than minimal.

37. Which of the following is an example of how the principle of beneficence is applied to a study involving human subjects?

    A. Ensuring that risks are reasonable in relationship to anticipated benefits
    B. Providing detailed information about the study to potential subjects
    C. Ensuring that the selection of subjects is fair
    D. Ensuring that subjects understand that participation is voluntary

38. According to the federal regulations in the United States and the World Health Organization's guidelines, which of the following studies meets the definition of research with human subjects?

    A. A university designs an in-house study to improve the mentoring of female students in its global health department with the proposed outcome consisting of a report of recommendations for the department.
    B. A researcher receives anonymized data for secondary analysis from a survey about gender-related differences in stress levels conducted by a colleague at a university in another country.
    C. A world organization for female academics in public health asks a country's agency to provide the number of female investigators funded by that agency to include in a report for its membership.
    D. An experiment is proposed on the relationship between gender-related stereotypes in global health and the subsequent performance by males and females on competency tests.

39. An electronic medical record is an example of

    A. Private behavior
    B. Public information
    C. Public behavior
    D. Private information

40. In addition to pregnant women, fetuses, and neonates, additional protections are stipulated for which of the following vulnerable populations?

    A. Prisoners
    B. College students
    C. Adults with decisional impairments
    D. The elderly

41. What statement about risks in global health research is most accurate?

    A. If a study offers potential benefits, it is not necessary to minimize risks.
    B. There are never any risks.
    C. Risks are specific to time, situation, and culture.
    D. Anonymizing data effectively manages the risk of creating emotional distress.

42. A researcher in South Africa is examining the quality of life for diamond miners who are HIV-positive using surveys followed by interview. The institutional review board must ensure that

    A. The survey instrument is standardized.
    B. A medical doctor serves as coinvestigator.

C. All miners receive HIV testing.

D. Confidentiality of the miners' health status is maintained.

43. A global health researcher is studying women who have been admitted to the hospital because of damage by female genital mutilation. All potential subjects must have children under the age of 5. Research subjects will be given a basket of toys to use at their children's first visit that the children can then take home. In assessing this proposal, the institutional review board (IRB) needs to determine that the toys are

A. Educational

B. Age appropriate

C. Not an excessive incentive

D. Of high quality

44. A U.S. global health researcher plans to conduct a clinical trial of feeding genetically engineered "golden rice" to cure vitamin-A deficiency syndrome in children in Bangladesh. Which of the following statements most accurately describes the requirement for the U.S. federal documentation of minors' assent to participate in research?

A. To protect minors documentation is always required.

B. Documentation is required unless waived by an institutional review board (IRB).

C. U.S. federal regulations do not require the documentation of minors' assent.

D. Parents must approve written documentation.

45. Researchers wish to evaluate a new treatment for eclampsia (a life-threatening condition in pregnant women) in Tanzanian women who are 30 to 50 years of age. The research is intended to directly benefit the pregnant woman who is otherwise healthy and competent. The investigator must obtain consent from whom?

A. The father of the fetus only

B. The pregnant woman only

C. The pregnant woman and her legally authorized representative

D. The pregnant woman and the father of the fetus

46. A professor of global health at UC Irvine proposes to study attitudes about obesity in Chile by giving human subjects in Chile surveys to complete. Which is a question that the UC Irvine institutional review board (IRB) should ask the researcher in order to determine if this study should be reviewed by a local Chilean IRB or ethics committee, as well as the UC Irvine IRB?

A. Is the survey more than minimal risk?

B. Does the potential subject population include children?

C. Will the researchers have collaborators at the research site abroad?

D. Does the professor speak Spanish fluently?

47. A global health researcher from UCLA proposes a study and wants to recruit subjects from healthcare clinics in Jamaica. The survey will be conducted by the U.S. researchers at the clinic. The nurses at the clinic will inform prospective subjects about the availability of the research but will not consent the subjects nor

perform any research procedures (even screening procedures). Are the nurses engaged in the research according to U.S. federal regulations?

A. No, they are not engaged because the research is not taking place at their clinic.

B. No, they are not engaged because they are only informing the subjects and not consenting or performing any research procedures, or receiving or sharing any private, identifiable information.

C. Yes, they are engaged because the research is taking place at the clinic and they work there.

D. Yes, they are engaged because they are interacting with potential research subjects and informing them about the study.

48. The age of majority in international research is determined by

A. The laws, customs, and norms in the area in which the research will be conducted

B. Legal drinking age in Jamaica where the research will take place

C. The research funding agency or sponsor

D. Laws in the state (California) where the researchers' institution resides

49. Which of the following online research strategies raises the most concerns regarding the ethical principle of respecting the autonomy of research subjects and the corresponding federal regulations requiring informed consent?

A. A global health researcher copies portions of postings on a health policy blog to document the use of cultural icons, health disparities, and the use of anti-vaccination statements in the postings.

B. A global health researcher posts a notice on an open online support group for immigrant adoptees asking anyone who would be interested in being interviewed for her study to contact her.

C. A researcher observes the communications in an HIV/AIDS open support group without announcing her presence. She is interested in observing how long members participate and how the membership shifts over time.

D. A researcher proposes to join a moderated support group for cancer survivors posing as a survivor. She plans to insert comments to see how the members respond.

50. Which of the following examples of using the Internet to conduct research meets the federal definition of research with human subjects?

A. Conducting an online focus group with cancer survivors to determine familial support systems. The researcher also invites subjects' significant others to be a part of the focus group.

B. Gathering data to supplement an oral history project about a global health rights activist. The activist passed away while the researcher was in the process of conducting in-person interviews with the individual's social network.

C. Downloading a publicly available dataset that includes high school students' academic achievement rates. The data are in aggregate and were derived from multiple school districts from different states.

D. Analyzing a website visitor report from several proanorexia blogs to determine the popularity of each blog. Access to the blogs is not restricted.

51. Which of the following statements is false?

    A. Global health researchers and professionals never carry stigmatizing attitudes.
    B. Global health researchers and professionals sometimes fail to get tested for HIV owing to the fear of being stigmatized.
    C. Increased contact with individuals who are affected may be a way of dealing with stigma.
    D. Self-stigma may foster a decline of self-esteem and self-efficacy.

52. In Pakistan, both men and women experience considerably high levels of associated stigma and discrimination due to their mental illness. In general, research results in this and other parts of the world have shown that women

    A. Have innate ability to resist stigmatization
    B. Are less subject to discrimination experience than men
    C. Are less prone to social withdrawal as a result of stigmatization than men
    D. Are less likely to commit suicide than men

53. The standard of care in cases of medical negligence is measured against

    A. The most recent medical research evidence available
    B. What is expected of a reasonable medical doctor
    C. What the majority of doctors would recommend
    D. The standard of experts in the field

54. Nonmaleficence is associated with

    A. Risks and costs of research in global health research and practice
    B. Self-governance in global health
    C. Doing no intentional harm in global health research and practice
    D. Promotion of the profession of global health research and practice

55. Randomized controlled trials (RCTs)

    A. Are not required to be based on the concept of equipoise
    B. Always have a control arm that uses placebo
    C. Are considered to be the "gold standard" for determining efficacy and safety in clinical research
    D. Are always "double blinded"

56. The "Mexico City Policy," a United States government policy that blocks U.S. federal funding for nongovernmental organizations that provide abortion counseling or referrals; that advocate to decriminalize abortion; or that promote expansion of abortion services, is applicable

    A. In all 50 U.S. States and Territories
    B. Only in States where abortion is illegal
    C. Only in States where abortion is legal
    D. Worldwide

57. According to the World Health Organization, during a pandemic, difficult choices will have to be made about how to secure the best health outcomes for

individuals, groups and communities; hence, it is critical that ethical consider-ations remain central to decision-making. The following are essential and/or desirable elements of an ethics framework in pandemic preparedness EXCEPT

A. Establish ethics committees to advise on pandemic preparedness and response activities, coordinating with existing national ethics structures
B. Review existing and proposed pandemic policies and interventions to take ethical concerns into consideration
C. Review legislation and policies on research-related data sharing, to ensure adequate protection of patient confidentiality and identifiable data
D. In an emergency, decision-making must proceed as needed, and considera-tion for ethical issues should occur only after the emergency has subsided

58. The International Health Regulations grew from the International Sanitary Conference of 1851, recognizing the following EXCEPT

A. Free movement of people and goods will increase the risk of cross-border transmission.
B. Quarantine is an impediment to free trade, and public health arguments can justify trade barriers.
C. International Health Regulations (1950) responsibility of WHO: Member states agree to notify other countries of specific infectious diseases outbreaks and abide by measures allowed by countries to protect themselves.
D. Quarantine is an impediment to free trade, and public health arguments cannot justify trade barriers because economic productivity is the precursor to good public health.

59. The 2005 version of the International Health Regulations stipulates that its implementation shall be the following EXCEPT

A. With full respect for the dignity, human rights, and fundamental freedom of persons
B. Guided by the Charter of the United Nations and the Constitution of the World Health Organization
C. Guided by the goal of their universal application for the protection of all people of the world from the international spread of disease
D. Guided by the fact that wealthier countries pay the most for international health security and their population should be prioritized in global health emergencies

60. The International Health Regulations of 2005 defines a "Public Health Emergency of International Concern" as "an extraordinary event which is deter-mined to constitute a public health risk to other States through the interna-tional spread of disease and to potentially require a coordinated international response." This definition requires situations that meet the following criteria EXCEPT

A. Serious, sudden, unusual, or unexpected
B. Carries implications for public health beyond the affected State's national border
C. Will not require too much money to implement interventions
D. May require immediate international action

■ ANSWERS

1. **C.** Three items are included in policy development.

   - Inform, educate, and empower people about environmental health issues
   - Mobilize community partnerships and actions to identify and solve environmental health problems
   - Develop policies and plans that support individual and community environmental health efforts

   See: https://www.cdc.gov/nceh/ehs/ephli/core_ess.htm

2. **D.** The missile offense program is a military activity likely to lead to war with high mortality and morbidity.

   In the 20th century, 72 million deaths (nearly half of which were civilians) occurred in 25 conflicts worldwide.

   - From 1987 to 1997, 2 million children were killed and 4 to 5 million children were seriously injured during armed conflict.
   - Each year in Afghanistan (one of the most heavily land-mined countries in the world), 2,000 to 3,000 people are killed or injured by landmines and unexploded ordnance (UXO); about two people per 1,000 are permanently disabled.
   - In recent years, frequency of rape and sexual violence has increased during and after conflicts. During the conflict in Bosnia in the early 1990s, estimates of the number of women raped ranged from 10,000 to 25,000.

   See: https://www.cdc.gov/nceh/publications/factsheets/War-related InjuryPrevention.pdf

3. **A.** Quarantine separates and restricts the movement of people who were exposed to a contagious disease to see if they become sick. Isolation separates sick people with a contagious disease from people who are not sick. Isolation and quarantine help protect the public by preventing exposure to people who have or may have a contagious disease.

   See: https://www.cdc.gov/quarantine/index.html

4. **D.** Stipulating moral standards is not part of the code of ethics because doing so may lead to cultural conflicts. For example, sexual practices in different cultures and subcultures are often linked to moral arguments and debates. A code of ethics for public health clarifies the distinctive elements of public health and the ethical principles that follow from or respond to those distinct aspects . . . . A code of ethics thus serves as a goal to guide public health institutions and practitioners and as a standard to which they can be held accountable.

   See: https://www.apha.org/-/media/files/pdf/membergroups/ethics/ethics_brochure.ashx

   https://www.cdc.gov/od/science/integrity/phethics/resources.htm

5. **C.** It may be desirable under many circumstances to prioritize the opinion of experts in public health intervention programs, but it is just as important if

not more so to solicit input from the community and population targeted by the intervention.

See: https://commed.vcu.edu/Chronic_Disease/2016/updatedroleforPH -JamaJAN.pdf

Stefanak, M., Frisch, L., & Palmer-Fernandez, G. (2007). An organizational code of public health ethics: Practical applications and benefits. *Public Health Reports, 122*(4), 548–551. doi:10.1177/003335490712200417

6. **A.** Corporations may be protected through some laws governing confidentiality, but in the general sense if a corporation is involved in a practice of product that threatens public health, public institutions are not bound to protect their identity. Instead, laws protect confidentiality of information for individuals.

Federal law, good statistical practice, and our ethical obligations to the American people all require that any personal information collected by public health professionals be treated with the utmost concern for the privacy of those who provide it. An Assurance of Confidentiality is a formal confidentiality protection authorized under Section 308(d) of the Public Health Service Act. It is used for projects conducted by the Centers for Disease Control and Prevention (CDC) staff or contractors that involve the collection or maintenance of sensitive identifiable or potentially identifiable information. This protection allows CDC programs to assure individuals and institutions involved in research or nonresearch projects that those conducting the project will protect the confidentiality of the data collected. The legislation states that no identifiable information may be used for any purpose other than the purpose for which it was supplied unless such institution or individual has consented to that disclosure.

See: https://www.cdc.gov/nchs/about/policy/confidentiality.htm

https://www.cdc.gov/od/science/integrity/confidentiality/index .htm

7. **D.** The Code of Federal Regulations (45 CFR 46) does not include research on plants, except under conditions that plants are provided to humans as part of their diet or medication.

See: https://www.hhs.gov/ohrp/sites/default/files/ohrp/policy/ ohrpregulations.pdf

8. **B.** In 1932, the Public Health Service, working with the Tuskegee Institute, began a study to record the natural history of syphilis in hopes of justifying treatment programs for Blacks. It was called the "Tuskegee Study of Untreated Syphilis in the Negro Male."

The study initially involved 600 Black men—399 with syphilis, 201 who did not have the disease. The study was conducted without the benefit of patients' informed consent. Researchers told the men they were being treated for "bad blood," a local term used to describe several ailments, including syphilis, anemia, and fatigue. In truth, they did not receive the proper treatment needed to cure their illness.

In the summer of 1973, a class-action lawsuit was filed on behalf of the study participants and their families. In 1974, a $10 million out-of-court settlement was reached. As part of the settlement, the U.S. government promised to give lifetime medical benefits and burial services to all living participants.

After the Syphilis Study at Tuskegee was exposed, the Senate Committee on Labor and Human Resources held hearings on this study and other alleged healthcare abuses. The outcomes of these hearings were

- The enactment of the National Research Act of 1974 requiring the Department of Health, Education, and Welfare to codify its policy for the protection of human subjects into regulations; and
- The formation of the National Commission for the Protections of Human Subjects of Biomedical and Behavioral Research, which drafted the Belmont Report.

See: https://grants.nih.gov/sites/default/files/PHRP_Archived_Course_
    Materials_English.pdf

   https://www.cdc.gov/tuskegee/timeline.htm

9. **C.** The importance of demonstrating respect for research participants is reflected in the principles used to define ethical research and the regulations, policies, and guidance that describe the implementation of those principles. Human subjects are essential to the conduct of research intended to improve human health. As such, the relationship between investigators and human subjects is critical and should be based on honesty, trust, and respect. The Belmont Report identified three principles essential to the ethical conduct of research with humans

1. Respect for persons
2. Beneficence
3. Justice

These three basic principles serve as the foundation of the current Health and Human Services (HHS) regulations and guidelines for the ethical conduct of human subjects research supported by HHS.

See: https://grants.nih.gov/sites/default/files/PHRP_Archived_Course_
    Materials_English.pdf

10. **A.** The Health and Human Services (HHS) regulations (45 CFR 46.116) require that investigators obtain legally effective informed consent from prospective participants in a way that allows them to consider whether or not to participate and that minimizes the possibility for coercion or undue influence.

The challenges in applying the Belmont principle of respect for persons are in

- Making sure that potential participants comprehend the risks and potential benefits of participating in research
- Avoiding influencing potential participants' decisions either through explicit or implied threats (coercion) or through excessive compensation (undue influence)

See: https://grants.nih.gov/sites/default/files/PHRP_Archived_Course_
    Materials_English.pdf

11. **D.** Passive or active observation of human participants refers to research in which the investigator observes and documents individuals or group

behavior. Some public health research poses minimal risk to subjects (i.e., no more risk than one would encounter in daily life) and are therefore ruled "exempt" from review if the research falls into one of the specified categories, including surveys, interviews, observation of public behavior, or benign behavioral intervention.

The Belmont principle of respect for persons is primarily applied by requiring that all human subject research participants provide voluntary informed consent to participate in research.

The three fundamental aspects of informed consent are

1. Voluntariness
2. Comprehension
3. Disclosure

The Health and Human Services (HHS) regulations (45 CFR 46.116) require that investigators obtain legally effective informed consent from prospective participants in a way that allows them to consider whether or not to participate and that minimizes the possibility for coercion or undue influence. Potential participants must understand that enrolling in the research is voluntary and that they may withdraw from the study at any time without penalty or loss of benefits (45 CFR 46.116(a)).

Fox, E. E., Bulger, E., Dickerson, A., del Junco, D., Klotz, P., Podbielski, J., . . . Rahbar, M. (2013). Waiver of consent in noninterventional, observational emergency research: The PROMMTT experience. *The Journal of Trauma and Acute Care Surgery, 75*(1 Suppl. 1), S3–S8. doi:10.1097/TA.0b013e31828fa3a0

12. **D.** Mobile phones are not necessarily equipped with protective technology like encryption, firewalls, and antivirus software that will secure health information to guarantee confidentiality.

Risks for using a mobile device include physical loss or theft of the phone and transmitting data via text or email through an unsecured Internet.

Bromwich, M., & Bromwich, R. (2016). Privacy risks when using mobile devices in health care. *CMAJ: Canadian Medical Association Journal, 188*(12), 855–856. doi:10.1503/cmaj.160026 https://www.cdc.gov/nchhstp/programintegration/data-security.htm

13. **D.** Investigators should incorporate cultural norms into the research process whenever possible and appropriate. Examples of cultural norms include community consent and informed consent from family representatives.

- If community consent is the cultural norm, it may be appropriate to obtain community consent in advance of obtaining informed consent from individuals. Community consent cannot replace the informed consent from individuals.
- If cultural norms require permission from a family member before an individual may enroll in research, it may be appropriate to obtain permission from the family member in addition to informed consent from the prospective research participant.

See: https://grants.nih.gov/sites/default/files/PHRP_Archived_Course_Materials_English.pdf

14. **D.** "Exceptional" review is not one of the categories of research with human participants.

Protocols may be reviewed either at a meeting of the full institutional review board (IRB) or by "expedited review."

For "certain types of research involving no more than minimal risk and for minor changes to existing research," an IRB may choose to use an expedited review procedure. The expedited review may be conducted by the IRB chair or by designated experienced IRB member(s) (45 CFR 46.110). Investigators should understand that expedited review is conducted by fewer individuals, but is no less stringent and not necessarily faster than a full IRB review. If any individual reviewer who conducts an expedited review is unable to approve a proposed study, the study must be discussed by the full IRB.

The Health and Human Services (HHS) regulations describe categories of human subjects research that may be exempt from requirements described in the HHS regulations including IRB oversight.

Studies proposing only research that falls under one or more of the exempt categories of research do not require IRB review and approval, but the HHS Office for Human Research Protections (OHRP) has stated that: "Institutions should have a clear policy in place on who shall determine what research is exempt under 46.101(b)" and that investigators should not be able to determine whether or not their own research is exempt. This authority should rest with the IRB or other entity designated by the institution.

The exemptions can be found at 45 CFR 46.101(b).

See: https://grants.nih.gov/sites/default/files/PHRP_Archived_Course_Materials_English.pdf

15. **D.** There is no such thing as genetic license or permanent waiver of rights to use of individual genetic information.

The Belmont Report identified three principles essential to the ethical conduct of research with humans: respect for persons (autonomy and confidentiality), beneficence, and justice. These three basic principles serve as the foundation of the current Health and Human Services (HHS) regulations and guidelines for the ethical conduct of human subjects' research supported by HHS, including genetic counseling.

See: https://grants.nih.gov/sites/default/files/PHRP_Archived_Course_Materials_English.pdf

https://www.nsgc.org/p/cm/ld/fid=12

16. **A.** The Office for Human Research Protections (OHRP) provides leadership in the protection of the rights, welfare, and well-being of human subjects involved in research conducted or supported by the U.S. Department of Health and Human Services (HHS). OHRP is part of the Office of the Assistant Secretary for Health in the Office of the Secretary of HHS.

OHRP provides clarification and guidance, develops educational programs and materials, maintains regulatory oversight, and provides advice on ethical and regulatory issues in biomedical and behavioral research. OHRP also supports the Secretary's Advisory Committee on Human Research Protections

(SACHRP), which advises the HHS Secretary on issues related to protecting human subjects in research.

See: https://www.hhs.gov/ohrp

17. **B.** Research means a systematic investigation, including research development, testing, and evaluation, designed to develop or contribute to generalizable knowledge. Activities which meet this definition constitute research for purposes of this policy, whether or not they are conducted or supported under a program which is considered research for other purposes. For example, some demonstration and service programs may include research activities.

Research on samples or data about deceased individuals does not qualify as human subjects research, although some other regulations may apply.

See: https://www.hhs.gov/ohrp/regulations-and-policy/guidance/ research-involving-coded-private-information/index.html

18. **C.** Institutionally designated authority such as the institutional review board (IRB) is a committee within a university or other organization receiving federal funds to conduct research that reviews research proposals. The IRB reviews the proposals before a project is submitted to a funding agency to determine if the research project follows the ethical principles and federal regulations for the protection of human subjects. The IRB has the authority to approve, disapprove, or require modifications of these projects.

See: https://www.apa.org/advocacy/research/defending-research/ review-boards

https://www.fda.gov/regulatory-information/search-fda-guidance -documents/institutional-review-boards-frequently-asked-questions

https://www.niehs.nih.gov/about/boards/irb/index.cfm

19. **B.** In seeking informed consent, all study participants must be informed that participation is voluntary, refusal to participate will involve no penalty or loss of benefits to which the subject is otherwise entitled, and the subject may discontinue participation at any time without penalty or loss of benefits to which the subject is otherwise entitled.

See: https://www.hhs.gov/ohrp/sites/default/files/ohrp/policy/ ohrpregulations.pdf

20. **A.** In seeking informed consent, all study participants must be informed that participation is voluntary, refusal to participate will involve no penalty or loss of benefits to which the subject is otherwise entitled, and the subject may discontinue participation at any time without penalty or loss of benefits to which the subject is otherwise entitled.

See: https://www.hhs.gov/ohrp/sites/default/files/ohrp/policy/ ohrpregulations.pdf

21. **A.** During the informed consent process, survey participants are assured that data collected will be used only for stated purposes and will not be disclosed or released to others without the consent of the individual or the establishment in accordance with section 308(d) of the Public Health Service Act

(42 U.S.C. 242m). During the study, study participants may raise questions, and at each stage the informed consent must be renegotiated, not just at the beginning.

See: https://www.cdc.gov/nchs/nhanes/genetics/genetic_participants .htm

https://www.hhs.gov/ohrp/sites/default/files/ohrp/policy/ohrpreg ulations.pdf

22. **C.** By definition, children are unable to provide informed consent to participate in research, although they might be able to give their assent. The institutional review board (IRB) should determine that unless parental permission can be waived, adequate provisions are made for soliciting the permission of the parent(s) or legal guardian(s).

See: https://www.hhs.gov/ohrp/regulations-and-policy/guidance/faq/ children-research/index.html

23. **D.** The Code of Federal Regulations outlines specific requirements to enhance protections for three groups:

- Pregnant women, human fetuses, and neonates
- Children
- Prisoners

It is important for researchers to keep in mind that risks may vary for particular groups, depending on the nature of the research being conducted. In addition to the groups specified in 45 CFR 46, consider what protections or additional steps may be needed to minimize risk for your study population, such as outlining procedures for consenting individuals with diminished decision-making capacity, or specifying a plan to address incidental findings from your research.

See: https://grants.nih.gov/policy/humansubjects/policies-and -regulations/vulnerable-populations.htm

24. **B.** "Prisoner" means any individual involuntarily confined or detained in a penal institution. The term is intended to encompass individuals sentenced to such an institution under a criminal or civil statute, individuals detained in other facilities by virtue of statutes or commitment procedures which provide alternatives to criminal prosecution or incarceration in a penal institution, and individuals detained pending arraignment, trial, or sentencing (45 CFR 46.303(c)).

Respect for persons incorporates at least two other fundamental ethical principles, namely

- Autonomy, which requires that those who are capable of deliberation about their personal goals should be treated with respect for their capacity for self-determination; and
- Protection of persons with impaired or diminished autonomy, which requires that those who are dependent or vulnerable be afforded security against harm or abuse.

In addition to the requirements of subpart A, subpart C of the Health and Human Services (HHS) regulations at 45 CFR part 46 identifies more requirements for research involving prisoners. The exemptions that generally apply to certain types of research involving human subjects do not apply to research involving prisoners. In order to approve research involving prisoners, the institutional review board (IRB) must find that the proposed research falls into one of the permissible categories of research, and make six other findings; the institution must certify to the Office for Human Research Protections (OHRP) that an IRB has reviewed the proposal and made seven required findings, and receive OHRP authorization prior to initiating any research involving prisoners. The IRB must include a prisoner or prisoner representative, and meet a membership requirement concerning the number of IRB members not associated with a prison involved in the research. Secretarial waiver of informed consent in certain emergency research is not applicable to research involving prisoners.

See: https://www.hhs.gov/ohrp/regulations-and-policy/guidance/faq/prisoner-research/index.html

https://www.who.int/ethics/indigenous_peoples/en/index13.html

25. **B.** Risks cannot be completely eliminated, though they should be minimized. Protection of Human Subjects includes an assessment of risk, the steps taken to protect the subjects from risk, potential benefits from the study to the subjects and others, and the importance of the knowledge to be gained from these studies.

See: https://acd.od.nih.gov/documents/reports/Red_Team_draft_report.pdf

26. **C.** It is the policy of the National Institutes of Health (NIH) that each Institute and Center (IC) should have a system for the appropriate oversight and monitoring of the conduct of clinical trials to ensure the safety of participants and the validity and integrity of the data for all NIH-supported or conducted clinical trials. The establishment of the data safety monitoring boards (DSMBs) is required for multisite clinical trials involving interventions that entail potential risk to the participants. The data and safety monitoring functions and oversight of such activities are distinct from the requirement for study review and approval by an institutional review board (IRB).

See: https://grants.nih.gov/policy/humansubjects/policies-and-regulations/data-safety.htm

27. **A.** Equipoise means that there is uncertainty in the expert medical community over whether a treatment will be beneficial; this should be considered in designing and reviewing to justify clinical trials of new interventions.

See: https://www.nejm.org/doi/full/10.1056/NEJMsb1011301

28. **B.** Minimal risk to human participants in research requires review and approval by an institutional review board (IRB), which may be expedited. Minimal risk generally means that the probability and magnitude of physical or psychological harm anticipated in the research are not greater in and of themselves than those ordinarily encountered in daily life, or in routine healthcare examinations.

See: http://irb.ucsf.edu/sites/hrpp.ucsf.edu/files/tip-sheet-minimal-risk
.pdf

29. **A.** It is important to develop a plan so that participants in developing countries who volunteer to participate in an HIV antiretroviral treatment trial have the option to continue to receive antiretroviral treatment following their completion of the trial. Without such a plan, there is an increased possibility that trial participants may not receive posttrial antiretroviral treatment. This would end the benefits of treatment they received during the trial and could affect their ability to use certain antiretrovirals in the future. Therefore, National Institutes of Health (NIH)-funded investigators, working with host countries' authorities and other stakeholders, are expected to identify sources available in the countries for the provision of antiretroviral treatment to trial participants following their completion of the trial.

See: https://grants.nih.gov/grants/policy/antiretroviral/QandA.htm

30. **C.** National Institutes of Health (NIH) policy (NOT-OD-18-116) requires individuals of all ages, including children, to be included in NIH-supported research unless there is a scientific or ethical reason not to include them. There are also specific requirements that apply to research involving children in 45 CFR 46 Subpart D. NIH defines a child as an individual under the age of 18. Note that children is defined in 45 CFR 46 as "persons who have not attained the legal age for consent to treatments or procedures involved in the research, under the applicable law of the jurisdiction in which the research will be conducted." The following are important points from 45 CFR 46 regarding research with children.

Exemption 2 does not apply to research with children except for research involving observations of public behavior when the investigator(s) do not participate in the activities being observed.

Research with children may require assent from the child in addition to permission from a parent(s).

Research involving greater than minimal risk is permitted with children only under specific conditions, and requirements depend on the prospect or absence of direct benefit to the individual participants.

When children are wards of the State or other agency/institution/entity, an advocate may be required in addition to an individual acting on behalf of the child as a guardian or in *loco parentis*.

See: https://grants.nih.gov/grants/guide/notice-files/not-98-024.html

31. **B.** When research covered by 45 CFR 46 policy takes place in foreign countries, procedures normally followed in the foreign countries to protect human subjects may differ from those set forth in this policy. In these circumstances, if a department or agency head determines that the procedures prescribed by the institution afford protections that are at least equivalent to those provided in this policy, the department or agency head may approve the substitution of the foreign procedures in lieu of the procedural requirements provided in this policy. Except when otherwise required by statute, executive order, or the department or agency head, notices of these actions as they occur will be published in the Federal Register or will be otherwise published as provided in department or agency procedures.

See: https://www.federalregister.gov/documents/2017/01/19/2017-01058/federal-policy-for-the-protection-of-human-subjects

https://www.hhs.gov/ohrp/sites/default/files/ohrp/policy/ohrpregulations.pdf

32. **D.** Obtaining the agreement of local community leadership for the proposed research is almost always good research practice and is mandatory in some communities.

- Agreement from the community leadership is obtained prior to, but does not replace, the consent and/or assent of individual participants.
- Community consent is generally obtained through a process of dialogue with the community leadership and often does not require written agreement.
- There are, however, some countries and communities which require written evidence of consent and of the nature of any collaboration between the community and the proposed research. It is the researchers' responsibility to become aware of, and respect, these requirements.
- While support from the community leadership can lead to research practices which are collaborative, culturally sensitive, and which facilitate a more supportive research environment, researchers should be aware that what constitutes community leadership is not always clear, nor always ethically supportable, and that consultation does not necessarily result in agreement.

Investigators should incorporate cultural norms into the research process whenever possible and appropriate. Examples of cultural norms include community consent and informed consent from family representatives.

- If community consent is the cultural norm, it may be appropriate to obtain community consent in advance of obtaining informed consent from individuals. Community consent cannot replace the informed consent from individuals.
- If cultural norms require permission from a family member before an individual may enroll in research, it may be appropriate to obtain permission from the family member in addition to informed consent from the prospective research participant.

See: https://grants.nih.gov/sites/default/files/PHRP_Archived_Course_Materials_English.pdf

https://cioms.ch/wp-content/uploads/2017/01/WEB-CIOMS-Ethical Guidelines.pdf

33. **A.** The voluntary consent of the human subject is absolutely essential. This means that the person involved should have legal capacity to give consent; should be so situated as to be able to exercise free power of choice, without the intervention of any element of force, fraud, deceit, duress, over-reaching, or other ulterior form of constraint or coercion; and should have sufficient knowledge and comprehension of the elements of the subject matter involved, as to enable him to make an understanding and enlightened decision. This latter element requires that, before the acceptance of an affirmative decision by the experimental subject, there should be made known to him the nature,

duration, and purpose of the experiment; the method and means by which it is to be conducted; all inconveniences and hazards reasonably to be expected; and the effects upon his health or person, which may possibly come from his participation in the experiment. The duty and responsibility for ascertaining the quality of the consent rests upon each individual who initiates, directs, or engages in the experiment. It is a personal duty and responsibility which may not be delegated to another with impunity.

See: https://history.nih.gov/research/downloads/nuremberg.pdf

https://www.hhs.gov/ohrp/international/ethical-codes-and-research
-standards/index.html

34. **C.** Research can be approved as "exempt" if it is no more than "minimal risk" and fits one of the exempt review categories as defined by federal regulation 45 CFR 46. Studies that may qualify for "exempt" must be submitted to the institutional review board (IRB) for review. Exempt reviews are conducted by a member of the IRB.

See: https://grants.nih.gov/policy/hs/faqs.htm

35. **C.** Institutional review boards (IRBs) provide ethical and regulatory oversight of research that involves human subjects according to federal policy as specified in 45 CFR 46.

IRBs are specifically charged with protecting the rights and welfare of human subjects, not with conductive inquiries into scientific misconduct, reviewing research manuscripts for publication, or minimum wage specifications.

See: https://www.hhs.gov/ohrp/regulations-and-policy/regulations/
common-rule/index.html

https://www.niehs.nih.gov/about/boards/irb/index.cfm

36. **A.** Beneficence means persons are treated in an ethical manner not only by respecting their decisions and protecting them from harm, but also by making efforts to secure their well-being. Such treatment falls under the principle of beneficence. The term "beneficence" is often understood to cover acts of kindness or charity that go beyond strict obligation. In this document, beneficence is understood in a stronger sense, as an obligation. Two general rules have been formulated as complementary expressions of beneficent actions in this sense: (a) do not harm and (b) maximize possible benefits and minimize possible harms.

See: https://www.hhs.gov/ohrp/regulations-and-policy/belmont-report/
read-the-belmont-report/index.html#xbenefit

37. **A.** Beneficence—Persons are treated in an ethical manner not only by respecting their decisions and protecting them from harm, but also by making efforts to secure their well-being. Such treatment falls under the principle of beneficence. The term "beneficence" is often understood to cover acts of kindness or charity that go beyond strict obligation. In this document, beneficence is understood in a stronger sense, as an obligation. Two general rules have been formulated as complementary expressions of beneficent actions in this sense: (a) do not harm and (b) maximize possible benefits and minimize possible harms.

The principle of beneficence often occupies a well-defined justifying role in many areas of research involving human subjects. An example is found in research involving children. Effective ways of treating childhood diseases and fostering healthy development are benefits that serve to justify research involving children—even when individual research subjects are not direct beneficiaries. Research also makes it possible to avoid the harm that may result from the application of previously accepted routine practices that on closer investigation turn out to be dangerous. But the role of the principle of beneficence is not always so unambiguous. A difficult ethical problem remains, for example, about research that presents more than minimal risk without immediate prospect of direct benefit to the children involved. Some have argued that such research is inadmissible, while others have pointed out that this limit would rule out much research promising great benefit to children in the future. Here again, as with all hard cases, the different claims covered by the principle of beneficence may come into conflict and force difficult choices.

See: https://www.hhs.gov/ohrp/regulations-and-policy/belmont-report/read-the-belmont-report/index.html#xbenefit

38. **D.** According to 45 CFR 46 Link to Non-U.S. Government Site—Click for Disclaimer, a human subject is "a living individual about whom an investigator (whether professional or student) is conducting research through obtaining, using, studying, analyzing, or generating identifiable private information or identifiable biospecimens."

See: https://grants.nih.gov/policy/humansubjects/research.htm

39. **D.** Electronic health records (EHRs) are electronic versions of the paper charts in your doctor's or other healthcare provider's office. An EHR may include your medical history, notes, and other information about your health including your symptoms, diagnoses, medications, lab results, vital signs, immunizations, and reports from diagnostic tests such as x-rays. Providers are working with other doctors, hospitals, and health plans to find ways to share that information. The information in EHRs can be shared with other organizations involved in your care if the computer systems are set up to talk to each other. Information in these records should only be shared for purposes authorized by law or by you. Privacy rights are relevant to whether an individual's information is stored as a paper record or stored in an electronic form. The same federal laws that already protect health information also apply to information in EHRs.

See: https://www.hhs.gov/sites/default/files/ocr/privacy/hipaa/understanding/consumers/privacy-security-electronic-records.pdf

40. **A.** The Code of Federal Regulations (CFR) outlines specific requirements to enhance protections for three groups:

- Pregnant women, human fetuses, and neonates
- Children
- Prisoners

It is important for researchers to keep in mind that risks may vary for particular groups, depending on the nature of the research being conducted. In addition to the groups specified in 45 CFR 46, consider what protections or additional steps may be needed to minimize risk for your study population, such as outlining procedures for consenting individuals with diminished decision-making capacity, or specifying a plan to address incidental findings from your research.

See: https://grants.nih.gov/policy/humansubjects/policies-and
-regulations/vulnerable-populations.htm

41. **C.** In global health, risks are defined by place, time, situation, and cultural opportunities or constraints. Traditionally, global health research focused on the crippling burden of infectious disease in developing countries. Infectious diseases led to high rates of childhood mortality and morbidity, as well as low life expectancy rates. In addition, the health research expertise needed to confront these challenges was primarily concentrated in high-income countries. Past scientific advances have played a critical role in combating the infectious disease burden; for example, smallpox eradication and the use of oral rehydration therapy contributed to significant reductions in morbidity and mortality around the globe.

See: https://www.who.int/healthinfo/global_burden_disease/Global
HealthRisks_report_full.pdf

Lavery, J. V., Green, S. K., Bandewar, S. V. S., Bhan, A., Daar, A., Emerson, C. I., . . . Singer, P. A. (2013). Addressing ethical, social, and cultural issues in global health research. *PLoS Neglected Tropical Diseases, 7*(8), e2227. doi:10.1371/journal.pntd.0002227

42. **D.** Certificates of Confidentiality (CoCs) protect the privacy of research subjects by prohibiting disclosure of identifiable, sensitive research information to anyone not connected to the research except when the subject consents or in a few other specific situations. Learn about the NIH Policy for issuing CoCs; its purpose, scope and applicability; disclosure requirements; and responsibilities of CoC recipients.

See: https://grants.nih.gov/policy/humansubjects/coc.htm

43. **C.** The Health and Human Services (HHS) regulations state that "An investigator shall seek such consent only under circumstances that provide the prospective subject or the representative sufficient opportunity to consider whether or not to participate and that minimize the possibility of coercion or undue influence" (45 CFR 46.116). This requirement applies to all nonexempt human subjects research not eligible for a waiver of the consent requirements. Coercion occurs when an overt or implicit threat of harm is intentionally presented by one person to another in order to obtain compliance. For example, an investigator might tell a prospective subject that he or she will lose access to needed health services if he or she does not participate in the research. Undue influence, by contrast, often occurs through an offer of an excessive or inappropriate reward or other overture in order to obtain compliance. For example, an investigator might promise psychology students extra credit if they participate in the research. If that is the only way a student can earn extra

credit, then the investigator is unduly influencing potential subjects. If, however, she offers comparable nonresearch alternatives for earning extra credit, the possibility of undue influence is minimized.

Paying research subjects in exchange for their participation is a common and, in general, acceptable practice. However, difficult questions must be addressed by the institutional review board (IRB). For example, how much money should research subjects receive, and for what should subjects receive payment—their time, inconvenience, discomfort, or some other consideration? IRBs must be sensitive to whether any aspect of the proposed remuneration will be an undue influence, thus interfering with the potential subjects' ability to give voluntary informed consent.

See: https://www.hhs.gov/ohrp/regulations-and-policy/guidance/faq/informed-consent/index.html

44. **C.** The institutional review board (IRB) must determine, to the extent required by 45 CFR 46.116, that adequate provisions are made for soliciting the assent of the children—when in the judgment of the IRB the children are capable of providing assent—as well as the permission of the parents (45 CFR 46.408). Permission means the agreement of the parent(s) or guardian to the participation of the child or ward in research (45 CFR 46.402(c)).

By regulatory definition, children are "persons who have not attained the legal age for consent to treatments or procedures involved in the research, under the applicable law of the jurisdiction in which the research will be conducted" (45 CFR 46.402(a)). In the United States, the legal age of adulthood is a matter of state and local law. This means that who is legally considered a child may vary from state to state; in a large majority of states, 18 years of age is the legal age of adulthood, but this is not true in every state, locality, or territory. State law also may address specific circumstances in which a person younger than the age of adulthood is legally authorized to consent to medical procedures: for example, some states allow children younger than the legal age of adulthood to consent to the provision of contraceptive services. Certain states provide a mechanism for the emancipation of minors, through which a child younger than the legal age of adulthood may gain certain civil rights, which might include the legal ability to consent to research participation.

See: https://www.hhs.gov/ohrp/regulations-and-policy/guidance/faq/informed-consent/index.html

45. **D.** If the research holds out the prospect of direct benefit solely to the fetus then the consent of the pregnant woman and the father is obtained in accord with the informed consent provisions, except that the father's consent need not be obtained if he is unable to consent because of unavailability, incompetence, or temporary incapacity or the pregnancy resulted from rape or incest.

See: https://grants.nih.gov/policy/humansubjects/policies-and-regulations/vulnerable-populations.htm

46. **C.** When research covered by 45 CFR 46 policy takes place in foreign countries, procedures normally followed in the foreign countries to protect human subjects may differ from those set forth in this policy. In these circumstances, if a department or agency head determines that the procedures prescribed by the institution afford protections that are at least equivalent to those provided

in this policy, the department or agency head may approve the substitution of the foreign procedures in lieu of the procedural requirements provided in this policy. Except when otherwise required by statute, Executive Order, or the department or agency head, notices of these actions as they occur will be published in the Federal Register or will be otherwise published as provided in department or agency procedures.

See: https://www.federalregister.gov/documents/2017/01/19/2017-01058 /federal-policy-for-the-protection-of-human-subjects

https://www.hhs.gov/ohrp/sites/default/files/ohrp/policy/ ohrpregulations.pdf

47. **B.** Research as a systematic investigation, including research development, testing, and evaluation, is designed to develop or contribute to generalizable knowledge. According to 45 CFR 46, a human subject is "a living individual about whom an investigator (whether professional or student) conducting research, in which an investigator obtains information or biospecimens through intervention or interaction with the individual, and uses, studies, or analyzes the information or biospecimens; or obtains, uses, studies, analyzes, or generates identifiable private information or identifiable biospecimens."

See: https://grants.nih.gov/policy/humansubjects/research.htm

https://www.research.uci.edu/compliance/human-research -protections/researchers/activities-irb-review.html

48. **A.** Research ethics govern the standards of conduct for scientific researchers. It is important to adhere to ethical principles in order to protect the dignity, rights, and welfare of research participants. As such, all research involving human beings should be reviewed by an ethics committee to ensure that the appropriate ethical standards are being upheld. Discussion of the ethical principles of beneficence, justice, and autonomy are central to ethical review. For global health research, the World Health Assembly further urges member states to "establish governance mechanisms for research for health, to ensure rigorous application of good research norms and standards, including protection for human subjects involved in research."

See: https://apps.who.int/iris/bitstream/handle/10665/44783/9789241502 948_eng.pdf;jsessionid=2232DEDFCB466E3D73457F626D5E7DD8? sequence=1

https://www.who.int/ethics/topics/research/en

49. **D.** Deception and incomplete disclosure raise concern as they may interfere with the ability of the subject to make a fully informed decision about whether or not to participate in the research. Deception and incomplete disclosure may be valuable research methodologies, yet their use presents special challenges to ensure that the research is conducted ethically. Sometimes, deception or incomplete disclosure may be necessary to avoid study bias or test a hypothesis that requires the participant's misdirection. However, the regulations for obtaining informed consent from research participants (§45 CFR 46.116) in general require full disclosure of all elements relevant to the subject's participation in the research.

Golder, S., Ahmed, S., Norman, G., & Booth, A. (2017). Attitudes toward the ethics of research using social media: A systematic review. *Journal of Medical Internet Research, 19*(6), e195. doi:10.2196/jmir.7082

https://www.hhs.gov/ohrp/regulations-and-policy/regulations/45-cfr-46/index.html#46.116

Smith, K. V., Thew, G. R., & Graham, B. (2018). Conducting ethical Internet-based research with vulnerable populations: A qualitative study of bereaved participants' experiences of online questionnaires. *European Journal of Psychotraumatology, 9*(Suppl. 1), 1506231. doi:10.1080/20008198.2018.1506231

50. **A.** Research means a systematic investigation, including research development, testing, and evaluation, designed to develop or contribute to generalizable knowledge. Activities that meet this definition constitute research for purposes of this policy, whether or not they are conducted or supported under a program that is considered research for other purposes. For example, some demonstration and service programs may include research activities. For purposes of this part, the following activities are deemed not to be research.

    1. Scholarly and journalistic activities (e.g., oral history, journalism, biography, literary criticism, legal research, and historical scholarship), including the collection and use of information, that focus directly on the specific individuals about whom the information is collected.
    2. Public health surveillance activities, including the collection and testing of information or biospecimens, conducted, supported, requested, ordered, required, or authorized by a public health authority. Such activities are limited to those necessary to allow a public health authority to identify, monitor, assess, or investigate potential public health signals, onsets of disease outbreaks, or conditions of public health importance (including trends, signals, risk factors, patterns in diseases, or increases in injuries from using consumer products). Such activities include those associated with providing timely situational awareness and priority setting during the course of an event or crisis that threatens public health (including natural or man-made disasters).
    3. Collection and analysis of information, biospecimens, or records by or for a criminal justice agency for activities authorized by law or court order solely for criminal justice or criminal investigative purposes.
    4. Authorized operational activities (as determined by each agency) in support of intelligence, homeland security, defense, or other national security missions.

    Written, or in writing, for purposes of this part, refers to writing on a tangible medium (e.g., paper) or in an electronic format.

    See: https://www.ecfr.gov/cgi-bin/retrieveECFR?gp=&SID=83cd09e1c0f5c6937cd9d7513160fc3f&pitd=20180719&n=pt45.1.46&r=PART&ty=HTML#se45.1.46_1102

51. **A.** All researchers are vulnerable to attitudes that may stigmatize conditions, individuals, or socioeconomic status, level of education, and other determinants of health in different countries. Training in cultural sensitivity is one of

the ways to cultivate ethical conduct that prevents stigmatization in research. The Fogarty International Center's Stigma and Global Health Research Program aimed to stimulate interdisciplinary, investigator-initiated research on the role of stigma in health, and how to intervene to prevent or mitigate its negative effects on the health and welfare of individuals, groups, and societies worldwide. This program encouraged research across a variety of scientific disciplines including the biomedical, social, and behavioral sciences, to elucidate the etiology of stigma in relation to public health, and to develop and test interventions to mitigate the negative effects of stigma on health outcomes. Studies examined stigma and public health in domestic, international, and cross-cultural contexts, with an emphasis on studies relevant to global health issues.

See: https://www.fic.nih.gov/Programs/Pages/stigma.aspx

52. **D.** In general, suicide ideation is equally common in both women and men, and women are more likely to attempt suicide than men, but men complete suicide more frequently than women. World Mental Health Day, observed on October 10, is an opportunity to raise awareness of mental health issues and to mobilize efforts in support of mental health. In 2019, the theme is suicide prevention. Every year close to 800,000 people take their own life and there are many more people who attempt suicide. Every suicide is a tragedy that affects families, communities, and entire countries and has long-lasting effects on the people left behind. Suicide occurs throughout life and is the second-leading cause of death among 15- to 29-year-olds globally.

See: https://www.who.int/news-room/events/detail/2019/10/10/
default-calendar/world-mental-health-day-2019-focus-on-suicide
-prevention

53. **B.** The medical standard of care is typically defined as the type and level of healthcare that a reasonably competent and skilled healthcare professional, with a similar background and in the same medical community, would have provided under the circumstances of interaction between the patient and provider. This definition is often used in alleged malpractice decisions.

Standard of treatment is accepted by medical experts as a proper treatment for a certain type of disease and is widely used by healthcare professionals. It is also called best practice, standard medical care, and standard therapy.

See: https://www.cancer.gov/publications/dictionaries/cancer-terms/def
/standard-of-care

Moffett, P., & Moore, G. (2011). The standard of care: Legal history and definitions: The bad and good news. *The Western Journal of Emergency Medicine, 12*(1), 109–112. Retrieved from https://www.ncbi.nlm.nih.gov/
pmc/articles/PMC3088386

54. **C.** Nonmaleficence ("first do no harm"), beneficence (doing good), and trust are fundamental ethical principles at the core of clinical care and public health.

See: https://apps.who.int/iris/bitstream/handle/10665/164576/978924069
4033_eng.pdf;jsessionid=E148503E2374EF0B706C597E8B7CA425?
sequence=1

55. C. Randomized clinical trials are studies in which the participants are divided by chance into separate groups that compare different treatments or other interventions. Using chance to divide people into groups means that the groups will be similar and that the effects of the treatments they receive can be compared more fairly. At the time of the trial, it is not known which treatment is best.

See: https://www.cancer.gov/publications/dictionaries/cancer-terms/def /randomized-clinical-trial

56. D. The Mexico City policy, sometimes referred to as the global gag rule, is a U.S. government policy that blocks U.S. federal funding for nongovern-mental organizations that provide abortion counseling or referrals, advocate to decriminalize abortion, or expand abortion services. On 23 January 2017, President Donald J. Trump issued a presidential memorandum regarding the Mexico City Policy.

See: https://www.whitehouse.gov/presidential-actions/presidential-mem orandum-regarding-mexico-city-policy

57. D. Ethical issues are paramount in all public and global health proce-dures. Responses to epidemics, emergencies, and disasters raise many ethical issues for the people involved, including public health specialists and policy makers.

See: https://www.who.int/ethics/publications/epidemics-emergencies -research/en

58. D. Isolation and quarantine help protect the public by preventing exposure to people who have or may have a contagious disease.

Isolation separates sick people with a contagious disease from people who are not sick.

Quarantine separates and restricts the movement of people who were exposed to a contagious disease to see if they become sick.

The International Health Regulations recognize that

Free movement of people and goods will increase the risk of cross-border transmission.

and

Quarantine is an impediment to free trade; public health arguments can justify trade barriers.

See: https://www.cdc.gov/quarantine/index.html

https://www.who.int/trade/distance_learning/gpgh/gpgh8/en/ index7.html

59. D. The stated purpose and scope of the International Health Regulations (IHR) are "to prevent, protect against, control and provide a public health response to the international spread of disease in ways that are commensu-rate with and restricted to public health risks, and which avoid unnecessary interference with international traffic and trade."

There is no provision to prioritize wealthy countries in the IHR.

See: https://www.who.int/ihr/publications/9789241596664/en

60. **C.** Financial cost is not included explicitly in the criteria for emergency declaration, although it is implicitly considered in decision-making processes. For example, during the 2019 Ebola outbreak in Congo, WHO faced criticism about unnecessary delay in the declaration of an emergency.

Some serious public health events that endanger international public health may be determined under the Regulations to be public health emergencies of international concern (PHEIC). The term "public health emergency of international concern" is defined in the IHR (2005) as "an extraordinary event which is determined, as provided in these Regulations:

- To constitute a public health risk to other States through the international spread of disease; and
- To potentially require a coordinated international response." This definition implies a situation that: is serious, unusual or unexpected; carries implications for public health beyond the affected State's national border; and may require immediate international action.

See: https://www.who.int/ihr/publications/9789241596664/en

5

Public Health Biology and Human Disease Risk

■ INTRODUCTION

Life on Earth is subject to the principles of evolution by natural selection. Humans and all organisms alive today, including notorious pathogenic viruses, bacteria, fungi, and protozoa, represent the outcome of billions of years of evolutionary strategies. We are witnessing only a very slim snapshot of this process in the temporal dimension. Yet, it is human nature to try hard to control the fate of our evolution by keeping pathogens at bay. We do this through scientific investigations into the molecular nature of infection and immunity. We have successfully created effective vaccines against deadly pathogens, and even managed to eradicate disfiguring diseases such as smallpox. The goal of eradication of other heartbreaking diseases such as poliomyelitis remain elusive. Diseases which we thought we had kept under control, such as measles, continue to reemerge. Preventable diseases such as malaria and diarrhea continue to kill millions of people because we have not yet mastered how to translate scientific results into various international contexts where diseases remain endemic. We are learning more and more that human ingenuity and pathogen genetics are constantly waging battles, as the emergence of antibiotic resistance in bacterial populations is showing us. We are also witnessing the influence of global environmental conditions such as climate change on disease burden. The demarcation of chronic and infectious diseases is breaking down as we understand more deeply that the human microbiome plays a role in diseases such as cancer and diabetes. Environmental pollution with chemicals contributes significantly to the societal burden of disease, yet preventing such diseases demands that public health professionals collaborate with materials scientists, product designers, and waste management agencies to enable full control of the life cycle of chemicals that have made modern lifestyles possible.

The questions on public health biology and human disease risk are designed to examine broad knowledge of the biological basis of health and disease. Practicing with these questions should enable you to

- Apply evidence-based biological concepts to inform public health laws, policies, and regulations
- Assess how biological agents affect human health
- Identify risk factors and modes of transmission for infectious diseases and how these diseases affect both personal and population health
- Identify risk factors for noninfectious diseases and how these issues affect both personal and population health

■ QUESTIONS

1. The following are examples of the influence of the study of medical geology on public health issues, EXCEPT
   A. Selenium deficiency and Keshan disease
   B. Iodine deficiency and mental retardation
   C. Mercury deficiency and anemia
   D. Niacin deficiency and pellagra

2. In 2016, an estimated 339.4 million people worldwide suffered from asthma, which is a lung disease that affects respiration. The symptoms are repeated episodes of wheezing, breathlessness, chest tightness, and coughing. Ozone is one of the most common asthma triggers. Which of the following is NOT true about ozone in the atmosphere?
   A. In the stratosphere, ozone forms a protective layer that absorbs the wavelength of solar radiation known as ultraviolet-B.
   B. Tropospheric ozone pollution is a concern primarily during the summer months when the weather conditions to form it (lots of sun and hot temperatures) normally occur.
   C. Peak concentrations of ozone typically occur in midafternoon after both the morning traffic rush and several hours of bright sunlight.
   D. Ozone levels are often highest in the inner large cities rather than the downwind suburban regions.

3. Widespread scientific consensus exists that the world's climate is changing. Some changes that could negatively affect health include more variable weather patterns, heat waves, heavy precipitation events, flooding, droughts, more intense storms, sea level rise, and air pollution. Greenhouse gases trap heat within the surface-troposphere system, causing heating at the surface of the planet. Greenhouse gases include which of the following?
   A. Carbon dioxide, methane, nitrous oxide, fluorinated gases
   B. Oxygen, nitrogen, helium
   C. Nitrous oxide, chlorofluorocarbons, and ozone
   D. Carbon dioxide, ozone, hydrogen sulfide, chlorine

4. Asbestos materials have been used for insulation in buildings and in various products such as roofing materials, water supply lines and clutches, brake linings, gaskets, and pads for automobiles. Today, chrysotile—the only commercial asbestos still in use—is mostly used in fiber cement boards. Individuals who are occupationally exposed to asbestos have developed several types of life-threatening diseases, including asbestosis, lung cancer, and mesothelioma. Which of the following statements is true about lead and asbestos pollution?

   A. Both lead and asbestos are commonly used in home building in the United States today.
   B. Both pollutants are difficult to recognize by sight and identification by special testing is needed.
   C. Asbestos is highly regulated today, but not lead.
   D. Drinking water contributes most to lead and asbestos exposure in the general U.S. population.

5. In 2014, the drinking water supply in Flint, Michigan, contained leached lead (Pb) causing a public health disaster. There are approximately half a million U.S. children ages 1 to 5 with blood lead levels above 5 micrograms per deciliter (mcg/dL), the reference level at which the Centers for Disease Control and Prevention (CDC) recommends public health actions be initiated. No safe blood lead level in children has been identified. Which part of the human body usually contains the highest amount of lead?

   A. Bones
   B. Blood
   C. Brain
   D. Liver

6. In the United States, exposure to radon is the second leading cause of lung cancer after smoking and is estimated to cause over 20,000 deaths each year, according to the U.S. Environmental Protection Agency. What is the predominant entry route of radon into the residential homes in the general U.S. population?

   A. Well water supply
   B. Soil gas
   C. Building materials
   D. Rocks

7. In May 2019, the state of California banned the controversial pesticide chlorpyrifos, a widely used organophosphate pesticide. Which of the following is true about pesticide pollution?

   A. Pesticide exposure has been associated with birth defects, miscarriage, and fetal death, but not diseases related to the nervous system.
   B. Pesticides usually kill undesirable insects or plants and have no impact on desirable insects or plants.
   C. Concentrations of pesticides can be high in an agricultural application field, but the concentrations are usually low at residential homes because there are no indoor sources.

D. Many pesticides can bioaccumulate in the human body, including dichlorodiphenyltrichloroethane (DDT) and polychlorinated biphenyl compound (PCB).

8. During natural disasters such as the 2005 Hurricane Katrina or the 2017 Hurricane Maria that hit Puerto Rico, raw sewage overflows and inadequately controlled stormwater discharges from municipal sewer systems introduced a variety of harmful pollutants, including disease-causing organisms, metals, and nutrients that threatened community water quality and contributed to disease outbreaks, beach and shellfish bed closings, fishing advisories, and basement backups of sewage. *Escherichia coli* has been used as a principal indicator of fecal pollution in water by the U.S. Environmental Protection Agency (EPA) because of the following EXCEPT

A. All *E. coli* strains are harmful pathogens.
B. Direct pathogen detection from environmental samples is usually technically demanding, slow to produce results, and expensive.
C. It is impossible to monitor for all pathogens.
D. *E. coli* is an indicator microorganism that is relatively simple to detect and commonly present in higher numbers in intestines of warm-blooded animals including human beings.

9. Identifying sources of pollution is important for prevention of adverse impacts on people and the environment. Point sources and nonpoint sources are the two broad source categories of water pollution. Which of the following is NOT one of the main nonpoint sources of water pollution?

A. Coal-fired power plant
B. Acid rain
C. Urban street runoff
D. Fallout of airborne pollutants

10. Mercury (Hg) has been used in human societies for many centuries. The human health effects from exposure to low environmental levels of elemental mercury are unknown. Very high mercury vapor concentrations can quickly cause severe lung damage. At low vapor concentrations over a long time, neurological disturbances, memory problems, skin rash, and kidney abnormalities may occur. The organic mercury poisoning outbreak in the 1950s in Minamata, Japan, was caused by the contamination of

A. Soil
B. Ocean water and seafood
C. Air
D. Seed grain

11. When two or more people get the same illness from the same contaminated food or drink, the event is called a foodborne disease outbreak. Since 1973 the Centers for Disease Control and Prevention (CDC) has maintained a collaborative surveillance program for collection and periodic reporting of data on the occurrence and causes of foodborne disease outbreaks (FBDOs). However, only a fraction of FBDOs are routinely reported. This underreporting problem is mainly because of the following reasons EXCEPT

A. Most household infections are not recognized or reported.
B. Emerging pathogens are unidentifiable.
C. Same pathogens are present in water and person-to-person contact.
D. The CDC has not established a convenient reporting pathway.

12. In 2017, the per capita consumption of seafood was 7.25 kg. Fish and shellfish are of substantial concern as contaminated food sources. This is because some of the environmental contaminants may be bio-concentrated in the aquatic food chain. Which of the following contaminant(s) may NOT have elevated concentrations in fish meat?

A. Heavy metals (e.g., mercury)
B. Light metals (e.g., sodium)
C. Lipophilic substances (e.g., polychlorinated biphenyl compounds [PCBs])
D. Pathogenic viruses

13. Electromagnetic radiation takes many forms. Ionizing radiation is a form of energy that acts by removing electrons from atoms and molecules of materials that include air, water, and living tissue. Ionizing radiation can pass through these materials. Humans and other mammals are more sensitive to ionizing radiation relative to other animals; therefore, higher doses of ionizing radiation may cause which of the following health effects in humans?

A. Cancers
B. Cardiovascular disease
C. Asthma
D. Indigestion

14. In the United States, approximately 9,500 people are diagnosed with skin cancer every day. Which of the following statements is false about the ultraviolet radiation and skin cancer?

A. Ultraviolet A rays (UVA) have a shorter wavelength than ultraviolet B rays (UVB); thus, they are more dangerous than UVB.
B. Melanoma is the worst kind of skin cancer because it is deadly.
C. One of the main reasons for the rising incidences of melanoma is the depletion of the ozone layer.
D. The sun's ultraviolet (UV) rays can damage skin in as little as 15 minutes.

15. Globally, approximately 2.01 billion metric tons of municipal solid waste are generated annually, leading to pollution crises such as the plastic contamination of the oceans. Solid waste is any garbage or refuse, as well as sludge from a wastewater treatment plant, water supply treatment plant, or air pollution control facility, and other discarded material resulting from industrial, commercial, mining, and agricultural operations, as well as from community activities. The best way to manage solid waste is to

A. Incinerate it
B. Dump it
C. Bury it
D. Reduce it, reuse it, and recycle it

16. In the United States, the Resource Conservation and Recovery Act (RCRA) was implemented in 1976 to create a framework for managing hazardous and non-hazardous waste. Materials regulated by RCRA are known as "solid wastes." Solid waste disposal with mass burning may be cheap because there is no sorting of waste required, but the process often causes greater problems with

  A. Nothing; there are no problems with mass burning
  B. Soil, water, and air contamination with toxic residual ash
  C. Ozone layer depletion in the troposphere
  D. Release of biogas

17. Most urban populations in the world now live under conditions of perpetual lighting, both indoors and outdoors. Which of the following is true about light pollution?

  A. Overlighting at night can reduce the rates of car accidents.
  B. Excessive light has been proven to reduce crime rates.
  C. Animals generally adapt to artificial lights more easily than humans; therefore, excessive light is not a problem for animals such as birds.
  D. Excessive light is a waste of energy and is associated with environmental pollution.

18. Many hazardous materials are used in human societies, but damage is prevented through limiting exposure. Exposure assessment is a branch of environmental science and occupational hygiene that focuses on the processes at the interface between the environment containing hazardous substances and organisms. Which of the following is true about uncertainty and variability in exposure assessment?

  A. Variability arises from incomplete knowledge, and uncertainty arises from natural stochasticity or true heterogeneity across people, places, or time.
  B. Uncertainty is not reducible by empirical effort, but can be better understood.
  C. Uncertainty can lead to inaccurate or biased estimates, whereas variability can affect the precision of the estimates and the degree to which they can be generalized.
  D. Uncertainty and variability can easily be separated in exposure assessment studies.

19. Environmental risk factors such as cigarette smoke, heavy metals, and chemical pesticides are known to be carcinogenic. Which of the following is TRUE about biotransformation of these xenobiotic chemicals in the human body?

  A. Phase II reactions introduce polar groups into the molecule, which makes electrophilic intermediate species that may be more toxic than the original pollutant.
  B. Phase II reactions involve conjugation of a chemical to form highly water-soluble metabolites that can be easily excreted by the liver, kidney, or gill.
  C. Phase I and Phase II biotransformation reactions usually work separately to convert xenobiotics into more readily excretable metabolites.
  D. Phase I reactions involve conjugation of a chemical to form highly water-soluble metabolites that can be easily excreted by the liver, kidney, or gill.

20. The attribution of risk factors to the concept of "causation" is very contentious in public health. Who among the following provided some guidelines for understanding causality in population health?

A. Sir William Richard Doll
B. Sir Austin Bradford Hill
C. Sir Richard Charles Branson
D. Sir Austin Danger Powers

21. Which of the following is not one of the guidelines for investigating causality in public health?

A. Prescience
B. Dose–response
C. Plausibility
D. Specificity

22. Which of the following terms describes the phenomenon of generally favorable biological responses to low exposures to toxins and other stressors?

A. Homeostasis
B. Heterogeneity
C. Hormesis
D. Homologous

23. Robert Koch was awarded the 1905 Nobel Prize in Medicine for his work on tuberculosis. His name is also associated with "Koch's Postulates," which state that, to establish an organism as the cause of a disease, the following criteria must be met, EXCEPT

A. The organism must be found in all cases of the disease examined.
B. It must be possible to prepare and maintain the organism in a pure culture.
C. The organisms must be capable of producing the original infection, even after several generations in culture.
D. The organism must be capable of eliciting an immune response in the infected host.

24. *"Ring around the rosy*
A pocketful of posies
Ashes, ashes
We all fall down"
The childhood song reproduced in the previous text emerged out of the experience of Western European populations devastated by the plague, caused by *Yersinia pestis* (formerly *Pasteurella pestis*), which is now easily controlled with antibiotic therapy. Louis Pasteur, for whom the discoverer originally named the pathogen, is best known for

A. Discovering the causative agent of the plague
B. Developing a vaccine for rabies
C. Developing a vaccine for smallpox
D. Discovering the causative agent of cholera

25. Our world regularly faces threats of pandemic infections, the latest being H1N1 flu. Molecular biology aids in the rapid development of vaccines necessary for controlling infectious epidemics. What do the "H" and "N" stand for in H1N1?

    A. Hydrogen and nitrogen
    B. Hydrocarbon and nitrosamine
    C. Hydrocarbon and neuraminidase
    D. Hemagglutinin and neuraminidase

26. The publication of a questionable research article in the 1990s instigated parental concerns about the possible effects of the Measles–Mumps–Rubella (MMR) vaccine and other vaccines used to prevent once threatening diseases on childhood diseases such as autism. What content of these vaccines provoked the concerns?

    A. Live viruses in the vaccines
    B. Attenuated viruses in the vaccines
    C. Genetically engineering organisms in the vaccines
    D. Mercury preservative in the vaccines

27. *"The history of child lead poisoning in the past century in this country is a good example of how powerful economic interests can prevent the implementation of a 'useful Truth'."* –Benjamin Franklin (1706–1790).
    Although exposure to lead (Pb) has been known as a risk factor to public health and well-being for the past two centuries, the recent use of policy instruments to reduce lead poisoning is considered one of the key milestone achievements in public health. Despite the successes, exposure to lead in commercial products remains a problem in many societies. People can still be exposed to toxic Pb directly or indirectly through the following pathways EXCEPT

    A. Energy resources
    B. Food resources
    C. Electronic products
    D. Linen

28. Despite numerous strategies to eliminate the use of lead (Pb) from commercial products such as gasoline and paint, lead poisoning remains a major threat to children's health worldwide. The symptoms of lead (Pb) poisoning include the following, EXCEPT

    A. Anemia
    B. Blindness
    C. Reduction in IQ
    D. Pain during urination

29. The eradication of deadly diseases in the human population is a goal of global health. Which of the following diseases has been eradicated in human populations?

    A. Measles
    B. Chickenpox
    C. Smallpox
    D. Bubonic plague

30. The Lady Mary Wortley Montagu (15 May 1689 – 21 August 1762) was an English aristocrat and writer who lived in the Ottoman Empire (modern day Turkey) and is credited with bringing what public health innovation to the Western world?

    A. Water chlorination
    B. A method of vaccination
    C. A method for preventing drug addiction
    D. Water filtration

31. There is a lot of controversy over the widespread use of chemicals such as dibromobiphenyl ethers as fire retardants. In recent history, fire retardation was accomplished through the widespread use of asbestos fibers, which has been demonstrated to be harmful to human health. Societies seem to keep replacing one source of hazard for another in our quest for a "safe" commerce-based society. The linkage of asbestos exposure to disease seemed straightforward because of the specificity and rarity of the disease, unlike the wide range of physiological effects associated with polybrominated diphenyl ethers. To what disease is asbestos exposure associated?

    A. Gout
    B. Mesothelioma
    C. Rare form of cognitive deficit
    D. Chronic dermatitis

32. *"For each of us, as for the robin in Michigan, or the Salmon in the Miramichi, this is a problem of ecology, of interrelationships, of interdependence . . .. We spray our elms and following springs are silent of robin song . . ."*
–Rachel Carson (1907–1964)
The Swiss chemist Paul Hermann Müller was awarded the Nobel Prize in Physiology or Medicine in 1948 "for his discovery of the high efficiency of dichlorodiphenyltrichloroethane (DDT)." Rachel Carson's observations laid the foundation for an ecological model of public health, and the publication of her book, *Silent Spring*, led to the clamor to ban dichlorodiphenyltrichloroethane (DDT). The banning of DDT in 1972 is considered the first major environmental victory in the United States. In a demonstration of the complexity of the ecological model of public health, there is a recent clamor to lift the ban on DDT in certain regions. What is the reason for this reversal?

    A. DDT is essential for the control of tuberculosis.
    B. DDT has recently been shown as an effective treatment for prolonging the lives of AIDS patients in Africa.
    C. DDT is effective against vector-borne diseases.
    D. There is no hard evidence that DDT actually causes cancer.

33. HIV, the causative agent of AIDS, has killed more than 25 million people since it was discovered. Why has it been difficult to develop a vaccine against HIV?

    A. Most effective vaccines consist of nonantigenic components of pathogens, and killed HIV does not retain antigenicity.
    B. Classic vaccines such as the vaccine against smallpox mimic natural immunity against reinfection generally seen in individuals who have recovered after illness. However, there are almost no such recoveries from AIDS.

C. Most vaccines protect against infection, not against disease, whereas HIV infection remains latent for very short periods before causing disease.

D. The use of killed retrovirus vaccine raises safety concerns.

34. The life expectancy at birth for Californians has increased by approximately 5 years over the past two decades. The California Department of Public Health is responsible for collecting and organizing data to assess the performance of the State in meeting the goals established by the national program, "Healthy People-2010." Cancer mortality has declined in the State, which may be responsible in part for the overall increase in life expectancy, but the burden of other diseases remains difficult to control. What is the leading cause of mortality in California?

A. Neuropsychiatric diseases
B. Cardiovascular diseases
C. Diabetes
D. HIV infection and AIDS

35. Aggressive diseases associated with community-acquired methicillin-resistant *Staphylococcus aureus* (MRSA) are increasingly a source of concern for public health. This development and others related to antibiotic resistance among pathogens threaten to reverse the gains associated with the discovery of penicillin and other antibiotics less than a century ago. Strategies to reduce the impact of MRSA and similar pathogens involve biological and behavior-change approaches. To combat this scourge, the Centers for Disease Control and Prevention (CDC) developed a Campaign to Prevent Antimicrobial Resistance. The strategies of the campaign include the following, EXCEPT

A. Prescribe antibiotics only against confirmed cases of virus infections
B. Minimize the use of broad-spectrum antibiotics
C. Perform handwashing hygiene regularly
D. Avoid chronic or long-term antibiotic prophylaxis

36. Mary Lasker lobbied strongly for the National Cancer Act of 1971, with the mandate to support basic research and the applications of the results of the basic research to reduce the incidence, mortality, and morbidity from cancer. Since then, billions of dollars have been spent and the burden of certain cancers has declined, whereas others have grown. Prevention and early detection remain the most successful approaches, although controversy persists on the best way to accomplish these goals. The following are known to be preventable, specific cancer risk factors, EXCEPT

A. Exposure to second-hand tobacco smoke
B. Human papillomavirus infection
C. Exposure to ultraviolet radiation
D. Low-fat diet

37. It is estimated that more than 100,000 people in the United States die each year because of air pollution. What are the major criteria air pollutants regulated by the U.S. Environmental Protection Agency (EPA) in the Clean Air Act?

A. CO, NOx, particulate matter, O3, Pb, and SO2
B. CO, NOx, particulate matter, O3, Pb

C. CO, NOx, particulate matter, O3

D. NOx, particulate matter, O3

38. The World Health Organization estimates that approximately 3% of the environmental burden of diseases is attributable to climate change, and the contribution is likely to increase given the trajectory of climate change. The U.S. Environmental Protection Agency also recently ruled that global warming has impacts on public health, clearing the way for the regulation of atmospheric carbon dioxide as a pollutant. The following are recognized effects of climate change on morbidity and mortality, EXCEPT

A. Exacerbation of cardiovascular diseases

B. Exacerbation of pulmonary diseases such as asthma

C. Hyperthermia

D. Exacerbation of diabetes

39. *Escherichia coli* O157:H7 is

A. A brand of food additive that causes cancer, and is being regulated by the FDA

B. A naturally occurring virus found in soils

C. The causative agent of tissue necrosis

D. A bacterial pathogen that contaminates beef

40. Since about 1982, U.S. maternal mortality has reached a plateau at 7 to 8 maternal deaths per 100,000 live births. The formal definition of maternal mortality is

A. Deaths that occur during a pregnancy, and for which the cause of death is listed as a complication of pregnancy, childbirth, or the puerperium

B. Deaths that occur within 150 days of the end of pregnancy, and for which the cause of death is listed as a complication of pregnancy, childbirth, or the puerperium

C. Death of a mother who is still breastfeeding

D. Death of a mother regardless of number or age of children

41. In the United States, the decline in infant mortality rates is unparalleled by any other mortality reduction in the 20th century. Infant mortality is defined in public health as

A. The number of infant deaths (1 year of age or younger) per 1,000 live births

B. The number of infant deaths (5 years of age or younger) per 1,000 live births

C. The number of infant deaths (1 year of age or younger) per 10,000 live births

D. The number of infant deaths (5 years of age or younger) per 10,000 live births

42. A birth defect is an abnormality of structure, function, or metabolism present at birth that results in physical or mental disability. Birth defects can be fatal and are the leading cause of infant mortality in the United States, accounting for more than 20% of all infant deaths. The following are undisputed causes of birth defects, EXCEPT

A. Mercury exposure

B. Alcohol consumption

C. Radiation exposure

D. Maternal age of 30 years or over

43. Amniocentesis is

A. A prescription of amino acids to boost the immune system

B. The analysis of amniotic fluid to determine chromosomal or genetic defects

C. Ammonium therapy for pregnant women who exhibit certain risk factors

D. Amine synthesis in the liver as a result of toxic exposures

44. Which of the following is NOT a common type of food additive?

A. Antioxidants

B. Emulsifiers

C. Dioxin

D. Preservatives

45. Mercury (Hg) poisoning is a global health problem that requires international collaboration to solve because

A. It only affects people in Minamata, and they cannot solve the problem alone.

B. Mercury pollution is widespread globally and people can be exposed to the toxic effects even if they do not live near a hot spot of mercury contamination.

C. Mercury poisoning contributes the largest burden of disease in developing countries.

D. Preventing mercury poisoning requires a large-scale vaccination campaign.

46. The global burden of disease attributed to neuropsychiatric conditions is very high because of the following, EXCEPT

A. The disability weight assigned to neuropsychiatric conditions is heavy.

B. In general, people live with neuropsychiatric conditions for a long period of time before they die.

C. Neuropsychiatric disorders affect mostly people in developing countries.

D. A large number of people suffer from neuropsychiatric illnesses.

47. Antimicrobial resistance is a global health problem for the following reasons, EXCEPT

A. Drug-resistance genes can be transferred across pathogens and cannot be stopped by national boundaries.

B. Humans can acquire drug-resistance infections through international travel.

C. The pace of discovery of new effective drugs is not keeping up with the pace of development of resistance among pathogens.

D. Resistance is found only in hospitals that take international patients through health tourism.

48. Abrupt global climate change is a risk factor for the future of global health because of the potential impacts on which of the following?

A. Increase in human population on the planet

B. Reduced migration of people

C. Increased prevalence of vector-borne diseases

D. Decreased prevalence of noncommunicable diseases

49. The Human Genome Project is

A. A project to determine the nature of genomes and their role in human affairs

B. A scientific effort to determine the genetic superiority of certain ethnic groups

C. A scientific project to determine the sequence of nucleotides in all human chromosomes

D. A scientific project to confirm the number of chromosomes in the human germ cell lines

50. Excess nutrition is a risk factor for the following EXCEPT

A. Obesity

B. Type 2 diabetes

C. Cardiovascular diseases

D. Asthma

51. Iodized salt supplies led to a rapid decline in which of the following?

A. Incidence of goiter

B. Incidence of gout

C. Incidence of heart disease

D. Incidence of irregular gait

52. Medical geology and public health researchers demonstrated that iodine deficiency

A. Occurs especially in areas close to the sea

B. Is unlikely to be seen in mountainous areas

C. Only results from the lack of iodine in drinking water

D. Can result in permanent mental retardation

53. Meat is the best source of addressing the following nutritional deficiencies EXCEPT

A. Iron

B. Vitamin A

C. Zinc

D. Vitamin C

54. Childhood obesity is of concern to public health professionals because

A. Type 2 diabetes, one result of obesity, is now seen in children.

B. Prevalence studies of obesity indicate that it is more prevalent in sub-Saharan Africa than in South America.

C. The prevalence has been increasing in many industrialized countries but not in poor, developing countries.

D. Childhood obesity typically precedes tobacco smoking behavior.

55. Breastfeeding for infants is important because

A. It is not affected by the mother's nutritional status.
B. It transfers immunity against certain infectious diseases.
C. It decreases the mother's chances of getting pregnant.
D. It reduces conflict between the infant and siblings.

56. In 2019, the three leading causes of death in the United States are

A. Heart disease, cancer, and stroke (CBV)
B. Heart disease, stroke (CBV), and Alzheimer's disease
C. Lower respiratory disease, heart disease, and unintentional injuries, especially hip fractures
D. Cancer, heart disease, and diabetes

57. The epidemiologic transition is defined as

A. The elimination of infectious diseases and the decrease in chronic diseases as the major problem in developing countries
B. The continuing problem of infectious diseases plus the rapid decrease in chronic diseases in developing countries
C. The development of epidemiology as a major discipline in developing countries
D. The process by which the pattern of mortality and disease is transformed from one of high mortality among infants and children to one of degenerative and chronic diseases

58. The U.S. President's Emergency Plan for AIDS Relief is touted to be one of the most successful public health intervention projects in the world. The highest incidence of HIV infections globally is occurring in which of the following regions?

A. North and South America
B. The Eastern Mediterranean area
C. South and Southeast Asia
D. Sub-Saharan Africa

59. The major mode of HIV transmission globally is

A. Male-to-male sex
B. Injection drug use
C. Unsafe blood and plasma procedures
D. Male–female sex

60. What does it mean to say that race is a *social construct*?

A. It is based on social group behavior.
B. It is based on genetic determinants.
C. It is defined by a society of molecular biologists.
D. It is perceived.

■ ANSWERS

1. **C.** Medical geology is an Earth science specialty that concerns how geologic materials and Earth processes affect human health. Geologic materials such as rocks, soils, dusts, and volcanic emissions can contain naturally elevated levels of elements, minerals, other compounds, or microbes that harm or benefit human health. They can also contain human-related chemical, mineral, or pathogen contaminants. Medical geologists work with Earth, biological, physical, and health scientists to help improve public health.

   Mercury is not used in any human physiological processes; therefore, there is no "deficiency" of mercury nor any linkage to anemia.

   See: https://www.usgs.gov/news/earthword—medical-geology

2. **D.** Life on Earth depends on a thin layer of ozone in the stratospheric section of the atmosphere, where ozone settles after being formed by the action of ultraviolet (UV) radiation from the sun photolyzing naturally occurring oxygen molecules (O_2) into highly reactive oxygen atoms (O), which then combine with oxygen to create ozone. Ozone at this level blocks UV light from reaching Earth's surface, thereby protecting life from mutation-inducing UVB radiation (important, e.g., in the causation of skin cancer). In the lower tropospheric layer, ozone (within 8 miles of the Earth's surface) is not a natural occurrence, but it is formed by human industrial activities, particularly the burning of fossil fuels to drive automobiles. Breathing too much tropospheric ozone is hazardous to the lungs in part because of the formation of radical oxygen atoms that damage tissue. Tropospheric ozone is subject to wind movement, which is why it is not only harmful to urban centers where it is formed by traffic congestion, but can affect people living further away in rural or suburban locations. Therefore, the correct answer is "D," which is not generally true.

3. **A.** Gases that trap heat in the atmosphere are referred to as "greenhouse" gases because they prevent the natural radiative heat from the Earth from leaving for outer space. Carbon dioxide, methane, nitrous oxides, and fluorinated gases are the most important anthropogenic greenhouse gases. Water vapor is a strong greenhouse gas, but it is formed naturally.

   See: https://www.epa.gov/ghgemissions/overview-greenhouse-gases

4. **B.** Asbestos and lead have been largely phased out of new home building materials in the United States. Internationally, both lead paint and asbestos roofing materials are still used in some countries. Lead solder remains in many drinking water distribution systems in the United States, and has caused poisoning of many populations, for example, in Flint, Michigan. Asbestos fibers can still be found in some drinking water supplies. The EPA's Maximum Contaminant Level for asbestos in drinking water is 7 MFL greater than 10 um in length (million fibers per liter) of drinking water. The Maximum Contaminant Level Goal for Pb in drinking water is zero, and the maximum Contaminant Level with Treatment Technique Action Level is 0.015 mg/L.

   Testing for the presence of lead and asbestos requires special chemical methods, and they cannot be identified with unaided senses.

See: https://www.atsdr.cdc.gov/csem/csem.asp?csem=29&po=8

https://www.atsdr.cdc.gov/csem/csem.asp?csem=34&po=0

5. **A.** The absorption and biological fate of lead once it enters the human body depends on a variety of factors. The blood carries only a small fraction of total lead body burden, and serves as the initial receptacle of absorbed lead, distributing it throughout the body, making it available to other tissues. Absorbed lead that is not excreted is exchanged primarily among three compartments: blood; mineralizing tissues (bones and teeth), which typically contain the vast majority of the lead body burden; and soft tissue (liver, kidneys, lungs, brain, spleen, muscles, and heart). Lead is predominantly stored in the human body in calcified tissues; 90% to 95% of the total lead burden is contained within bone in nonoccupationally exposed adults. The bone in a typical 70-year-old male contains about 200 mg of Pb.

See: https://www.atsdr.cdc.gov/csem/csem.asp?csem=34&po=9

6. **A.** Radon is a naturally occurring radioactive gas that is odorless and tasteless. It is formed from the radioactive decay of uranium. Uranium is found in small amounts in most rocks and soil. It slowly breaks down to other products such as radium, which breaks down to radon. Radon also undergoes radioactive decay. Radon and radon progeny are normally found in surface and groundwater and are expected to be in drinking water from these sources. They are also found in drinking water from wells that contain radon. Radon in water can become airborne especially when the water is used for cooking or showering.

The correct answer is "A"—Well water supply.

See: https://www.atsdr.cdc.gov/substances/toxsubstance.asp?toxid=71

7. **D.** Pesticide toxicity can affect all parts of human physiology. For example, organophosphates such as malathion directly target nervous tissue. Although pesticides can be selectively toxic, many have an impact on desirable organisms (nontargets). Indoor use of pesticides is high in some homes due to insect control, including ants, cockroaches, and spiders. Pesticide toxicity is often linked to disease because of the bioaccumulation in the food chain or bioconcentration in human tissues from repeat exposures.

See: https://www.psr-la.org/files/pesticides_and_human_health.pdf

8. **A.** *E. coli* and enterococci levels are used as indicators of the presence of fecal material in drinking and recreational waters. Both indicate the possible presence of disease-causing bacteria, viruses, and protozoans. Such pathogens may pose health risks to people fishing and swimming in a water body. Sources of bacteria include improperly functioning wastewater treatment plants, leaking septic systems, storm water runoff, animal carcasses, and runoff from animal manure and manure storage areas.

The human intestine contains *E. coli* cells as commensals, and most strains of *E. coli* are not pathogenic.

See: https://www.epa.gov/dwreginfo/total-coliform-rule-tcr-federal
-register-notice

9. **A.** The U.S. Environmental Protection Agency (EPA) as the U.S EPA defines point source pollution as any single identifiable source of pollution from which pollutants are discharged, such as a pipe, ditch, ship, or factory smokestack.

Factories and sewage treatment plants are two common types of point sources. Factories, including oil refineries, pulp and paper mills, and chemical, electronics and automobile manufacturers, typically discharge one or more pollutants in their discharged waters (called effluents). Some factories discharge their effluents directly into a water body. Others treat it themselves before it is released, and still others send their wastes to sewage treatment plants for treatment. Sewage treatment plants treat human wastes and send the treated effluent to a stream or river.

See: https://oceanservice.noaa.gov/education/kits/pollution/03point source.html

https://www.epa.gov/nps/basic-information-about-nonpoint-source -nps-pollution

10. **B.** The United Nations' 2017 landmark Minamata Convention on Mercury was named for Minamata Bay in Japan, where water contamination and fish harvested from the ocean caused extensive human exposure and disfiguring disability outcomes in children born to exposed mothers.

See: http://www.mercuryconvention.org

11. **D.** The Centers for Disease Control and Prevention (CDC) publishes annual summaries of domestic foodborne disease outbreaks based on reports provided by state, local, and territorial health departments. These summaries help public health practitioners better understand the germs, foods, settings, and contributing factors (e.g., food not kept at the right temperature) involved in these outbreaks. They also can help identify emerging foodborne disease threats and can be used to shape and assess outbreak prevention measures. FDOSS is CDC's program for collecting and reporting data about foodborne disease outbreaks in the United States. It is a part of the National Outbreak Reporting System (NORS), which also includes data on illnesses resulting from contact with animals, environmental contamination, spread by person-to-person, waterborne transmission, and other enteric illness outbreaks.

See: https://www.cdc.gov/fdoss/annual-reports/index.html

https://www.cdc.gov/fdoss/faq.html#whycdc

https://www.cdc.gov/foodsafety/outbreaks/index.html

12. **B.** Many light metals, including sodium (as sodium chloride), occur naturally and are essential in human physiology. Heavy metals such as mercury have no use in human physiology, nor anthropogenic industrial pollutants such as polychlorinated biphenyl compounds (PCBs).

13. **A.** Ionizing radiation has sufficient energy to affect the atoms in living cells and thereby damage their genetic material (DNA). Fortunately, the cells in our bodies are extremely efficient at repairing this damage. However, if the damage is not repaired correctly, a cell may die or eventually become cancerous. Exposure to very high levels of radiation, such as being close to an atomic blast, can cause acute health effects such as skin burns and acute radiation syndrome ("radiation sickness"). It can also result in long-term health

effects such as cancer and cardiovascular disease. Exposure to low levels of radiation encountered in the environment does not cause immediate health effects but is a minor contributor to our overall cancer risk.

See: https://www.epa.gov/radiation/radiation-health-effects

14. **A.** The sun's energy reaches Earth in different ways: visible light, infrared radiation that is felt as heat, and rays of ultraviolet (UV) radiation that humans cannot sense directly. The Earth's atmosphere protects living things from most UV radiation. Exposure to sunlight is needed to synthesize vitamin D in humans, but too much UV is mutagenic. There are three types of UV rays

Ultraviolet A rays (UVA): Most UVA radiation reaches Earth's surface. UVA rays cause skin aging and eye damage, and can compromise immune response. UVA rays also contribute to the risk of skin cancer.

Ultraviolet B rays (UVB): The Earth's atmosphere blocks most UVB rays— the amount of UVB rays that reach the Earth's surface depends on latitude, altitude, and season. UVB rays cause sunburns, skin cancer, skin aging, and snow blindness (a sunburn to your cornea that causes a temporary loss of vision) and can compromise immune response.

Ultraviolet C rays (UVC): UVC rays do not reach the Earth's surface because they are completely absorbed by the atmosphere. Harmful effects from UVC rays are minimal.

See: https://www.epa.gov/radtown/ultraviolet-uv-radiation-and-sun
-exposure

https://www.epa.gov/sunsafety/health-effects-uv-radiation

15. **D.** Proper waste management is an essential part of society's public and environmental health. The Resource Conservation and Recovery Act (RCRA), passed in 1976, created the framework for America's hazardous and non-hazardous waste management programs. Materials regulated by RCRA are known as "solid wastes." Only materials that meet the definition of solid waste under RCRA can be classified as hazardous wastes, which are subject to additional regulation. The Environmental Protection Agency (EPA) developed detailed regulations that define what materials qualify as solid wastes and hazardous wastes. Understanding the definition of a solid waste is an important first step in the process EPA set up for generators of hazardous waste to follow when determining if the waste they generated is a regulated hazardous waste.

See: https://www.epa.gov/facts-and-figures-about-materials-waste-and
-recycling

https://www.epa.gov/hw/criteria-definition-solid-waste-and-solid
-and-hazardous-waste-exclusions

16. **B.** Municipal Solid Waste (MSW)—more commonly known as trash or garbage—consists of everyday items we use and then throw away, such as product packaging, grass clippings, furniture, clothing, bottles, food scraps, newspapers, appliances, paint, and batteries. This comes from homes, schools, hospitals, and businesses. Each year the EPA produces a report called *Advancing Sustainable Materials Management: Facts and Figures 2015* (year for which data are available), formerly called *Municipal Solid Waste in the United States:*

Facts and Figures. It includes information on MSW generation, recycling, and disposal.

After 30 years of tracking MSW, the report has been expanded to include additional information on source reduction (waste prevention) of MSW, information on historical landfill tipping fees for MSW, and information on construction and demolition debris generation, which is outside of the scope of MSW. The new name also emphasizes the importance of sustainable materials management (SMM). SMM refers to the use and reuse of materials in the most productive and sustainable ways across their entire life cycle. SMM practices conserve resources, reduce wastes, slow climate change, and minimize the environmental impacts of the materials we use.

In 2015, Americans generated about 262.4 million tons of trash and recycled and composted about 67.8 million tons of this material, equivalent to a 25.8% recycling rate. On average, we recycled and composted 1.51 pounds of our individual waste generation of 4.40 pounds per person per day. EPA encourages practices that reduce the amount of waste needing to be disposed of, such as waste prevention, recycling, and composting. Backyard burning of solid waste produces various compounds toxic to the environment including nitrogen oxides, volatile organic compounds (VOCs), carbon monoxide, and particle pollution.

See: https://www.epa.gov/facts-and-figures-about-materials-waste-and -recycling/national-overview-facts-and-figures-materials#National Picture

https://www.epa.gov/rcra/final-rule-reconsideration-and-final-amen dments-non-hazardous-secondary-materials-are-solid#rule-summary

17. **D.** Light pollution is increasing globally, in both developed and developing countries. Most of the data on the growth of light pollution comes from a handful of weather satellite images and computer modeling using population trends.

Chepesiuk, R. (2009). Missing the dark: Health effects of light pollution. *Environmental Health Perspectives, 117*(1), A20–A27. doi:10.1289/ehp.117-a20. Retrieved from https://www.ncbi.nlm.nih.gov/pmc/articles/PMC2627884/

See: https://www.lightpollutionmap.info/#zoom=4&lat=5759860&lon=161 9364&layers=B0FFFFFTFFFF

https://www.nps.gov/subjects/nightskies/growth.htm

https://www.nps.gov/subjects/nightskies/lightpollution.htm

https://www.washingtonexaminer.com/epa-chief-light-pollution-in -our-portfolio

18. **C.** Variability refers to the inherent heterogeneity or diversity of data in an assessment. It is "a quantitative description of the range or spread of a set of values" and is often expressed through statistical metrics such as variance, standard deviation, and interquartile ranges that reflect the variability of the data. Variability cannot be reduced, but it can be better characterized.

Uncertainty refers to a lack of data or an incomplete understanding of the context of the risk assessment decision. It can be either qualitative or quantitative. Uncertainty can be reduced or eliminated with more or better data.

See: https://www.epa.gov/expobox/uncertainty-and-variability

19. **B.** Biotransformation reactions are categorized not only by the nature of their reactions, for example, oxidation, but also by the normal sequence with which they tend to react with a xenobiotic. They are usually classified as Phase I and Phase II reactions.

Phase I reactions are generally reactions which modify the chemical by adding a functional structure. This allows the substance to "fit" into a second, or Phase II, enzyme, so that it can become conjugated (joined together) with another substance.

Phase II reactions consist of those enzymatic reactions that conjugate the modified xenobiotic with another substance. The conjugated products are larger molecules than the substrate and generally polar in nature (water soluble). Thus, they can be readily excreted from the body. Conjugated compounds also have poor ability to cross cell membranes.

In some cases, the xenobiotic already has a functional group that can be conjugated and the xenobiotic can be biotransformed by a Phase II reaction without going through a Phase I reaction.

For example, phenol can be directly conjugated into a metabolite that can then be excreted. The biotransformation of benzene requires both Phase I and Phase II reactions. Benzene is biotransformed initially to phenol by a Phase I reaction (oxidation). Phenol has a structure including a functional hydroxyl group that is then conjugated by a Phase II reaction (sulfation) to phenyl sulfate.

See: https://toxtutor.nlm.nih.gov/12-002.html

20. **B.** "Environmental diseases are those illnesses for which cause-and-effect can be reasonably associated through epidemiological studies, preferably verified through laboratory experiments. Therefore, the recognition of environmental diseases draws upon two traditional postulates regarding causation in the study of human diseases, one ascribed to Robert Koch (1843–1910) and the other ascribed to Austin Bradford Hill (1897–1991). The more important set of guidelines for environmental diseases is generally known in epidemiology as Hill's criteria of causation, based on his landmark 1965 publication entitled 'The Environment and Disease: Association or Causation?' Hill warned in the article that cause-effect decisions should not be based on a set of rules. Instead, he supported the view that cost-benefit analysis is essential for policy decisions on controlling environmental quality in order to avoid diseases. It is arguable that Hill's treatise initiated current trends characterized by the precautionary principle in environmental health science. Nevertheless, Hill's nine viewpoints for exploring the relationship between environment and disease are worth emphasizing. They are precedence, correlation, dose-response, consistency, plausibility, alternatives, empiricism, specificity, and coherence."

See: https://www.who.int/bulletin/volumes/83/10/792.pdf

Ogunseitan, O. A. (2007). Environmental diseases. In B. C. Auday, M. A. Buratovich, & G. F. Marrocco (Eds.), *Magill's medical guide* (4th rev. ed., p. 827). Pasadena, CA: Salem Press. Retrieved from https://www.salempress.com/Magills-Medical-Guide

21. **A.** Hill's nine viewpoints for exploring the relationship between environment and disease are worth emphasizing. They are precedence, correlation, dose–response, consistency, plausibility, alternatives, empiricism, specificity, and coherence.

Hill, A. B. (1965). The environment and disease: Association or causation? *Proceedings of the Royal Society of Medicine, 58,* 295–300. Retrieved from https://www.ncbi.nlm.nih.gov/pmc/articles/PMC1898525. A classic publication on causality in environmental epidemiology.

22. **C.** Hormesis describes a theoretical phenomenon of dose–response relationships in which something (as a heavy metal or ionizing radiation) that produces harmful biological effects at moderate to high doses may produce beneficial effects at low doses. The physiological mechanisms underpinning hormesis can vary. For example, a single cellular receptor, which interacts with the chemical agent, is responsible for both stimulating and inhibiting the biological response when the chemical is at a low dose and a high dose, respectively. Corticosterone and estradiol, both hormones, have been shown to act via this mechanism; A cellular receptor may respond to low doses of an agent by stimulating a biological response, while a different cellular receptor responds to high doses of an agent by inhibiting a biological response. Histamine, an inflammatory mediator, has been shown to act via this mechanism. Thirdly, a cellular receptor may stimulate a low-dose response, but the cause of the high-dose inhibition is unknown, for example, nitric oxide effects.

Calabrese, E. J. (2013). Hormetic mechanisms. *Critical Reviews in Toxicology, 43*(7), 580–606. doi:10.3109/10408444.2013.808172

23. **D.** On March 24, 1882, Robert Koch announced to the Berlin Physiological Society that he had discovered the cause of tuberculosis. Three weeks later, on April 10, he published an article entitled "The Etiology of Tuberculosis". In 1884, in a second paper with the same title, he first expounded "Koch's Postulates," which have since become basic to studies of all infectious diseases. He had observed the bacillus in association with all cases of the disease, had grown the organism outside the body of the host, and had reproduced the disease in a susceptible host inoculated with a pure culture of the isolated organism.

Koch continued his studies on tuberculosis, hoping to find a cure. In 1890, he announced the discovery of tuberculin, a substance derived from tubercle bacilli, which he thought was capable of arresting bacterial development *in vitro* and in animals. This news gave rise to tremendous hope throughout the world, which was soon replaced by disillusionment when the product turned out to be an ineffective therapeutic agent. Tuberculin later proved to be a valuable diagnostic tool.

In 1905, when Koch was awarded the Nobel Prize in medicine, he devoted his acceptance speech to promoting greater understanding of tuberculosis and its causative agent. Koch died in 1910, leaving the scientific community and the world in general with a valuable inheritance of knowledge and understanding resulting from his seminal work on anthrax, cholera, trypanosomiasis, and especially tuberculosis.

See: https://www.cdc.gov/mmwr/preview/mmwrhtml/00000222.htm

KOCH'S POSTULATES

Three rules for experimental proof of the pathogenicity of an organism were presented in 1883 by the German bacteriologist, Robert Koch. A fourth was appended by E. F. Smith in 1905. Briefly, these rules state

1. The suspected causal organism must be constantly associated with the disease.
2. The suspected causal organism must be isolated from an infected plant and grown in pure culture.
3. When a healthy susceptible host is inoculated with the pathogen from pure culture, symptoms of the original disease must develop.
4. The same pathogen must be reisolated from plants infected under experimental conditions.

These rules of proof are often referred to as "Koch's Postulates."

See: https://www.osti.gov/servlets/purl/924019

24. **B.** Modern research approaches to cultivate microorganisms isolated from natural environments owe much to the pioneering work of Louis Pasteur (1822–1895), who is best known for demonstrating that microorganisms are not spontaneously generated in liquid broth cultures. Pasteur's work also illuminated the current models of microbial nutrition by demonstrating the differences in culture byproducts when yeasts are cultivated under various conditions of aeration. On July 6, 1885, Louis Pasteur and his colleagues injected the first of 14 daily doses of rabbit spinal cord suspensions containing progressively inactivated rabies virus into 9-year-old Joseph Meister, who had been severely bitten by a rabid dog 2 days before. This was the beginning of the modern era of immunization, which had been presaged by Edward Jenner nearly 100 years earlier. Pasteur's decision to treat the child followed 4 years of intensive research, culminating in the development of a vaccine capable of protecting experimentally challenged rabbits and dogs. His decision was difficult: "The child's death appeared inevitable. I decided not without acute and harrowing anxiety, as may be imagined, to apply to Joseph Meister the method which I had found consistently successful with dogs." The immunization was successful; and the Pasteur rabies immunization procedure was rapidly adopted throughout the world. By 1890, there were rabies treatment centers in Budapest, Madras, Algiers, Bandung, Florence, Sao Paulo, Warsaw, Shanghai, Tunis, Chicago, New York, and many other places throughout the world.

See: https://www.cdc.gov/mmwr/preview/mmwrhtml/00000572.htm

Ogunseitan, O. A. (2005). *Microbial diversity* (p. 308). Oxford, England: Blackwell Publishing.

25. **D.** The 2009 H1N1 influenza virus (referred to as "swine flu" early on) was first detected in people in the United States in April 2009. This virus was originally referred to as "swine flu" because laboratory testing showed that its

gene segments were similar to influenza viruses that were most recently identified in and known to circulate among pigs. The Centers for Disease Control and Prevention (CDC) believes that this virus resulted from reassortment, a process through which two or more influenza viruses can swap genetic information by infecting a single human or animal host. When reassortment does occur, the virus that emerges will have some gene segments from each of the infecting parent viruses and may have different characteristics than either of the parental viruses, just as children may exhibit unique characteristics that are like both of their parents. In this case, the reassortment appears most likely to have occurred between influenza viruses circulating in North American pig herds and among Eurasian pig herds. Reassortment of influenza viruses can result in abrupt, major changes in influenza viruses, also known as "antigenic shift." When shift happens, most people have little or no protection against the new influenza virus that results.

See: https://www.cdc.gov/h1n1flu/information_h1n1_virus_qa.htm

There are four types of influenza viruses: A, B, C, and D. Human influenza A and B viruses cause seasonal epidemics of disease almost every winter in the United States. The emergence of a new and very different influenza A virus to infect people can cause an influenza pandemic. Influenza type C infections generally cause a mild respiratory illness and are not thought to cause epidemics. Influenza D viruses primarily affect cattle and are not known to infect or cause illness in people.

Influenza A viruses are divided into subtypes based on two proteins on the surface of the virus: the hemagglutinin (H) and the neuraminidase (N). There are 18 different hemagglutinin subtypes and 11 different neuraminidase subtypes. (H1 through H18 and N1 through N11, respectively.)

Influenza A viruses can be further broken down into different strains. Current subtypes of influenza A viruses found in people are influenza A (H1N1) and influenza A (H3N2) viruses. In the spring of 2009, a new influenza A (H1N1) virus (CDC 2009 H1N1 Flu website) emerged to cause illness in people. This virus was very different from the human influenza A (H1N1) viruses circulating at that time. The new virus caused the first influenza pandemic in more than 40 years. That virus (often called "2009 H1N1") has now replaced the H1N1 virus that was previously circulating in humans.

Influenza B viruses are not divided into subtypes but can be further broken down into lineages and strains. Currently circulating influenza B viruses belong to one of two lineages: B/Yamagata and B/Victoria. The CDC follows an internationally accepted naming convention for influenza viruses. This convention was accepted by WHO in 1979 and published in February 1980 in the Bulletin of the World Health Organization, 58(4): 585–591 (1980; see A Revision of the System of Nomenclature for Influenza Viruses: a WHO Memorandum). The approach uses the following components

- The antigenic type (e.g., A, B, C)
- The host of origin (e.g., swine, equine, chicken, etc. For human-origin viruses, no host of origin designation is given)
- Geographical origin (e.g., Denver, Taiwan, etc.)
- Strain number (e.g., 15, 7, etc.)
- Year of isolation (e.g., 57, 2009, etc.)

- For influenza A viruses, the hemagglutinin and neuraminidase antigen description in parentheses (e.g., [H1N1], [H5N1]

See: https://www.cdc.gov/flu/about/viruses/types.htm

26. **D.** Thimerosal is a mercury-based preservative that has been used for decades in the United States in multidose vials (vials containing more than one dose) of medicines and vaccines. There is no evidence of harm caused by the low doses of thimerosal in vaccines, except for minor reactions like redness and swelling at the injection site. However, in July 1999, the Public Health Service agencies, the American Academy of Pediatrics, and vaccine manufacturers agreed that thimerosal should be reduced or eliminated in vaccines as a precautionary measure.

Research does not show any link between thimerosal in vaccines and autism, a neurodevelopmental disorder. Many well conducted studies have concluded that thimerosal in vaccines does not contribute to the development of autism. Even after thimerosal was removed from almost all childhood vaccines, autism rates continued to increase, which is the opposite of what would be expected if thimerosal caused autism.

See: https://www.cdc.gov/vaccinesafety/concerns/thimerosal/index.html

27. **D.** Today almost everyone is exposed to environmental lead. Exposure to lead and lead chemicals can occur through inhalation, ingestion, dermal absorption, absorption from a retained or embedded leaded foreign body, and transplacental (endogenous) routes. Most human exposure to lead occurs through ingestion or inhalation. In the United States, the public is not as likely to encounter lead that readily enters the human body through the skin (dermal exposure), especially now that leaded gasoline is banned for on-road vehicles, although leaded fuel is still used in aviation, posing threats of exposure to those living near airports. Lead pollution from recycling processes (e.g., lead–acid batteries and electronic waste remain problematic sources), retained shrapnel, bullets, or other embedded leaded foreign bodies can be a source of ongoing lead exposure. Inhalation may be the major contributor for workers in lead-related occupations and "do-it-yourself" home renovators and persons with hobbies (stained glass making/soldering, etc.). Lead exposure is a global issue. Lead mining and lead smelting are common in many countries, where children and adults can receive substantial lead exposure from often unregulated sources at high levels that are uncommon today in the United States. Most countries have discontinued or are in the process of phasing out the use of leaded gasoline for all uses.

See: https://www.atsdr.cdc.gov/csem/csem.asp?csem=34&po=6

Ogunseitan, O. A. (2016). Power failure: The battered legacy of leaded batteries. *Environmental Science & Technology, 50,* 8401–8402. doi:10.1021/acs.est.6b03174

28. **D.** The continuum of signs and symptoms of ongoing lead (Pb) exposure are demarcated by dose.

Lowest exposure dose signs and symptoms

- Impaired cognitive abilities/subclinical neuro/psychoneuro/neurobehavioral findings (patient may appear asymptomatic)
- Decreased learning and memory

- Decreased verbal ability
- Early signs of hyperactivity or ADHD
- Impaired speech and hearing functions
- Lowered IQ

Low exposure dose signs and symptoms

- Irritability
- Lethargy
- Mild fatigue
- Myalgia or paresthesia
- Occasional abdominal discomfort

Moderate exposure dose signs and symptoms

- Arthralgia
- Constipation
- Difficulty concentrating/Muscular exhaustibility
- Diffuse abdominal pain
- General fatigue
- Headache
- Tremor
- Vomiting
- Weight loss

High exposure dose signs and symptoms

- Colic (intermittent, severe abdominal cramps)
- Encephalopathy—may abruptly lead to seizure, change in consciousness, coma, and death
- Paresis or paralysis

See: https://www.atsdr.cdc.gov/csem/csem.asp?csem=34&po=12

29. **C.** The eradication of smallpox from the world in 1977 proved the feasibility of infectious disease eradication. The International Task Force for Disease Eradication (ITFDE) is assessing the potential for global eradication of other infectious diseases. This report summarizes the ITFDE's findings on the potential to eradicate eight diseases based on draft versions of criteria under development. Four factors and conditions enabled the eradication of smallpox: (a) no reservoir of the virus existed except in humans; (b) nearly all persons infected with smallpox had an obvious, characteristic rash and were infectious for a relatively short period; (c) the natural infection conferred lifelong immunity; and (d) a safe, effective (even in newborns), and inexpensive vaccine was available that was also highly stable in tropical environments.

See: https://www.cdc.gov/mmwr/preview/mmwrhtml/00001590.htm

30. **B.** The English aristocrat and writer Lady Mary Wortley Montagu (1689–1762) is today remembered particularly for her letters from Turkey, an early example of a secular work by a Western woman about the Muslim Orient. When Lady Mary was in the Ottoman Empire, she discovered the local practice of variolation, the inoculation against smallpox. Unlike Jenner's later vaccination, which used cowpox, variolation used a small measure of smallpox itself.

Lady Mary, who had suffered from the disease, encouraged her own children to be inoculated while in Turkey. On her return to London, she enthusiastically promoted the procedure, but encountered a great deal of resistance. However, her example certainly popularized the practice of inoculation with smallpox in British high society. The numbers inoculated remained small, and medical effort throughout the 18th century was concentrated on reducing the risks and side-effects of the inoculation process.

Grundy, I. (2001). *Lady Mary Wortley Montagu: Comet of the enlightenment.* Oxford, England: Oxford University Press.

See: http://muslimheritage.com/article/lady-montagu-and-introduction -smallpox-inoculation-england

31. **B.** Malignant mesothelioma is a neoplasm associated with inhalation exposure to asbestos fibers and other elongate mineral particles (EMPs). The median survival after malignant mesothelioma diagnosis is approximately 1 year. The latency period between the first exposure to asbestos fibers or other EMPs and mesothelioma development ranges from 20 to 71 years. Occupational exposure has occurred in industrial operations including mining and milling, manufacturing, shipbuilding and repair, and construction. Current occupational exposure occurs predominantly during maintenance and remediation of asbestos-containing buildings. The projected number of malignant mesothelioma deaths was expected to increase to 3,060 annually by 2001 to 2005; after 2005, mortality was projected to decrease.

See: https://www.cdc.gov/mmwr/volumes/66/wr/mm6608a3.htm

32. **C.** Dichlorodiphenyltrichloroethane (DDT) is an insecticide used in agriculture. The United States banned the use of DDT in 1972, but some countries still use the chemical. DDT has also been used in the past for the treatment of lice. It is still in use outside the United States for the control of mosquitoes that spread malaria. DDT and its related chemicals persist for a long time in the environment and in animal tissues. People are most likely to be exposed to DDT from foods, including meat, fish, and dairy products. DDT can be absorbed by eating, breathing, or touching products contaminated with DDT. In the body, DDT is converted into several breakdown products called metabolites, including the metabolite dichlorodiphenyldichloroethylene (DDE). DDT and DDE are stored in the body's fatty tissues. In pregnant women, DDT and DDE can be passed to the fetus. Both chemicals are found in breast milk, resulting in exposure to nursing infants.

See: https://www.cdc.gov/biomonitoring/DDT_FactSheet.html

33. **B.** There is currently no vaccine available that will prevent HIV infection or treat those who have it. However, scientists are working to develop one. Building on the findings of an earlier study that found for the first time, albeit modestly, that a vaccine could prevent HIV infection in 2016, an NIH-supported clinical trial was launched to test a modified HIV vaccine. This current vaccine trial, called HVTN 702, is testing whether an experimental vaccine regimen safely prevents HIV infection among South African adults.

See: https://www.hiv.gov/hiv-basics/hiv-prevention/potential-future -options/hiv-vaccines

Vaccines protect people from diseases such as chickenpox, influenza (flu), and polio. Vaccines are given by needle injection (a shot), by mouth, or sprayed into the nose. The process of getting a vaccine is called vaccination or immunization.

When a person gets a vaccine, the body responds by mounting an immune response against the particular disease. (An immune response includes all the actions of the immune system to defend the body against the disease.) In this way, the immune system learns to defend the body if the person is later exposed to the disease. Most vaccines are designed so that a person never gets a particular disease or only gets a mild case of the disease.

Vaccines not only protect individuals from disease, they protect communities as well. When most people in a community get immunized against a disease, there is little chance of a disease outbreak.

See: https://aidsinfo.nih.gov/understanding-hiv-aids/fact-sheets/21/57/hiv-and-immunizations

34. **B.** Nearly one in three adults—over eight million Californians—are living with at least one of the most common forms of cardiovascular disease (CVD), which are heart disease, heart failure, stroke, or hypertension (high blood pressure). In California, the burden of CVD mirrors that of the nation. CVD accounts for one in three of all deaths in the state with over 78,000 deaths in 2014. The majority of CVD deaths were from heart disease (24% of all deaths) and stroke (6% of all deaths), making them the second and third leading causes of death, respectively.

The California Department of Public Health has a number of ongoing initiatives and activities to improve cardiovascular health in the state by supporting evidence-based programs that promote health behaviors and healthy communities; they also improved the prevention, diagnosis, and management of chronic disease.

The Chronic Disease Control Branch conducts CVD prevention activities with funding from the Centers for Disease Control and Prevention (CDC) Prevention First, Lifetime of Wellness: Communities in Action, California Preventive Health and Health Services Block Grant, and the California Stroke Registry/-Paul Coverdell Program.

See: https://www.cdph.ca.gov/Programs/CCDPHP/DCDIC/CDCB/Pages/HeartDiseasePrevention.aspx

35. **A.** "REDUCE methicillin-resistant *Staphylococcus aureus* (MRSA)," which stands for Randomized Evaluation of Decolonization versus Universal Clearance to Eliminate MRSA, was designed to find a simple solution to prevent healthcare-associated infections (HAIs). HAIs, including those caused by MRSA, are a leading cause of preventable illness and death. Reducing MRSA is a priority because these bacteria can cause severe disease, are resistant to treatment, and are increasingly common in healthcare settings, particularly among ICU patients.

The REDUCE MRSA study was designed to assess the comparative effectiveness of three principal strategies for the prevention of MRSA in ICUs. The research was conducted in partnership with the Hospital Corporation of America (HCA) and nearly four dozen of its affiliated facilities. The study concept and design was created by experts at the Centers for Disease Control and Prevention (CDC) and the CDC Prevention Epicenter Programs at the University of California, Irvine and Harvard Pilgrim Health Care Institute. The study, published in the *New England Journal of Medicine*, was funded by and conducted through research programs at two U.S. Department of Health and Human Services agencies: the Agency for Healthcare Research and Quality (AHRQ) and the CDC.

Researchers have evaluated the effectiveness of three common MRSA prevention practices

Prevention strategy one: Routine care

This strategy involved screening (testing) patients for MRSA when they were admitted to the ICU. Healthcare providers used gloves and gowns when caring for patients who tested positive for MRSA. Among patients in ICUs that applied this prevention strategy, neither the presence of MRSA nor bloodstream infections were significantly reduced.

Prevention strategy two: Bathing and treating patients who carry MRSA

This strategy involved screening (testing) patients for MRSA upon entering the ICU. Healthcare providers used gloves and gowns when caring for patients who tested positive for MRSA, and these patients were bathed daily with a 2% chlorhexidine (an antiseptic that is safe for the skin)-containing cloth, and had an antibiotic ointment called mupirocin applied twice daily inside their nose (the body site most commonly colonized with *S. aureus*) for 5 days. Among patients in ICUs applying this strategy, bloodstream infections caused by all germs combined were reduced by 23%.

Prevention strategy three: Bathing and treating all ICU patients (universal decolonization)

This strategy involved not testing patients for MRSA when they entered the ICU. Instead, all patients were bathed daily with a 2% chlorhexidine cloth and received mupirocin ointment twice daily inside their nose for 5 days. Gloves and gowns continued to be used when treating patients who tested positive for MRSA. Among patients in these ICUs, the presence of MRSA was reduced 37%, and bloodstream infections caused by all germs were decreased by 44%. Of the three strategies studied, this strategy was found to be the most effective at reducing infections.

See: https://www.cdc.gov/hai/epicenters/reduce_mrsa.html

36. **D.** Cancer prevention is action taken to lower the risk of getting cancer. This can include maintaining a healthy lifestyle, avoiding exposure to known cancer-causing substances, and taking medicines or vaccines that can prevent cancer from developing. Cancer prevention is action taken to lower the chance of getting cancer. In 2019, more than 1.7 million people will be diagnosed with cancer in the United States. In addition to the physical problems and emotional distress caused by cancer, the high costs of care are also a burden to patients, their families, and to the public. By preventing cancer, the number of new cases of cancer is lowered. Hopefully, this will reduce the burden of cancer and lower the number of deaths caused by cancer.

Factors that are known to increase the risk of cancer

- Cigarette smoking and tobacco use
- Infections

- Radiation
- Immunosuppressive medicines after organ transplant

Factors that may affect the risk of cancer

- Diet
- Alcohol
- Physical activity
- Obesity
- Diabetes
- Environmental risk factors

See: https://www.cancer.gov/about-cancer/causes-prevention/patient-prevention-overview-pdq#_199

37. **A.** The Clean Air Act requires the Environmental Protection Agency (EPA) to set National Ambient Air Quality Standards (NAAQS) for six common air pollutants (also known as "criteria air pollutants"). These pollutants are found all over the United States. They can harm human health and the environment, and cause property damage. The Standards were established by the EPA for maximum allowable concentrations of six "criteria" pollutants in outdoor air. The six pollutants are carbon monoxide, lead, ground-level ozone, nitrogen dioxide, particulate matter, and sulfur dioxide. The standards are set at a level that protects public health with an adequate margin of safety.

See: https://www.epa.gov/criteria-air-pollutants

38. **D.** Widespread scientific consensus exists that the world's climate is changing. Some changes that could negatively affect health include more variable weather patterns, heat waves, heavy precipitation events, flooding, droughts, more intense storms, sea level rise, and air pollution. The Centers for Disease Control and Prevention (CDC)'s Climate and Health Program is the national leader in empowering communities to protect human health from a changing climate. While climate change is a global issue, the particular health effects will vary across geographic regions and populations. For this reason, our climate and health program is helping states, cities, territories, and tribes prepare for the specific climate-related health impacts their communities will face.

The CDC program's mission is to

- Lead efforts to identify populations vulnerable to climate change
- Help communities prevent and adapt to the current and anticipated health impacts of climate change
- Ensure effective systems are in place to detect and respond to these health threats

The CDC pursues this mission by building the climate science evidence base, expanding community adaptation capacity, and telling the story of how these efforts are helping communities prepare for and adapt to the health effects of climate change.

See: https://www.cdc.gov/climateandhealth/default.htm

So far (2019) no studies have directly linked climate change to progeria, a genetic disorder.

See: https://www.genome.gov/Genetic-Disorders/Progeria

39. D. *Escherichia coli* (abbreviated as *E. coli*) are bacteria found in the environment, foods, and intestines of people and animals. *E. coli* are a large and diverse group of bacteria. Although most strains of *E. coli* are harmless, others can make you sick. Some kinds of *E. coli* can cause diarrhea, while others cause urinary tract infections, respiratory illness and pneumonia, and other illnesses. To find cases in an outbreak of *Escherichia coli* O157 (*E. coli* O157) infections, public health laboratories perform a kind of "DNA fingerprinting" on *E. coli* O157 laboratory samples. Investigators determine whether the "DNA fingerprint" pattern of *E. coli* O157 bacteria from one person is the same as that from other people in the outbreak and from the contaminated food, water, or infected animal. Bacteria with the same "DNA fingerprint" are likely to come from the same source. Public health officials conduct intensive investigations, including interviews with ill people, to determine if people whose infecting bacteria match by "DNA fingerprinting" are part of a common-source outbreak.

See: https://www.cdc.gov/ecoli/index.html

https://www.cdc.gov/ecoli/reporting-timeline.html

40. A. According to the World Health Organization, maternal death is the death of a woman while pregnant or within 42 days of termination of pregnancy, irrespective of the duration and site of the pregnancy, from any cause related to or aggravated by the pregnancy or its management but not from accidental or incidental causes. To facilitate the identification of maternal deaths in circumstances in which cause of death attribution is inadequate, a new category has been introduced: Pregnancy-related death is defined as the death of a woman while pregnant or within 42 days of termination of pregnancy, irrespective of the cause of death.

See:https://www.who.int/healthinfo/statistics/indmaternalmortality/en

According to the U.S. Centers for Disease Control and Prevention, a pregnancy-related death is defined as the death of a woman while pregnant or within 1 year of the end of a pregnancy—regardless of the outcome, duration, or site of the pregnancy—from any cause related to or aggravated by the pregnancy or its management, but not from accidental or incidental causes.

See: https://www.cdc.gov/reproductivehealth/maternalinfanthealth/pregnancy-mortality-surveillance-system.htm

41. A. Infant mortality is the death of an infant before his or her first birthday. The infant mortality rate is the number of infant deaths for every 1,000 live births. In addition to giving us key information about maternal and infant health, the infant mortality rate is an important marker of the overall health of a society. In 2017, the infant mortality rate in the United States was 5.8 deaths per 1,000 live births. Over 22,000 infants died in the United States in 2017. The five leading causes of infant death in 2017 were

Birth defects

Preterm birth and low birth weight

Maternal pregnancy complications

Sudden infant death syndrome

Injuries (e.g., suffocation)

See: https://www.cdc.gov/reproductivehealth/maternalinfanthealth/infa
ntmortality.htm

42. **D.** About one in every 33 babies is born with a birth defect. Not all birth
defects can be prevented. However, a woman can take steps to increase her
own chance of having a baby with the best health possible. Every 4½ minutes, a baby is born with a birth defect in the United States. That means nearly
120,000 babies are affected by birth defects each year. Birth defects are structural changes present at birth that can affect almost any part or parts of the
body (e.g., heart, brain, foot). They may affect how the body looks, works, or
both. Birth defects can vary from mild to severe. The well-being of each child
affected with a birth defect depends mostly on which organ or body part is
involved and how much it is affected. Depending on the severity of the defect
and what body part is affected, the expected life span of a person with a birth
defect may or may not be affected.

See: https://www.cdc.gov/ncbddd/birthdefects/facts.html

43. **B.** Amniocentesis is a test for fetal health whereby amniotic fluid is collected
from the area surrounding the fetus. The fluid is then tested to measure protein levels, which might indicate certain birth defects. Cells in the amniotic
fluid can be tested for chromosomal disorders, such as Down syndrome,
and genetic problems, such as cystic fibrosis or Tay–Sachs disease. Generally,
an amniocentesis is offered to women who received an abnormal result on
a screening test or to women who might be at higher risk. It is completed
between 15 and 18 weeks of pregnancy. Amniocentesis tests for the following
proteins.

Alpha-fetoprotein (AFP)

- AFP, a protein the unborn baby produces. A high level of AFP in the amniotic fluid might mean that the baby has a defect indicating an opening in
the tissue, such as a neural tube defect (anencephaly or spina bifida), or a
body wall defect, such as omphalocele or gastroschisis.

Acetylcholinesterase (AChE)

- AChE, an enzyme that the unborn baby produces. This enzyme can pass
from the unborn baby to the fluid surrounding the baby if there is an
opening in the neural tube.

See: https://www.cdc.gov/ncbddd/birthdefects/diagnosis.html

44. **C.** Dioxins are mainly by-products of industrial practices. They are produced
through a variety of incineration processes, including improper municipal
waste incineration and burning of trash, and can be released into the air during natural processes, such as forest fires and volcanoes. Almost every living
creature has been exposed to dioxins or dioxin-like compounds (DLCs). Strict
regulatory controls on major industrial sources of dioxin have reduced emissions into the air by 90%, compared to levels in 1987.

Today people are exposed to dioxins primarily by eating food, in particular
animal products, contaminated by these chemicals. Dioxins are absorbed and
stored in fat tissue and, therefore, accumulate in the food chain. More than
90% of human exposure is through food. Before safeguards and regulations

were introduced, dioxin releases were a major problem in the United States. The Polychlorinated Biphenyls (PCBs) worked with the industry to ban products containing dioxin and to curb dioxin emissions. In 1979, the EPA banned the manufacture of products containing PCBs, some of which are included under the term dioxin.

See: https://www.niehs.nih.gov/health/topics/agents/dioxins/index.cfm

45. **B.** The United Nations' Minamata Convention on Mercury is a global treaty to protect human health and the environment from the adverse effects of mercury. It was agreed at the fifth session of the Intergovernmental Negotiating Committee on Mercury in Geneva, Switzerland, at 7 a.m. on the morning of Saturday, January 19, 2013, and adopted later that year on October 10, 2013, at a Diplomatic Conference (Conference of Plenipotentiaries), held in Kumamoto, Japan. The Minamata Convention entered into force on August 16, 2017, on the 90th day after the date of deposit of the 50th instrument of ratification, acceptance, approval, or accession.

The Convention draws attention to a global and ubiquitous metal that, while naturally occurring, has broad uses in everyday objects and is released to the atmosphere, soil, and water from a variety of sources. Controlling the anthropogenic releases of mercury throughout its life cycle has been a key factor in shaping the obligations under the Convention.

Major highlights of the Minamata Convention include a ban on new mercury mines, the phase-out of existing ones, the phase-out and phase-down of mercury use in a number of products and processes, control measures on emissions to air and on releases to land and water, and the regulation of the informal sector of artisanal and small-scale gold mining. The Convention also addresses interim storage of mercury and its disposal once it becomes waste, sites contaminated by mercury, and health issues.

See: http://www.mercuryconvention.org/Convention/Text/tabid/3426/language/en-US/Default.aspx

https://www.atsdr.cdc.gov/toxprofiles/tp.asp?id=115&tid=24

46. **C.** The World Health Organization (WHO) estimates that follow in the provided link represent broad categories of diseases/disorders and the percentage that each category contributes to total global disability adjusted life years (DALYs). Neuropsychiatric disorders are the third leading cause of global DALYs. The neuropsychiatric disorders category includes: Mental and behavioral disorders, which account for 7.4% of total global DALYs; and neurological disorders, which account for 3% of total global DALYs.

See: https://www.nimh.nih.gov/health/statistics/global/global-leading-categories-of-diseases-disorders.shtml

47. **D.** Antimicrobial resistance (AMR) is the ability of a microorganism (like bacteria, viruses, and some parasites) to stop an antimicrobial (such as antibiotics, antivirals, and antimalarials) from working against it. As a result, standard treatments become ineffective, infections persist, and they may spread to others.

- AMR threatens the effective prevention and treatment of an ever-increasing range of infections caused by bacteria, parasites, viruses, and fungi.
- AMR is an increasingly serious threat to global public health that requires action across all government sectors and society.
- Without effective antibiotics, the success of major surgery and cancer chemotherapy would be compromised.
- The cost of healthcare for patients with resistant infections is higher than care for patients with nonresistant infections due to longer duration of illness, additional tests, and use of more expensive drugs.
- In 2016, 490,000 people developed multidrug resistant TB globally, and drug resistance is starting to complicate the fight against HIV and malaria, as well.

See: https://www.who.int/antimicrobial-resistance/en/

https://www.who.int/news-room/fact-sheets/detail/antimicrobial -resistance

48. C. Climate change poses a major, and largely unfamiliar, challenge. The World Health Organization (WHO) is addressing the process of global climate change, its current and future impacts on human health, and how our societies can lessen those adverse impacts, via adaptation strategies and by reducing greenhouse gas emissions.

Change in the world climate would influence the functioning of many ecosystems and their member species. Likewise, there would be impacts on human health. Some of these health impacts would be beneficial. For example, milder winters would reduce the seasonal winter-time peak in deaths that occurs in temperate countries, while in currently hot regions a further increase in temperatures might reduce the viability of disease-transmitting mosquito populations. Overall, however, scientists consider that most of the health impacts of climate change would be adverse.

Climatic changes over recent decades have probably already affected some health outcomes. Indeed, the WHO estimated, in its "World Health Report 2002," that climate change was estimated to be responsible in 2000 for approximately 2.4% of worldwide diarrhea, and 6% of malaria in some middle-income countries. However, small changes, against a noisy background of ongoing changes in other causal factors, are hard to identify. Once spotted, causal attribution is strengthened if there are similar observations in different population settings.

The first detectable changes in human health may well be alterations in the geographic range (latitude and altitude) and seasonality of certain infectious diseases—including vector-borne infections such as malaria and dengue fever, and foodborne infections (e.g., salmonellosis) which peak in the warmer months. Warmer average temperatures combined with increased climatic variability would alter the pattern of exposure to thermal extremes and resultant health impacts, in both summer and winter. By contrast, the public health consequences of the disturbance of natural and managed food-producing ecosystems, rising sea-levels, and population displacement for reasons of physical hazard, land loss, economic disruption, and civil strife may not become evident for up to several decades.

See: https://www.who.int/globalchange/summary/en

49. **C.** The Human Genome Project (HGP) was one of the great feats of exploration in history. Rather than an outward exploration of the planet or the cosmos, the HGP was an inward voyage of discovery led by an international team of researchers looking to sequence and map all of the genes—together known as the genome—of members of our species, *Homo sapiens*. Completed in April 2003, the HGP gave us the ability, for the first time, to read nature's complete genetic blueprint for building a human being.

The main goals of the Human Genome Project were first articulated in 1988 by a special committee of the U.S. National Academy of Sciences, and later adopted through a detailed series of 5-year plans jointly written by the National Institutes of Health (NIH) and the Department of Energy (DOE).

Congress funded both the NIH and the DOE to embark on further exploration of this concept, and the two government agencies formalized an agreement by signing a Memorandum of Understanding to "coordinate research and technical activities related to the human genome."

James Watson was appointed to lead the NIH component, which was dubbed the Office of Human Genome Research. The following year, the Office of Human Genome Research evolved into the National Center for Human Genome Research.

In 1990, the initial planning stage was completed with the publication of a joint research plan, "Understanding Our Genetic Inheritance: The Human Genome Project, The First Five Years, FY 1991 to 1995." This initial research plan set out specific goals for the first 5 years of what was then projected to be a 15-year research effort.

HGP researchers deciphered the human genome in three major ways: determining the order, or "sequence," of all the bases in our genome's DNA; making maps that show the locations of genes for major sections of all our chromosomes; and producing what are called linkage maps, through which inherited traits (such as those for genetic disease) can be tracked over generations.

See: https://www.genome.gov/human-genome-project/What

50. **D.** Americans are eating and drinking too much added sugars, which can lead to health problems such as weight gain and obesity, type 2 diabetes, and heart disease. To live healthier, longer lives, most need to move more and eat better, including getting fewer calories from added sugars. Obesity is a complex health issue to address. Obesity results from a combination of causes and contributing factors, including individual factors such as behavior and genetics. Behaviors can include dietary patterns, physical activity, inactivity, medication use, and other exposures. Additional contributing factors in our society include the food and physical activity environment, education and skills, and food marketing and promotion.

Obesity is a serious concern because it is associated with poorer mental health outcomes, reduced quality of life, and the leading causes of death in the United States and worldwide, including diabetes, heart disease, stroke, and some types of cancer.

See: https://www.cdc.gov/obesity/adult/causes.html

51. **A.** Iodine is essential for healthy brain development in the fetus and young child. Iodine deficiency negatively affects the health of women, as well as economic productivity and quality of life. Most people need an additional source of iodine as it is found in relatively small amounts in the diet. Iodization is the process of fortifying salt for human consumption with iodine and is an effective strategy to increase iodine intake at the population level.

The public health goals of reducing salt and increasing iodine intake through salt iodization are compatible as the concentration of iodine in salt can be adjusted as needed. Monitoring the levels of iodine in salt and the iodine status of the population are critical for ensuring that the population's needs are met and not exceeded.

See: https://www.who.int/elena/titles/salt_iodization/en

52. **D.** Iodine, a trace element found in soil, is an essential component of the thyroid hormones involved in regulating the body's metabolic processes. Iodized salt and seafood are the major dietary sources of iodine. In the United States, salt is iodized with potassium iodide at 100 parts per million (76 milligrams [mg] of iodine per kilogram of salt). Iodized salt is chosen by about 50% to 60% of the U.S. population. Still, most ingested salt comes from processed food (approximately 70%), which is typically not iodized in the United States.

For the thyroid to synthesize thyroid hormones, iodine is essential. Iodine deficiency disorders include mental retardation, hypothyroidism, goiter, cretinism, and varying degrees of other growth and developmental abnormalities. Iodine deficiency is the most preventable cause of mental retardation in the world. Thyroid enlargement (goiter) is usually the earliest clinical feature of iodine deficiency. Thyroid hormone is particularly important in the development of the central nervous system during the fetal and early postnatal periods. In areas where iodized salt is common, iodine deficiency is rare.

The median intake of iodine from food in the United States is approximately 240 to 300 micrograms (mcg) per day for men and 190 to 210 mcg/day for women, largely owing to the iodization of salt. Iodine deficiency develops when iodide intake is less than 20 mcg/day. Most dietary iodine absorbed in the body eventually appears in the urine; thus, urinary iodine excretion is recommended for assessing recent dietary iodine intake worldwide. Excess iodine intake may also result in goiter, as well as in hyper- or hypothyroidism. High iodine intake has also been associated with increased risk for thyroid papillary cancer. For most people, iodine intake from usual foods and supplements is unlikely to exceed the tolerable upper intake level (1,100 mcg/day). The Institute of Medicine recommends iodine intake at 150 mcg per day for nonpregnant adults, 220 mcg per day for pregnant women, and 290 mcg per day during lactation.

See: https://www.cdc.gov/nutritionreport/99-02/pdf/nr_ch4a.pdf

53. **D.** Micronutrients are dietary components, often referred to as vitamins and minerals, which, although only required by the body in small amounts, are vital to development, disease prevention, and well-being. Micronutrients are not produced in the body and must be derived from the diet. Heme iron, which is found only in meat, poultry, and fish, is two to three times more

absorbable than nonheme iron, which is found in plant-based foods and iron-fortified foods. Vitamins A (retinol) and E (tocopherol) and the carotenoids are fat-soluble micronutrients that are found in many foods, including some vegetables, fruits, meats, and animal products. Fish-liver oils, liver, egg yolks, butter, and cream are known for their higher content of vitamin A. Vitamin A found in foods that come from animal sources is called preformed vitamin A.

A wide variety of foods contain zinc. Oysters contain more zinc per serving than any other food, but red meat and poultry provide the majority of zinc in the American diet.

See: https://www.cdc.gov/diabetes/ndep/pdfs/dietary_guidelines_slides .pdf

https://www.cdc.gov/mmwr/preview/mmwrhtml/00051880.htm

https://ods.od.nih.gov/factsheets/Zinc-HealthProfessional

54. **A.** More than 30 million Americans have diabetes (about 1 in 10), and 90% to 95% of them have type 2 diabetes. Type 2 diabetes most often develops in people over age 45, but more and more children, teens, and young adults are also developing it. Insulin is a hormone made by your pancreas that acts like a key to let blood sugar into the cells in your body for use as energy. If you have type 2 diabetes, cells do not respond normally to insulin; this is called insulin resistance. Your pancreas makes more insulin to try to get cells to respond. Eventually your pancreas cannot keep up, and your blood sugar rises, setting the stage for prediabetes and type 2 diabetes. High blood sugar is damaging to the body and can cause other serious health problems, such as heart disease, vision loss, and kidney disease. Type 2 diabetes symptoms often develop over several years and can go on for a long time without being noticed (sometimes there are not any noticeable symptoms at all). Because symptoms can be hard to spot, it is important to know the risk factors for type 2 diabetes and to see your doctor to get your blood sugar tested if you have any of them.

See: https://www.cdc.gov/diabetes/basics/type2.html

55. **B.** Breastfeeding is the best source of nutrition for most infants. It can also reduce the risk for some short- and long-term health conditions for both infants and mothers. Most mothers want to breastfeed but stop early due to a lack of ongoing support. Certain factors make the difference in whether and how long infants are breastfed.

See: https://www.cdc.gov/breastfeeding/index.htm

56. **A.** In 2017, the number of deaths attributable to the leading causes of death in the United States were

- Heart disease: 647,457
- Cancer: 599,108
- Accidents (unintentional injuries): 169,936
- Chronic lower respiratory diseases: 160,201
- Stroke (cerebrovascular diseases): 146,383
- Alzheimer's disease: 121,404
- Diabetes: 83,564

- Influenza and pneumonia: 55,672
- Nephritis, nephrotic syndrome, and nephrosis: 50,633
- Intentional self-harm (suicide): 47,173

See: https://www.cdc.gov/nchs/fastats/leading-causes-of-death.htm

57. D. *"The theory of epidemiologic transition begins with the major premise that mortality is a fundamental factor in population dynamics.* The clearest indication of mortality's dominant role in population dynamics is implicit in theories of population cycles. The cyclic rises and falls in population size that have been observed in animal and pre-modern human populations reflect sequential phases of population growth and decline; disregarding the possible selective influences of migration, these cyclic movements must ultimately be accounted for in terms of the range of variation in fertility and mortality."

Omran, A. R. (2005, December). The epidemiologic transition: A theory of the epidemiology of population change. *Milbank Quarterly, 83*(4), 731–757. doi:10.1111/j.1468-0009.2005.00398.x

58. D. HIV, the virus that causes AIDS, is one of the world's most serious public health challenges. But there is a global commitment to stopping new HIV infections and ensuring that everyone living with HIV has access to HIV treatment. There were approximately 36.9 million people worldwide living with HIV/AIDS in 2017. Of these, 19.6 million people living with HIV (53%) are in eastern and southern Africa, 6.1 million (16%) in western and central Africa, 5.2 million (14%) in Asia and the Pacific, and 2.2 million (6%) in western and central Europe and North America.

See: https://www.hiv.gov/hiv-basics/overview/data-and-trends/global
-statistics

59. D. HIV can be transmitted via the exchange of a variety of body fluids from infected individuals, such as blood, breast milk, semen, and vaginal secretions. Individuals cannot become infected through ordinary day-to-day contact such as kissing, hugging, shaking hands, or sharing personal objects, food, or water. Behaviors and conditions that put individuals at greater risk of contracting HIV include: having unprotected anal or vaginal sex; having another sexually transmitted infection such as syphilis, herpes, chlamydia, gonorrhea, or bacterial vaginosis; sharing contaminated needles, syringes, and other injecting equipment and drug solutions when injecting drugs; receiving unsafe injections, blood transfusions, tissue transplantation, or medical procedures that involve unsterile cutting or piercing; and experiencing accidental needlestick injuries, including among health workers.

See: https://www.who.int/hiv/data/en

60. D. Race is a sociobiologic concept denoting a single breeding population that varies in definable ways from other subpopulations. However, there is no effective operational definition of race among humans. A logical approach to defining racial identity has been derived from advances in molecular biology. Race as a scientific concept ultimately could be tested by determining the proportion of persons who, based on allele frequencies, could be assigned with an acceptable degree of certainty to a genetically defined population subgroup.

In practice, the designation of race is based on socially defined phenotypic traits as seen through the filter of individual and social perspective, while ethnicity is a category determined by genes, culture, and social class, a product of social evolution. An advantage of ethnicity (vs. race) as a concept for public health surveillance is the implicit recognition of social arrangements on health. Ethnicity is the inevitable response of the species to changing opportunities and challenges in the social environment; therefore, ethnicity will change over time.

Ethnicity may be a more appropriate classification than race for public health surveillance, research, and practice for two reasons. First, the potential impact of population differences in gene frequencies is subsumed under the category of ethnicity. Second, since population groups do not exist in a fixed array, the mutability implied by ethnicity represents a strength of this category. Because "the composition of U.S. ethnic groups is changing rapidly, public health surveillance systems must reflect these changes."

See: https://www.cdc.gov/mmwr/PDF/rr/rr4210.pdf. Perspective of a Health Scientist: Use of Race in Public Health Surveillance—Richard Cooper

https://www.scientificamerican.com/article/race-is-a-social-construct -scientists-argue

https://www.nytimes.com/roomfordebate/2015/06/16/how-fluid-is -racial-identity/race-and-racial-identity-are-social-constructs

6 Collaboration and Partnerships

◼ INTRODUCTION

At the 65th World Health Assembly held in Geneva, Switzerland, in May 2012, member states of the World Health Organization adopted the "Rio Political Declaration on Social Determinants of Health" through resolution WHA65.8.[1] The Social Determinants of Health (SDH) conceptual framework expands the scope of public health practice by recognizing that the root causes of population health status and disparities are located in sectors that have not been traditionally included in public health research and translational science. Thus, housing, transportation, employment, and political representation all have strong influences on the capacity of the public health sector to improve the health of populations. The solution is not to retrain public health professionals as experts in other disciplines that determine these root causes, but to enable public health professionals to gain competencies in how to collaborate and form partnerships with other sectors and with community stakeholders to advance the agenda of population health improvement. Competent public health professionals must acquire the skills needed to identify community stakeholders, health professionals, and governmental agencies and to develop partnerships with these organizations to address the needs of individuals and populations. Public health professionals must also be able to establish the roles, responsibilities, and action steps to manage these partnerships for shared accountability and effective performance.

The questions in this section focus on key components of public health collaboration and partnerships that are essential for effective programs. These components include opportunities to

- Identify opportunities to partner with health and public health professionals across sectors and related disciplines
- Identify key stakeholders

---

1 World Conference on Social Determinants of Health—https://www.who.int/sdhconference/background/en/.

- Develop collaborative and partnership agreements with various stakeholders on specific projects
- Establish roles, responsibilities, and action steps of key stakeholders in order to meet project goals and objectives
- Engage key stakeholders in problem-solving and policy development
- Access the knowledge, skills, and abilities of health professionals to ensure that policies, programs, and resources improve the public's health
- Use knowledge of the role of public health and the roles of other health professions to appropriately address the health needs of individuals and populations
- Manage partnerships with agencies within the national, state, or local levels of government that have authority over public health situations or with specific issues, such as emergency events
- Apply relationship-building values and principles of team dynamics to plan strategies and deliver population health services
- Develop procedures for managing health partnerships
- Implement methods of shared accountability and performance measurement with multiple organizations
- Implement strategies for collaboration and partnership among diverse organizations to achieve common public health goals
- Develop strategies for collaboration and partnership among diverse organizations to achieve common public health goals
- Identify critical stakeholders for the planning, implementation, and evaluation of health programs, policies, and interventions
- Engage community partners in actions that promote a healthy environment and healthy behaviors

▪ QUESTIONS

1. The World Health Organization (WHO) has the authority to declare "pandemics" to initiate a specific course of actions to control infectious diseases. The declaration considers several factors, including the coordination of infection rates reported from WHO Regional Offices. Which of the following is NOT a WHO Regional Office?
   - A. Region of the Americas, based in Washington, DC
   - B. Asia Region, based in Beijing
   - C. Africa Region, based in Brazzaville
   - D. Eastern Mediterranean Region, based in Cairo

2. Public announcement of putative geographical "origins" of epidemics often have negative impacts on populations and cultures, including social stigma and economic boycotts. For example, the "origin" of HIV in Africa, "origin" of the 2009 H1N1 in Mexico, and "origin" of mad cow disease in England. The integration of "diversity and culture," defined as the ability to interact with both diverse individuals and communities to produce or impact an intended public health outcome, is essential in professional practice. Which among the following is NOT included in the cultural competence of public health professionals?

   A. Explain why cultural competence alone cannot address health disparity
   B. Use the basic concepts and skills involved in culturally appropriate community engagement and empowerment with diverse communities
   C. Cite examples of situations where consideration of culture-specific needs resulted in a less effective health intervention
   D. Apply the principles of community-based participatory research to improve health in diverse populations

3. The National Health and Nutrition Examination Survey (NHANES) is a program of studies designed to assess the health and nutritional status of adults and children in the United States. The survey is unique in that it combines interviews and physical examinations. The following are among the major uses of NHANES data, EXCEPT

   A. Determination of the prevalence of major diseases and risk factors for diseases
   B. Assessment of nutritional status and its association with health promotion and disease prevention
   C. The basis for national standards for such measurements as height, weight, and blood pressure
   D. Epidemiological studies and health sciences research, which help develop sound public health policy between the years 1859 and 1961

4. The mission of the Centers for Disease Control and Prevention (CDC) is to collaborate to create the expertise, information, and tools that people and communities need to protect their health—through health promotion; prevention of disease, injury, and disability; and preparedness for new health threats. The CDC's expertise and resources support both domestic and internal challenges in public health. Under what agency is the CDC's programs organized?

   A. The World Health Organization
   B. The U.S. National Institutes of Health
   C. The U.S. Department of Health and Human Services
   D. The U.S. Department of Homeland Security

5. On November 4, 2016, President Barack Obama issued an Executive Order entitled "Advancing the Global Health Security Agenda to Achieve a World Safe and Secure From Infectious Disease Threats." The Order is a "multi-faceted, multi-country initiative intended to accelerate partner countries' measurable capabilities to achieve specific targets to prevent, detect, and respond to infectious disease threats (GHSA targets), whether naturally occurring, deliberate,

or accidental." The president specified that the roles, responsibilities, and activities described in the order will support the goals of the International Health Regulations (IHR) and will be conducted, as appropriate, in coordination with the following international organizations, EXCEPT:

A. The World Health Organization (WHO)
B. The Food and Agriculture Organization of the United Nations (FAO)
C. The World Organization for Animal Health (OIE)
D. The United Nations Education, Social, and Cultural Organization

6. According to the U.S. Centers for Disease Control and Prevention, the following are reasons why global health security matters EXCEPT

A. Disease threats can spread faster and more unpredictably than ever before.
B. Global health security provides protection from chronic disease threats.
C. Global health is economically smart.
D. The Global Health Security Agenda is effective as a unilateral strategy.

7. Under the Global Health Security Agenda, the Joint External Evaluation (JEE) is a voluntary, collaborative process to assess a country's capacity under the International Health Regulations to prevent, detect, and rapidly respond to public health threats whether occurring naturally or due to deliberate or accidental events. Of the 19 capacities and 48 indicators included in the United States' JEE, the following capacities score a perfect 5, EXCEPT

A. National legislation, policy, and financing
B. Linking public health and security authorities
C. Immunizations
D. Antimicrobial resistance

8. The International Health Regulations were established in 2005, and entered into force in 2007 as a legally binding instrument of international law to (a) assist countries to work together to save lives and livelihoods endangered by the international spread of diseases and other health risks, and (b) avoid unnecessary interference with international trade and travel. Member states of the World Health Organization (WHO) are required to assess all reports of urgent events within their territories within 48 hours, and to notify WHO within 24 hours after identifying a notifiable event according to decision criteria that include the following, EXCEPT

A. The seriousness of the health impact
B. The risk of international disease spread
C. The risk that travel or trade restrictions will be imposed by other countries
D. The magnitude of potential economic loss to the country

9. The "tasks to be done" are determined by which core public health function?

A. Assessment
B. Surveillance
C. Advocacy
D. Policy development

10. Which of the following activities is NOT within the scope of conventional public health practice?

    A. Promoting healthy behaviors
    B. Preparing against environmental hazards
    C. Providing comprehensive patient care
    D. Using vaccination campaigns as a cover for entrapment in international affairs

11. Public health policy development includes

    A. Conducting inspection of a restaurant
    B. Collecting data on a measles outbreak
    C. Developing goals and measurable objectives for the public health workforce
    D. Providing community health needs assessments

12. Public health regulatory functions include the following EXCEPT

    A. Sanitary codes
    B. Clean air standards
    C. Animal control
    D. Tax code reform

13. What question does NOT describe the core function of assurance?

    A. What should be done based on monitoring?
    B. What is the reason for the importance of the public health problem rationale?
    C. What will be done based on individual preferences and priorities?
    D. What is the best means to get priorities accomplished?

14. The essential services of public health assurance do NOT include which of the following?

    A. Enforce laws and regulations that protect health and ensure safety
    B. Link people to needed personal health services and assure the provision of healthcare when otherwise unavailable
    C. Assure a competent public health and personal healthcare workforce
    D. Develop policies and plans that support individual and community environmental public health efforts

15. The essential services of public health policy development include all of the following EXCEPT

    A. Inform, educate, and empower people about public health issues
    B. Mobilize community partnerships and actions to identify and solve public health problems
    C. Develop policies and plans that support individual and community environmental public health efforts
    D. Defer enforcement of laws and regulations that protect health and ensure safety to the military/police

16. The "Community-Campus Partnerships for Health," which identified elements for authentic partnerships, included all the following EXCEPT

    A. Guiding principles of partnerships
    B. Transformative experiences
    C. Quality processes
    D. Professor–student relationships

17. The definition of a stakeholder is

    A. An individual, a group of people, or an organization that can affect or be affected positively or negatively by a project
    B. The persons who hold the grounded stakes for marking the geographic limits of a territory
    C. The majority stockholder of a traded enterprise
    D. The minority stockholder of a traded enterprise

18. It is important to identify the right stakeholders for public health projects in order to

    A. Improve the quality of the project, as stakeholders can give vital information and make sure nothing important is missed
    B. Avoid delays by manipulating stakeholders to avoid obstacles to getting approval for the project
    C. Secure financial commitments from wealth stakeholders for projects that may be controversial in the community
    D. Secure authoritative clout from politician stakeholders for projects that may be controversial in the community

19. It is important to categorize stakeholders in order to ensure that the level of engagement is commensurate with the level of interest or influence of each stakeholder. The following are recommended categories of stakeholders, EXCEPT

    A. High Power/High Interest (Fully engage)
    B. High Power/Low Interest (Keep satisfied)
    C. Low Power/High Interest (Keep informed)
    D. Low Power/No Interest (Fully engage)

20. Stakeholder mapping is a collaborative process used to develop the structure and function of engagement with each stakeholder. The phases of stakeholder mapping include the following EXCEPT

    A. Identifying the most important stakeholders
    B. Analyzing stakeholder perspective and interests
    C. Mapping the relationship of stakeholder to specific objectives
    D. Prioritizing and ranking stakeholder relevance to objectives

21. When stakeholders are satisfied, they may exhibit which of the following behaviors?

    A. Demonstrate loyalty to the agency
    B. Leave the agency

C. Seek to change things in the agency
D. Ask for more financial support

22. What should public health agencies do with stakeholders who have high interest and high power?

A. Keep satisfied
B. Keep informed
C. Invest maximum effort
D. Invest minimal effort

23. What should public health agencies do with stakeholders who have high interest and low power?

A. Invest minimal effort
B. Keep informed
C. Invest maximum effort
D. Keep satisfied

24. In the "Power-Legitimacy-Urgency" model of stakeholder engagement, dormant stakeholders possess which of the following attributes?

A. Legitimacy
B. Power
C. Urgency
D. Integrity

25. In the "Power-Legitimacy-Urgency" model of stakeholder engagement, discretionary stakeholders possess which of the following attributes?

A. Legitimacy
B. Power
C. Urgency
D. Integrity

26. In the "Power-Legitimacy-Urgency" model of stakeholder engagement, demanding stakeholders possess which of the following attributes?

A. Legitimacy
B. Power
C. Urgency
D. Integrity

27. In the "Power-Legitimacy-Urgency" model of stakeholder engagement, dependent stakeholders possess which of the following attributes?

A. Legitimacy and urgency
B. Power and integrity
C. Urgency and power
D. Integrity and urgency

28. In the "Power-Legitimacy-Urgency" model of stakeholder engagement, definite stakeholders possess which of the following attributes?

    A. Legitimacy, power, and urgency
    B. Power, legitimacy, and integrity
    C. Urgency, power, and integrity
    D. Power, legitimacy, and intimacy

29. In the "Power-Legitimacy-Urgency" model of stakeholder engagement, dangerous stakeholders possess which of the following attributes?

    A. Legitimacy and power
    B. Power and urgency
    C. Urgency and legitimacy
    D. Integrity and Power

30. In the "Power-Legitimacy-Urgency" model of stakeholder engagement, dominant stakeholders possess which of the following attributes?

    A. Legitimacy and power
    B. Power and integrity
    C. Urgency and power
    D. Integrity and intimacy

31. Qualitative and quantitative strategies for identifying potential stakeholders in a public health program include

    A. Focus groups
    B. Population survey
    C. Workshops
    D. Telemarketing

32. Government-sponsored public health agencies sometimes have to collaborate with nongovernmental organizations to work in underserved communities. Review the following sentence: "The objective of improving the access of refugees to primary healthcare will be achieved through increased funding of NGO outreach activities." This sentence refers to an example of

    A. An official policy
    B. A contingency plan
    C. A strategy
    D. A benchmark

33. In an emergency, public health professionals must typically collaborate with other societal sectors, including law enforcement, urban planning, clinicians, and so on. Which of the following is the least likely feature of an emergency?

    A. Increased mortality
    B. High levels of violence against civilians
    C. High food insecurity
    D. High number of battle-deaths

34. In a public health emergency, collaborations and partnerships usually require rapid exchange of information across sectors. Which of the following is the least important issue to consider in a crisis health information exchange?

    A. Timeliness
    B. Precision
    C. Accuracy
    D. Validity

35. The donation of medication or vaccines is commonplace in public health crisis contexts, and existing collaboration and partnerships may facilitate quick deployment of such donations. Which one of the following statements MOST accurately describes disrupted health sectors?

    A. Such medicine donations are a vital component of an emergency response and should be encouraged.
    B. Without adequate controls, the negative effects of medicine donations are likely to offset their benefits.
    C. No major effort should be devoted to regulating medicine donations, because their weight is usually marginal.
    D. Recent research has highlighted the positive effects of medicine donations on healthcare provision in crisis-affected health sectors. Thus, international agencies are actively trying to promote them.

36. Which of the following processes characterizes the level of disease prevention known as tertiary prevention?

    A. Prevention of disease before its biological onset
    B. Prevention of disease progression and additional disease complications after overt clinical disease occurs
    C. Prevention of clinical illness through the early and asymptomatic detection and remediation of certain disease conditions
    D. Prevention of illness through appropriate individual and group behavior modification designed to minimize infection risk

37. Collaboration of public health agencies and school districts is important in preventing drug abuse among students. Which of the following instructional approaches is likely to be most effective in minimizing and preventing drug use, including use of alcohol and tobacco, among students?

    A. Familiarizing students with effective decision-making, resistance, and refusal techniques and engaging them in activities in which they practice using the techniques
    B. Emphasizing the connections between a drug-free lifestyle and academic success and showing students research studies and data that support these findings
    C. Referring students to a variety of digital and social media resources that promote alcohol, tobacco, and drug prevention strategies designed specifically for young people
    D. Having students study the mechanisms by which alcohol, tobacco, and drugs affect major body systems and discuss their short- and long-term health effects

38. In a meeting of public health stakeholders, pairs practice conflict-management and resolution skills. Stakeholder partners brainstorm a hypothetical interpersonal conflict situation and then practice the key steps used in conflict resolution models. Which of the following steps is typically carried out first in a conflict management and resolution process?

A. Taking turns explaining the factors that led to conflict.
B. Listening to a third party's advice about how to best resolve the situation.
C. Taking the time to calm down and think about the situation.
D. Brainstorming various solutions to the conflict until one is mutually agreed upon.

39. In promoting health behavior, public health professionals typically need to collaborate with other trusted sectors that engage the public. Which of the following sources of health-related information is MOST likely to present unbiased, accurate facts?

A. An article in a popular health magazine promoting a new drug that the author asserts will control weight without dieting
B. A peer-reviewed article in a professional medical journal announcing the development of a new treatment for skin cancer
C. A pharmaceutical company brochure promoting a new drug that reportedly alleviates all major symptoms of osteoarthritis
D. A dental office flyer provided by a toothbrush manufacturer praising the toothbrush's effectiveness against gum disease

40. Which of the following is NOT a key characteristic of not-for-profit public health organizations?

A. Multiple stakeholders
B. Economic profit orientation
C. Multiple objectives
D. Transparency

41. The model typically used to analyze and categorize stakeholders for public health agencies is based on the level of interest and on which of the following?

A. The level of threat
B. The number of trustees
C. The level of power
D. The level of activities

42. In 2019, the measles outbreak in the United States is an example of how public health agencies form partnerships with other government branches, for example, the legislature to promote vaccination. It is also an example of how some pressure groups campaign to resist change (e.g., the anti-vaccination coalition). Which of the following is important in pressure group campaigning?

A. Publicity
B. Fundraising activity
C. Philanthropist
D. Market segmentation

43. The practice of a public health agency contracting with external partners to handle specific functions on a permanent basis is referred to as

    A. Contract administration
    B. Payroll and benefits administration
    C. Hiring temporary employees
    D. Outsourcing

44. The Community Coalition Action Theory describes progressive stages of community engagement as

    A. Solicitation, recruitment, verification
    B. Solicitation, recruitment, retention
    C. Formation, maintenance, institutionalization
    D. Formation, engagement, investments

45. The Community Empowerment Model consists of the following dimensions.

    A. Power brokering, power deployment, power accountability
    B. Power structuring, power brokering, power deployment
    C. Powerful persons, powerful groups, powerful communities
    D. Person or group, environmental, empowerment capacity and outcome

46. The Framework for Collaborative Empowerment includes the following dimensions.

    A. Community planning, community action, community change
    B. Community profiling, community assessment, community empowerment
    C. Community profiling, community assessment, community engagement
    D. Community planning, community assessment, community empowerment

47. The Collective Impact Framework includes the following conditions.

    A. Common agenda, cost-benefit analysis, critical review
    B. Collective assessments, collective benefits, collective impacts
    C. Collective framework, collective social work, collective impact
    D. Common agenda, shared metrics, continuous communication

48. The Planned Approach to Community Health (PATCH) Model guides users through the following phases EXCEPT

    A. Mobilizing the community
    B. Collecting and organizing data
    C. Choosing health priorities
    D. Enforcing health disparities

49. The Mobilizing for Action through Planning and Partnership (MAPP) Model was developed by the

    A. Association of Schools and Programs of Public Health (ASPPH)
    B. American Public Health Association (APHA)
    C. National Association of County and City Health Officials (NACCHO)
    D. American Medical Association (AMA)

50. The Mobilizing for Action through Planning and Partnership (MAPP) Model is organized around the following themes EXCEPT

    A. Community themes and strength assessment
    B. Local public health system assessment
    C. Community health and status assessment
    D. Litigating public health violations

51. The Asset-Based Community Development (ABCD) Model recognizes the following assets EXCEPT

    A. Individuals
    B. Institutions
    C. Physical assets
    D. Fluency in English

52. During 2014 to 2017, the U.S. Centers for Disease Control and Prevention supported "Partnerships to Improve Community Health (PICH)" for which of the following purposes?

    A. To address the leading risk factors for the major causes of death and disability in the United States: tobacco use, poor nutrition, and physical inactivity
    B. To address the leading risk factors for the major causes of death and disability in the United States: traffic accidents, poor nutrition, and physical inactivity
    C. To address the leading risk factors for the major causes of death and disability in the United States: opioid addiction, poor nutrition, and physical inactivity
    D. To address the leading risk factors for the major causes of death and disability in the United States: tobacco use, suicides, and physical inactivity

53. Collaborations and partnerships are important to reduce disparities in public health. The U.S. Centers for Disease Control and Prevention's program "Racial and Ethnic Approaches to Community Health (REACH)" aims to reduce health disparities among racial and ethnic populations with the highest burden of which of the following chronic diseases?

    A. Hypertension
    B. Tuberculosis
    C. Hepatitis
    D. Valley fever

54. The following are examples of partnerships used by public health agencies EXCEPT

    A. Advisory boards or committees
    B. Task force
    C. Coalition
    D. Indentureship

55. A county's public health program to build community capacity should include the following, EXCEPT

A. Organization of community assets and resources
B. Assessment of how many patients the community clinic can keep hospitalized
C. Establishing partnerships to support decision-making
D. Identifying root causes of health problems

56. Achieving the goals set for "Healthy People 2020" requires collaborations and partnerships, particularly to address high-risk populations. One of the main goals of Healthy People 2020 is

A. To provide better insurance programs
B. To have collaboration among governmental agencies
C. To provide access to preventive healthcare services
D. To improve assessment of services

57. Through collaboration with a university's school of public health, a public health professional educates a class that the Predisposing, Reinforcing and Enabling factors, and Causes in Educational Diagnosis and Evaluation (PRECEDE) component of the PRECEDE-PROCEED begins with

A. An examination of administrative and organizational issues
B. A comprehensive community assessment
C. Preventative programs
D. The implementation of behavior change

58. Imagine that you are a public health professional using the Mobilizing for Action through Planning and Partnership (MAPP) model to conduct an assessment within the community and you have reached the third phase, the four assessments. You understand that analysis of the legislation, technology, and other external influences that have an impact on the promotion and protection of the public's health is called a

A. Community themes and strengths assessment
B. Forces of change assessment
C. Community health status assessment
D. Local Public Health System Assessment (LPHSA)

59. Public health professionals can help avoid cross-cultural misunderstandings during partnership meetings by

A. Cultivating cultural understanding of fellow members
B. Maintaining a professional appearance at all times
C. Interacting with others influenced by their own cultural beliefs
D. Not engaging directly with participants with whom they feel uncomfortable

60. Cultivating which of the following partnership environments will support increased knowledge and respect for public health team members for each other?

   A. Collaborative and aggressive
   B. Collaborative and passive
   C. Collaborative and reactive
   D. Collaborative and participative

61. Preserving long-term collaborations and partnerships in public health requires the following, EXCEPT

   A. Understanding the mission and strategic priorities
   B. Limiting transparency in communicating information
   C. Reaching out to stakeholders at the program onset
   D. Keeping an open communication flow exchange

■ ANSWERS

1. **B.** The Asia region based in Beijing is not a regional office of the World Health Organization (WHO). The regional offices are

- Africa; HQ: Brazzaville, Republic of Congo
- Western Pacific; HQ: Manila, Philippines
- Eastern Mediterranean; HQ: Cairo, Egypt
- South East Asia; HQ: New Delhi, India
- Europe; HQ: Copenhagen, Denmark
- Americas; HQ: Washington D.C., USA

See: https://www.who.int/about/who-we-are/regional-offices

2. **C.** Culture is defined by group membership, such as racial, ethnic, linguistic, or geographical groups, or as a collection of beliefs, values, customs, ways of thinking, communicating, and behaving specific to a group. Culture-specific needs evidently result in more effective, rather than less effective, public health interventions. "Cultural competence is an essential element of quality healthcare and can help improve health outcomes, increase clinic efficiency, and produce greater patient satisfaction."

See: https://www.cdc.gov/healthliteracy/culture.html

https://www.cdc.gov/tb/publications/guidestoolkits/ethnographic guides/SomaliTBBooklet.pdf

https://www.cdc.gov/tb/publications/guidestoolkits/ethnographic guides/china.pdf

3. **D.** The National Health and Nutrition Examination Survey (NHANES) did not exist before 1961. The NHANES is a program of studies designed to assess the health and nutritional status of adults and children in the United States. The survey is unique in that it combines interviews and physical examinations.

See: https://www.cdc.gov/nchs/nhanes/index.htm

4. **C.** The Centers for Disease Control and Prevention (CDC) is an operating division unit under the U.S. Department of Health and Human Services.

See: https://www.hhs.gov/about/agencies/orgchart/index.html

5. **D.** The United Nations Educational, Scientific and Cultural Organization (UNESCO) is not included in the Global Health Security Agenda (GHSA).

The GHSA was launched in February 2014 and is a growing partnership of over 64 nations, international organizations, and nongovernmental stakeholders to help build countries' capacity to help create a world safe and secure from infectious disease threats and elevate global health security as a national and global priority. GHSA pursues a multilateral and multisectoral approach to strengthen both the global capacity and nations' capacity to prevent, detect, and respond to human and animal infectious disease threats, whether naturally occurring or accidentally or deliberately spread.

UNESCO seeks to build peace through international cooperation in education, the sciences, and culture. UNESCO's programs contribute to the achievement of the Sustainable Development Goals defined in Agenda 2030, adopted by the UN General Assembly in 2015.

See: https://obamawhitehouse.archives.gov/the-press-office/2016/11/04/
executive-order-advancing-global-health-security-agenda-achieve
-world

https://www.ghsagenda.org

https://en.unesco.org

6. **D.** Global health security is most effective as a MULTILATERAL strategy.

More than 70% of the world remains underprepared to prevent, detect, and respond to a public health emergency. Through the Global Health Security Agenda (GHSA), the Centers for Disease Control and Prevention (CDC) works with countries to strengthen public health systems and contain outbreaks at the source, before they spread into regional epidemics or global pandemics. Public health threats, health emergencies, and infectious diseases do not recognize or respect boundaries. Effective and functional public health systems in all countries reduce the risk and opportunity for health threats to affect the United States.

See: https://www.cdc.gov/globalhealth/healthprotection/ghs/index.html

7. **D.** Bacteria and other microbial species evolve in response to their environment and inevitably develop mechanisms to resist being killed by antimicrobial agents. For many decades, the problem was manageable as the growth of resistance was slow and the pharmaceutical industry continued to create new antibiotics. Over the past decade, however, this problem has become a crisis. The evolution of antimicrobial resistance (AMR) is occurring at an alarming rate and is outpacing the development of new countermeasures capable of thwarting infections in humans. This situation threatens patient care, economic growth, public health, agriculture, economic security, and national security.

See: https://www.ghsagenda.org/docs/default-source/jee-reports/united
-states-jee-report.pdf

8. **D.** The magnitude of potential economic loss to the country is not included as a consideration in decision criteria. Under the International Health Regulations, states' parties are required to carry out an assessment of public health events arising in their territories utilizing the decision instrument contained in Annex 2 of the Regulations, and then to notify the World Health Organization (WHO) of all qualifying events within 24 hours of such an assessment. The purpose of the WHO guidance on Annex 2 is to help national authorities to use the decision instrument in assessing public health events that may require notification to WHO.

See: https://www.who.int/ihr/revised_annex2_guidance.pdf?ua=1

9. **D.** Policy development includes

- Inform, educate, and empower people about environmental health issues
- Mobilize community partnerships and actions to identify and solve environmental health problems

- Develop policies and plans that support individual and community environmental health efforts

See: https://www.cdc.gov/nceh/ehs/ephli/core_ess.htm

https://www.cdc.gov/publichealthgateway/publichealthservices/essentialhealthservices.html

10. **D.** It is never a good idea to use deception in vaccination campaigns. Some experts believe that this practice has complicated the eradication of polio in Pakistan because the U.S. agencies used a vaccination campaign as a cover for entrapment of wanted individuals.

See: https://news.nationalgeographic.com/2015/02/150225-polio-pakistan-vaccination-virus-health/

https://www.milbank.org/quarterly/articles/global-polio-eradication-espionage-disinformation-and-the-politics-of-vaccination/

11. **C.** The policy development core function of public health includes developing goals and measurable objectives for the public health workforce.

Inform, educate, and empower people about environmental health issues

Mobilize community partnerships and actions to identify and solve environmental health problems

Develop policies and plans that support individual and community environmental health efforts

See: https://www.cdc.gov/nceh/ehs/ephli/core_ess.htm

12. **D.** Tax code reform is not included in public health regulatory functions. Assurance function includes

Enforce laws and regulations that protect environmental health and ensure safety

Link people to needed environmental health services and assure the provision of environmental health services when otherwise unavailable

Assure a competent environmental health workforce

Evaluate the effectiveness, accessibility, and quality of personal and population-based environmental health services

Research for new insights and innovative solutions to environmental health problems

See: https://www.cdc.gov/nceh/ehs/ephli/core_ess.htm

13. **C.** Individual preferences and priorities are relevant but not the focus of public health, which emphasizes populations. Assurance function includes

Enforce laws and regulations that protect environmental health and ensure safety

Link people to needed environmental health services and assure the provision of environmental health services when otherwise unavailable

Assure a competent environmental health workforce

Evaluate the effectiveness, accessibility, and quality of personal and population-based environmental health services

Research for new insights and innovative solutions to environmental health problems

See: https://www.cdc.gov/nceh/ehs/ephli/core_ess.htm

14. **D.** Developing policies and plans that support individual and community environmental public health efforts is not included in assurance.

The essential services of the public health assurance function include

Enforce laws and regulations that protect environmental health and ensure safety

Link people to needed environmental health services and assure the provision of environmental health services when otherwise unavailable

Assure a competent environmental health workforce

Evaluate the effectiveness, accessibility, and quality of personal and population-based environmental health services

Research for new insights and innovative solutions to environmental health problems

See: https://www.cdc.gov/nceh/ehs/ephli/core_ess.htm

15. **D.** Deferment of enforcement of laws and regulations that protect health and ensure safety to the military/police is not included in policy development.

The policy development essential services include

Inform, educate, and empower people about environmental health issues

Mobilize community partnerships and actions to identify and solve environmental health problems

Develop policies and plans that support individual and community environmental health efforts

See: https://www.cdc.gov/nceh/ehs/ephli/core_ess.htm

16. **D.** Professor–student relationships are not included.

The mission of Community-Campus Partnerships for Health is to promote health equity and social justice through partnerships between communities and academic institutions.

See: https://www.ccphealth.org

17. **A.** Stakeholders are people or organizations invested in the program, interested in the results of the evaluation, and/or with a stake in what will be done with the results of the evaluation. Representing their needs and interests throughout the process is fundamental to good program evaluation.

See: https://www.cdc.gov/eval/guide/step1/index.htm

   https://www.cdc.gov/std/Program/pupestd/Identifying%20and%20 Determining%20Stakeholders.pdf

18. **A.** It is important to identify the right stakeholders for public health projects in order to improve the quality of the project, as stakeholders can give vital information and make sure nothing important is missed.

See: https://www.cdc.gov/eval/guide/step1/index.htm

19. D. Stakeholder management involves identifying and using the positive influences and minimizing negative influences through four stages: identify stakeholders, assess their interest and influence, develop communication management plans, and engage and influence stakeholders. Assessing interest and influence can be completed through a power/interest mapping. There is no need to fully engage a stakeholder with low power and no interest.

Brugha, R., & Varvasovszky, Z. (2000). Stakeholder analysis: A review. *Health Policy and Planning, 15*(3), 239–246.

> https://businessanalystlearnings.com/ba-techniques/2013/1/23/how -to-draw-a-stakeholder-matrix
>
> https://www.cdc.gov/eval/guide/step1/index.htm
>
> https://www.cdc.gov/std/Program/pupestd/Identifying%20and%20 Determining%20Stakeholders.pdf
>
> https://www.who.int/hac/techguidance/training/stakeholder%20 analysis%20ppt.pdf?ua=1
>
> https://www.who.int/workforcealliance/knowledge/toolkit/33.pdf

20. A. Identifying stakeholders is an important first step in stakeholder engagement. Each stakeholder should be important for the success of the project, and the mapping exercise serves to ensure a good match between project objectives and the stakeholder's interests and perspectives to inform the prioritization and engagement process.

Brugha, R., & Varvasovszky, Z. (2000). Stakeholder analysis: A review. *Health Policy and Planning, 15*(3), 239–246. doi:10.1093/heapol/15.3.239

> https://www.bsr.org/reports/BSR_Stakeholder_Engagement_Stake holder_Mapping.final.pdf
>
> https://www.cdc.gov/eval/guide/step1/index.htm

21. A. Loyalty is an outcome of good stakeholder engagement. Satisfied stakeholders will not leave, seek to change the agency, or ask for money to remain engaged.

Brugha, R., & Varvasovszky, Z. (2000). Stakeholder analysis: A review. *Health Policy and Planning, 15*(3), 239–246. doi:10.1093/heapol/15.3.239

> https://www.cdc.gov/eval/guide/step1/index.htm

22. C. Stakeholders who have high interest and high power should be engaged to the maximum extent possible.

Brugha, R., & Varvasovszky, Z. (2000). Stakeholder analysis: A review. *Health Policy and Planning, 15*(3), 239–246. doi:10.1093/heapol/15.3.239

> https://www.bsr.org/reports/BSR_Stakeholder_Engagement_Stake holder_Mapping.final.pdf
>
> https://www.cdc.gov/eval/guide/step1/index.htm
>
> https://www.ncbi.nlm.nih.gov/books/NBK50712/

Mitchell, R. K., Agle, B. R., & Wood, D. J. (1997). Toward a theory of stakeholder identification and salience: Defining the principle of who and what really counts. *The Academy of Management Review, 22*(4), 853–86. doi:10.2307/259247

23. **B.** Stakeholders who have high interest and low power should be kept informed, but their potential to take action is limited. They may serve as excellent testimonial advocates for the project.

Brugha, R., & Varvasovszky, Z. (2000). Stakeholder analysis: A review. *Health Policy and Planning, 15*(3), 239–246. doi:10.1093/heapol/15.3.239

> https://www.bsr.org/reports/BSR_Stakeholder_Engagement_Stake holder_Mapping.final.pdf
>
> https://www.cdc.gov/eval/guide/step1/index.htm
>
> https://www.ncbi.nlm.nih.gov/books/NBK50712/

Mitchell, R. K., Agle, B. R., & Wood, D. J. (1997). Toward a theory of stakeholder identification and salience: Defining the principle of who and what really counts. *The Academy of Management Review, 22*(4), 853–886. doi:10.2307/259247

24. **B.** The stakeholder salience model uses three variable criteria to rate stakeholders: power, legitimacy, and urgency. Dormant stakeholders possess power to impose their will through coercive, utilitarian, or symbolic means, but have little or no interaction/involvement as they lack legitimacy or urgency.

Brugha, R., & Varvasovszky, Z. (2000). Stakeholder analysis: A review. *Health Policy and Planning, 15*(3), 239–246. doi:10.1093/heapol/15.3.239

> https://www.atsdr.cdc.gov/communityengagement/pdf/PCE_ Report_508_FINAL.pdf

Mitchell, R., Agle, B., & Wood, D. (1997). Toward a theory of stakeholder identification and salience: Defining the principle of who and what really counts. *The Academy of Management Review, 22*(4), 853–886. doi:10.5465/amr.1997.9711022105

Stakeholder Salience https://www.stakeholdermap.com/stakeholder -analysis/stakeholder-salience.html

25. **A.** Discretionary or latent stakeholders have legitimate claims, but have no power to influence the organization nor urgent claims.

> https://requirementstechniques.wordpress.com/stakeholder -analysis/power-legitimacy-and-urgency-model/

Mitchell, R., Agle, B., & Wood, D. (1997). Toward a theory of stakeholder identification and salience: Defining the principle of who and what really counts. *The Academy of Management Review, 22*(4), 853–886. doi:10.5465/amr.1997.9711022105

26. **C.** Demanding stakeholders have urgent claims, but no power or legitimacy to enforce them.

See: https://requirementstechniques.wordpress.com/stakeholder-analysis/power-legitimacy-and-urgency-model/

Mitchell, R., Agle, B., & Wood, D. (1997). Toward a theory of stakeholder identification and salience: Defining the principle of who and what really counts. *The Academy of Management Review*, 22(4), 853–886. doi:10.5465/amr.1997.9711022105

27. **A.** Dependent stakeholders lack power, but have urgent and legitimate claims.

See: https://requirementstechniques.wordpress.com/stakeholder-analysis/power-legitimacy-and-urgency-model/

Mitchell, R., Agle, B., & Wood, D. (1997). Toward a theory of stakeholder identification and salience: Defining the principle of who and what really counts. *The Academy of Management Review*, 22(4), 853–886. doi:10.5465/amr.1997.9711022105

28. **A.** Definite stakeholders have power, legitimacy, and urgency, and therefore they need to be communicated with.

See: https://requirementstechniques.wordpress.com/stakeholder-analysis/power-legitimacy-and-urgency-model/

Mitchell, R., Agle, B., & Wood, D. (1997). Toward a theory of stakeholder identification and salience: Defining the principle of who and what really counts. *The Academy of Management Review*, 22(4), 853–886. doi:10.5465/amr.1997.9711022105

29. **B.** Dangerous stakeholders have power and urgency, but lack of legitimacy. They are seen as dangerous as they may resort to coercion and even violence.

See: https://requirementstechniques.wordpress.com/stakeholder-analysis/power-legitimacy-and-urgency-model/

Mitchell, R., Agle, B., & Wood, D. (1997). Toward a theory of stakeholder identification and salience: Defining the principle of who and what really counts. *The Academy of Management Review*, 22(4), 853–886. doi:10.5465/amr.1997.9711022105

30. **A.** Dominant stakeholders have both power and legitimate claims in the organization, giving them strong influence in the project.

See: https://requirementstechniques.wordpress.com/stakeholder-analysis/power-legitimacy-and-urgency-model/

Mitchell, R., Agle, B., & Wood, D. (1997). Toward a theory of stakeholder identification and salience: Defining the principle of who and what really counts. *The Academy of Management Review*, 22(4), 853–886. doi:10.5465/amr.1997.9711022105

31. **C.** The reliable way to combine qualitative and quantitative approaches for stakeholder identification is a workshop, where stakeholders are briefed on the project and activities. The workshop format provides an opportunity to assess stakeholder interests and concerns, identify roles and responsibilities, and share communication plans.

See: https://www.cdc.gov/std/Program/pupestd/Identifying%20and%20Determining%20Stakeholders.pdf

32. **C.** Strategy may be defined as "the unique set of activities and operating structures that an organization puts in place to deliver value to its customers."

    See: https://www.cdc.gov/ncbddd/disabilityandhealth/documents/foa_1603_2015_publichealthstrategies.pdf

    https://www.healthaffairs.org/do/10.1377/hblog20120312.017575/full/

33. **D.** Battle-deaths are not an emergency because war is often planned ahead, and casualties are expected.

    See: https://www.who.int/hac/techguidance/hbp/Conflict.pdf

34. **B.** Precision is the act, quality, condition, or fact of being exact. In an emergency, precision is less important than accuracy (correctness), validity (factual), and timeliness.

    See: https://www.cdc.gov/cpr/pubs-links/2018/documents/2018_Preparedness_Report.pdf

35. **B.** Without adequate controls, the negative effects of medicine donations are likely to offset their benefits.

    The 12 articles of the Guidelines for Drug Donations are based on four core principles. The first and paramount principle is that a drug donation should benefit the recipient to the maximum extent possible. This implies that all donations should be based on an expressed need and that unsolicited drug donations are to be discouraged. The second principle is that a donation should be made with full respect for the wishes and authority of the recipient, and be supportive of existing government health policies and administrative arrangements. The third principle is that there should be no double standards in quality: If the quality of an item is unacceptable in the donor country, it is also unacceptable as a donation. The fourth principle is that there should be effective communication between the donor and the recipient: Donations should be based on an expressed need and should not be sent unannounced.

    See: https://www.who.int/hac/techguidance/guidelines_for_drug_donations.pdf

36. **C.** Prevention activities are typically categorized by the following three definitions

    1. Primary prevention—intervening before health effects occur, through measures such as vaccinations, altering risky behaviors (poor eating habits, tobacco use), and banning substances known to be associated with a disease or health condition.
    2. Secondary prevention—screening to identify diseases in the earliest stages, before the onset of signs and symptoms, through measures such as mammography and regular blood pressure testing.
    3. Tertiary prevention—managing disease post-diagnosis to slow or stop disease progression through measures such as chemotherapy, rehabilitation, and screening for complications.

    See: https://www.cdc.gov/pictureofamerica/pdfs/picture_of_america_prevention.pdf

37. **A.** The most effective strategy is to familiarize students with effective decision-making, resistance, and refusal techniques and engaging them in activities in which they practice using the techniques. Academic success is an incentive, but not as effective.

    See: https://www.cdc.gov/features/teen-substance-use/index.html

    https://www.cdc.gov/media/releases/2017/p0925-rx-awareness
    -campaigns.html

38. **C.** Impulsive reactions often deepen conflict. Instead, putting distance in time and space to contemplate a response is a good strategy for conflict resolution.

    See: https://www.cdc.gov/bam/life/getting-along.html

    https://www.wfm.noaa.gov/workplace/ConflictResolution_
    QtrlyJune2014.pdf

39. **B.** A peer-reviewed article published in a professional medical journal is the least subject to bias and inaccuracies, although this is not guaranteed.

    The World Health Organization (WHO) publishes a peer-reviewed journal.

    The *Bulletin of the World Health Organization* is an international journal of public health with a special focus on developing countries. Since it was first published in 1948, it has become one of the world's leading public health journals. In keeping with its mission statement, the peer-reviewed monthly maintains an open-access policy so that the full contents of the journal and its archives are available online free of charge. As the flagship periodical of the WHO, the *Bulletin* draws on WHO experts as editorial advisers, reviewers, and authors, as well as on external collaborators. Anyone can submit a paper to the *Bulletin*, and no author charges are levied. All peer-reviewed articles are indexed, including in Institute for Scientific Information Web of Science and MEDLINE.

    The U.S. Centers for Disease Control and Prevention publishes a peer-reviewed journal, and commits to peer-review in other ways

    See: https://www.cdc.gov/maso/pdf/PeerReview.pdf

    https://www.cdc.gov/od/science/quality/support/peer-review.htm

    https://www.who.int/bulletin/about/en/

40. **B.** Not-for-profit organizations have a public service orientation, and any economic gains are expected to be used to improve services, instead of being distributed as income to stakeholders. They may have multiple objectives and are particularly transparent in their proceedings.

    See: https://healthfinder.gov/FindServices/SearchOrgType.aspx?OrgType
    ID=2&show=1

41. **C.** The power/interest model is used to gauge level of investment in stakeholder engagement. Investments could be the mode and frequency of communication, as well as expectations for active participation in program events.

    See: https://www.cdc.gov/eval/guide/step1/index.htm

    https://www.stakeholdermap.com/stakeholder-analysis.html

42. **A.** Pressure groups (or advocacy groups/coalitions in the United States) are usually organized to influence government policy or legislation. They are also referred to as special interest groups, lobbying groups, or protest groups. In

the United States, grantees of federal agencies such as the Centers for Disease Control and Prevention (CDC) must disavow lobbying.

See: https://www.apha.org/-/media/files/pdf/advocacy/171107_ advocacy_lobbying.ashx?la=en&hash=78AE848CCEC79E0833FFB431 AAB564835A239704

https://www.cdc.gov/grants/documents/anti-lobbying_restrictions_ for_cdc_grantees_july_2012.pdf

https://www.historylearningsite.co.uk/british-politics/pressure -groups/what-are-pressure-groups/

43. **D.** Outsourcing refers to obtaining goods or services from an outside or for- eign supplier, especially instead of an internal source.

For example, outsourcing occurs when state Medicaid agencies enter into agreements with contractors to perform administrative functions. Outsourc- ing can occur inside the United States (domestic outsourcing) or outside (off- shore outsourcing) and can be direct (when a Medicaid agency contracts with an offshore contractor) or indirect (when a Medicaid agency's contrac- tor subcontracts to an offshore contractor). There are no federal regulations that prohibit the offshore outsourcing of Medicaid administrative functions. However, the Health Insurance Portability and Accountability Act (HIPAA) requires covered entities to have business associate agreements (BAAs) to pro- tect personal health information (PHI).

See: https://oig.hhs.gov/oei/reports/oei-09-12-00530.asp

44. **C.** The Community Coalition Action Theory (CCAT) has 14 major constructs and 23 practice-proven propositions within the constructs. CCAT describes action-oriented partnerships and coalitions formed to prevent community problems by analysis, data collection, and assessment followed by an action plan with solutions identified, implementation of the solutions, monitoring outcomes, and ultimately creating social change.

Butterfoss, F., Goodman, R., & Wandersman, A. (1993). Community coalitions for prevention and health promotion. *Health Education Research, 8*(3), 315–330. doi:10.1093/her/8.3.315

Butterfoss, F., Lachance, L., & Orians, C. (2006). Building allies coali- tions: Why formation matters. *Health Promotion Practice, 7*(2), 23s–33s. doi:10.1177/1524839906287062

https://aspe.hhs.gov/report/literature-review-developing-conceptual -framework-assess-sustainability-community-coalitions-post-federal -funding/b-theories-community-coalitions

https://www.atsdr.cdc.gov/communityengagement/pce_mos_frame works.html

45. **C.** Persons, groups, and communities are the foundations of community empowerment, which refers to the process of enabling communities to increase control over their lives. "Communities" are groups of people that may or may not be spatially connected, but who share common interests, con- cerns, or identities. These communities could be local, national, or interna- tional, with specific or broad interests. "Empowerment" refers to the process by which people gain control over the factors and decisions that shape their

lives. It is the process by which they increase their assets and attributes and build capacities to gain access, partners, networks, and/or a voice, in order to gain control.

A six-step model for community empowerment incorporates a social ecological framework.

Gaining entry into the community

Identifying issues of interest or concern to the community

Prioritizing identified issues

Formulating a strategy to address a priority issue

Developing and implementing an action plan to resolve the priority issue

Transitioning to a new issue and leadership

See: https://aspe.hhs.gov/report/literature-review-developing-conceptual
-framework-assess-sustainability-community-coalitions-post-federal
-funding/b-theories-community-coalitions

https://journals.sagepub.com/doi/pdf/10.1177/1524839907307884

https://www.atsdr.cdc.gov/communityengagement/pce_models
.html

https://www.who.int/healthpromotion/conferences/7gchp/
track1/en/

46. **A.** Framework for collaborative empowerment describes the process of community empowerment in five interrelated elements of community empowerment: collaborative planning; community action; community change; community capacity and outcomes; and adaptation, renewal, and institutionalization.

Fawcett, S. B., Paine-Andrews, A., Francisco, V. T., Schultz, J. A., Richter, K. P., Lewis, R. K., . . . Lopez, C. M. (1995). Using empowerment theory in collaborative partnerships for community health and development. *American Journal of Community Psychology, 23*(5), 677–697. doi:10.1007/BF02506987

https://aspe.hhs.gov/report/literature-review-developing-conceptual
-framework-assess-sustainability-community-coalitions-post-federal
-funding/b-theories-community-coalitions

https://www.atsdr.cdc.gov/communityengagement/pce_models
.html

47. **D.** The collective impact framework describes an intentional way of working together and sharing information for the purpose of solving a complex problem. The framework demands common agenda, shared metrics, and continuous communication.

See: https://ssir.org/articles/entry/collective_impact

https://www.councilofnonprofits.org/tools-resources/collective
-impact

48. **D.** The Planned Approach to Community Health (PATCH) Model is a process that many communities use to plan, conduct, and evaluate health promotion and disease prevention programs. PATCH cannot be used to "enforce" disparities in health, which is not desirable.

See: http://www.lgreen.net/patch.pdf

    https://wonder.cdc.gov/wonder/prevguid/p0000064/P0000064.asp

49. C. Mobilizing for Action through Planning and Partnerships (MAPP) was developed by the National Association of City and County Officials (NAC-CHO). Members of the Association of Schools and Programs of Public Health (ASPPH), American Public Health Association (APHA), and American Medical Association (AMA) should be familiar with MAPP, and several collaborate to use the model for community health needs assessment and implementation of action plans.

See: https://www.naccho.org/programs/public-health-infrastructure/perf
    ormance-improvement/community-health-assessment/mapp

50. D. The Mobilizing for Action through Planning and Partnerships (MAPP) Model is not designed to litigate violations. The themes are

1. Organize for successful partnerships
2. Visioning
3. Assessments—Community Themes and Strengths Assessment, Local Public Health System Assessment, Community Health Status Assessment, Forces of Change Assessment
4. Strategic issues identification
5. Goals and strategies
6. Action cycle

See: https://www.naccho.org/programs/public-health-infrastructure/perf
    ormance-improvement/community-health-assessment/mapp

51. D. Fluency in English is not an asset in the Asset-Based Community Development (ABCD) Model.

ABCD is a strategy for sustainable community-driven development. Beyond the mobilization of a particular community, ABCD is concerned with how to link micro-assets to the macro-environment. The appeal of ABCD lies in its premise that communities can drive the development process themselves by identifying and mobilizing existing, but often unrecognized assets, and thereby responding to and creating local economic opportunity.

See: https://resources.depaul.edu/abcd-institute/resources/Documents/
    WhatisAssetBasedCommunityDevelopment.pdf

52. A. Partnerships to Improve Community Health (PICH) was a 3-year initiative that supported implementation of evidence-based strategies to improve the health of communities and reduce the prevalence of chronic disease. PICH built on a body of knowledge developed through previously funded Centers for Disease Control and Prevention (CDC) programs and encouraged collaborations with a multisectoral coalition to implement sustainable changes in communities where people live, learn, work, and play.

See: https://www.cdc.gov/nccdphp/dch/programs/partnershipstoimpro
    vecommunityhealth/index.html

53. A. Tuberculosis, hepatitis, and valley fever are infectious diseases.

Racial and Ethnic Approaches to Community Health (REACH) is a national program administered by the Centers for Disease Control and Prevention (CDC) to reduce racial and ethnic health disparities.

Through REACH, recipients plan and carry out local, culturally appropriate programs to address a wide range of health issues among African Americans, American Indians, Hispanics/Latinos, Asian Americans, Alaska Natives, and Pacific Islanders.

See: https://www.cdc.gov/nccdphp/dnpao/state-local-programs/reach/index.htm

54. D. Indentureship, the state or period of being a servant bound to service for a specified time in return for passage to a colony, is not a public health partnership.

See: https://www.cdc.gov/partners/index.html

55. B. Keeping people hospitalized is not a goal of public health and community engagement. The goals of Building Capacity of the Public Health System to Improve Population Health through National, Nonprofit Organizations include

Improved public health systems and organizational efficiencies

Improved public health workforce

Increased use of technology and better population data

Improved planning, implementation, and evaluation of evidence-based public health policies, laws, programs, and services

Increased use of results-driven partnerships

Increased availability and access to public health resources and materials

See: https://www.cdc.gov/publichealthgateway/funding/rfaot13.html

56. C. Healthy People provides science-based, 10-year national objectives for improving the health of all Americans. For three decades, Healthy People has established benchmarks and monitored progress over time in order to

Encourage collaborations across communities and sectors

Empower individuals toward making informed health decisions

Measure the impact of prevention activities

A specific goal is to improve access to comprehensive, quality healthcare services.

See: https://www.healthypeople.gov/2020/About-Healthy-People

https://www.healthypeople.gov/2020/topics-objectives/topic/Access-to-Health-Services

57. B. Predisposing, Reinforcing and Enabling factors, and Causes in Educational Diagnosis and Evaluation (PRECEDE) begins with a comprehensive community assessment including social, epidemiological, ecological, and administrative factors which predispose, reinforce, and enable implementation of interventions.

See: https://www.ruralhealthinfo.org/toolkits/health-promotion/2/
program-models/precede-proceed

58. **B.** Mobilizing for Action through Planning and Partnerships (MAPP) is a community-driven strategic planning process for improving community health. Facilitated by public health leaders, this framework helps communities apply strategic thinking to prioritize public health issues and identify resources to address them. MAPP is not an agency-focused assessment process; rather, it is an interactive process that can improve the efficiency, effectiveness, and ultimately the performance of local public health systems.

The forces of change assessment focuses on identifying forces such as legislation, technology, and other impending changes that affect the context in which the community and its public health system operate. This answers the questions: "What is occurring or might occur that affects the health of our community or the local public health system?" and "What specific threats or opportunities are generated by these occurrences?"

See: https://www.naccho.org/programs/public-health-infrastructure/perf
ormance-improvement/community-health-assessment/mapp/phase-3
-the-four-assessments

59. **A.** Cross-cultural misunderstanding can be achieved by cultivating cultural competence and sensitivity.

Cultural and linguistic competence is a set of congruent behaviors, attitudes, and policies that come together in a system, agency, or among professionals that enables effective work in cross-cultural situations. "Culture" refers to integrated patterns of human behavior that include the language, thoughts, communications, actions, customs, beliefs, values, and institutions of racial, ethnic, religious, or social groups. "Competence" implies having the capacity to function effectively as an individual and an organization within the context of the cultural beliefs, behaviors, and needs presented by consumers and their communities.

See: https://npin.cdc.gov/pages/cultural-competence

60. **D.** Collaborative and participative characteristics are essential. Partnerships, coalitions, and collaborations are necessary for the success of any public health program. Both partnerships and coalitions fulfill different roles and are able to accomplish different activities for the state oral health program.

See: https://www.cdc.gov/oralhealth/state_programs/infrastructure/
partnerships.htm

61. **B.** Transparency of operations, mission, and strategic priorities are essential for maintaining long-term partnerships and collaborations.

See: https://www.cdc.gov/globalhealth/countries/vietnam/pdf/thomasfr
iedeninterview.pdf

7 Program Planning and Evaluation

■ INTRODUCTION

Public health practice is quintessentially a collaborative endeavor, and prospectively planning the roles of collaborating stakeholders is essential for team success. The planning process begins with clearly articulated vision, mission, objectives, strategies, and actions for specific projects led by public health agencies or organizations. Good planning also demands continuous monitoring and evaluation of progress toward articulated goals, and strategies to change course if necessary in response to evaluation outputs. Several models have been developed for program planning and evaluation, and these can be adapted to support new public health projects, interventions, and health promotion initiatives. Competencies in program planning and evaluation are tested with questions designed to examine broad knowledge of planning and assessment of public health initiatives. Practicing with these questions should enable you to

- Develop and conduct formative evaluation plans
- Develop and conduct outcome evaluation plans
- Develop process evaluation plans
- Apply qualitative evaluation methods
- Apply quantitative evaluation methods
- Evaluate the benefits of qualitative or quantitative methods for use in evaluation
- Assess evaluation reports in relation to their quality, utility, and impact
- Assess program performance
- Utilize evaluation results to strengthen and enhance activities and programs
- Apply evidence-based practices to program planning, implementation, and evaluation

- Identify challenges to program implementation
- Ensure that program implementation occurs as intended
- Plan evidence-based interventions to meet established program goals and objectives
- Implement context-specific health interventions based on situation analysis and organizational goals
- Design context-specific health interventions based on situation analysis and organizational goals
- Plan and communicate steps and procedures for the planning, implementation, and evaluation of health programs, policies, and interventions
- Design action plans for enhancing community or population-based health
- Evaluate personnel and material resources
- Use available evidence to inform effective teamwork and team-based practices
- Prioritize individual, organizational, or community concerns and resources for health programs
- Design public health interventions that incorporate factors such as gender, race, poverty, history, migration, or culture within public health systems
- Develop a community health plan based on needs and resource assessments
- Apply evaluation frameworks to measure the performance and impact of health programs, policies, and systems

▣ QUESTIONS

1. "A model of health that emphasizes the linkages and relationships among multiple factors (or determinants) affecting health" is known as

   A. The preventive model of public health
   B. The integrative model of public health
   C. The ecological model of public health
   D. The multifactorial model of public health

2. Which of the following is NOT considered a core function of public health?

   A. Assurance
   B. Policy development
   C. Assessment
   D. Interrogation

3. The framework of public health performance requires the integration of core functions and essential services. Which of the following is NOT an essential service of public health?

   A. Diagnose and investigate health problems and health hazards in the community
   B. Enforce laws and regulations that protect health and ensure safety
   C. Prescribe medication in communities with prevalent public health problems
   D. Research for new insights and innovative solutions to health problems

4. Imagine that you are a public health professional assigned to the county health department to direct a new program for monitoring health status to identify and solve community health problems. Which of the following should you NOT expect to be included as part of your responsibilities?

   A. Monitor wastewater treatment and disposal
   B. Mosquito surveillance
   C. Screening for diabetes
   D. Screening for criminal record

5. In 1896, the first recorded fatal traffic accident occurred in London. The World Health Organization projects that by the year 2020, automobile accidents will become the third leading cause of mortality in the world. But there is a major disparity in this situation. Only 20% of automobiles in the world are driven in developing countries where 90% of the fatalities occur. Which among the following can explain the global disparity in mortality associated with automobile accidents?

   A. Drunk driving is less prevalent in developing countries.
   B. Seat belt laws are only enforced in developing countries.
   C. The quality of the roads and traffic infrastructure are weaker in developing countries.
   D. Government-issued driver's licenses are not available to immigrants.

6. One of the essential services of public health practice is to assure effectiveness through the development of innovative solutions to public health problems. The services under this function include the following, EXCEPT

   A. Participation in bio-exigency surveys
   B. Study of successful public health programs in other jurisdictions
   C. Customer service evaluations
   D. Health needs assessment

7. The need to prioritize investments in public health and to address the most burdensome health problems at the population level led to collaboration between the World Bank and the World Health Organization to develop composite measures of disease burden. Among the best known of the quantitative indexes of the burden of disease is the "Disability-Adjusted Life Year." This index includes which of the following data?

   A. Number of years of life lost from premature mortality
   B. Number of years of life lived in luxury according to the World Bank's luxury index

  C. Number of years of life lived with a partner

  D. Number of years of life lived in poverty according to the World Bank's poverty index

8. According to the most recent global burden of disease assessment using the Disability-Adjusted Life Year indicator, which of the following is the leading cause of mortality in the world?

  A. Diarrheal diseases

  B. Cardiovascular diseases

  C. Mental diseases

  D. Vector-borne diseases

9. According to the most recent global burden of disease assessment, one of the top five leading causes of years of life lived with disability is

  A. Unipolar depressive disorders

  B. Cardiovascular diseases

  C. Malaria

  D. Diarrheal diseases

10. The estimation of years of life lived with disability in the calculation of Disability-Adjusted Life Year includes the following, EXCEPT

  A. Number of incidence cases of disease in a given period

  B. Average duration of disease

  C. Life expectancy

  D. Disability weighting factor

11. The estimation of years of life lost in the calculation of Disability-Adjusted Life Year includes the following, EXCEPT

  A. Global standard life expectancy

  B. Age-weighting factor

  C. Time discounting factor

  D. Severity weight corresponding to the cause of death

12. The Disability-Adjusted Life Year index includes an assessment of the level of "severity" associated with different diseases, using a "person trade-off" protocol in an exercise that includes healthcare workers from different parts of the world. The following considerations are included in estimates of disease severity in different regions of the world, EXCEPT

  A. Socioeconomic status

  B. Cultural context

  C. Disabling sequelae of disease and injury

  D. Marital status

13. Among the uses of quantitative studies of disease burden is the projection of future trends of various categories of disease and disability to plan for adequate

healthcare provision for future generations. The following data are included in the estimates of future projections of disease burden, EXCEPT

A. Income per capita
B. Population growth rate
C. Human capital index
D. Behavior change index

14. Program planning, including anticipation of future disease burden in the population, is one of the major functions of public health professionals. Which among the following would NOT be among your responsibilities as a public health professional in charge of program planning for a local public health agency?

A. Differentiate between qualitative and quantitative evaluation methods in relation to their strengths, limitations, and appropriate uses, and emphasis on reliability and validity
B. Prepare a program budget with justification
C. In collaboration with others, prioritize individual, organizational, and community concerns and resources for public health programs
D. Provide immigration status of specific individuals visiting health clinics to the Department of Homeland Security

15. The responsibilities of the World Health Organization demonstrate one of the major examples of the need for systems thinking in public health. Systems thinking, defined as "the ability to recognize system level properties that result from dynamic interactions among human and social systems and how they affect the relationships among individuals, groups, organizations, communities, and environments," involves the following, EXCEPT

A. Prioritization of systemic diseases
B. Analysis of interrelationships among systems that influence the quality of life of people in their communities
C. Explanation of how the contexts of gender, race, poverty, history, migration, and culture are important in the design of interventions within public health systems
D. Explanation of how systems (e.g., individuals, social networks, organizations, and communities) may be viewed as systems within systems in the analysis of public health problems

16. The quantitative assessment of the global burden of disease facilitates the implementation of programs to prevent diseases by modifying the environment in which people live. This facilitation requires appropriate attribution of fractions of disease burden to specific risk factors. In the estimation of attributable risk, the following data are included, EXCEPT

A. Prevalence of exposure to the risk factor
B. Relative risk of disease for exposed versus unexposed group
C. Life expectancy at birth
D. Relative risk of injury for exposed versus unexposed group

17. Community-based approaches to prevent childhood lead (Pb) poisoning have proven to be effective, especially after the successes observed in Rhode Island where a disproportionate number of families live in older homes. The community-based approach model includes the following, EXCEPT

    A. Creation of a broad-based community coalition or advisory group
    B. Involvement of community members most at risk in all stages of the program
    C. Securing diverse and dedicated sources of funding for the program
    D. Working with dentists to remove lead (Pb) in tooth fillings

18. The transformation of countries from **high birth rates** and **high death rates** to **low** birth rates and **low** death rates as part of the **economic** development of a country from a preindustrial to an industrialized economy is known as

    A. Globalization
    B. Economic development
    C. Episodic burden conversion
    D. Demographic transition

19. The change in population development involving sudden increase in growth rates due to public health innovation in treating or preventing diseases, followed by a re-leveling of population growth from subsequent declines in procreation rates, is a public health theory known as

    A. Episodic burden transition
    B. Environmental risk transition
    C. Epidemiologic transition
    D. Demographic transition

20. The company "23andMe" now sells a personal genetic testing kit at a pharmacy store for about $199 per (health and ancestry kit). This controversial development is bringing to the public sphere decisions about genetic predisposition to deadly diseases such as breast cancer and Huntington's disease. From a public health perspective, which of the following is NOT a concern regarding public access and interpretation of genetic profile data?

    A. Health insurance costs
    B. Confidentiality issues
    C. Perfectly complete scientific understanding of gene–environment–behavior interactions
    D. Potential to base individual life decisions on incomplete information

21. Which of the following components of a strategic planning process in a public health agency has logical priority over the others?

    A. Setting strategic goals for a 3-year cycle
    B. Reviewing (and revising) the vision and mission statements for the agency
    C. Developing an operating budget and staffing plan for the agency
    D. Preparing an action plan for eradicating cryptosporidiosis in the municipal water system

22. Reasons to invest public funds in understanding the status and trends in human health at the global level exclude

    A. Single-disease global health initiatives, which are better than multiple-disease trends
    B. To address unmet needs for new drugs and vaccines
    C. The need to understand the root causes of ill health that arise in other sectors
    D. To develop a new breed of strategic research and development partnerships

23. The most relevant reason for using interdisciplinary approaches and methods to identify the determinants of global health is that

    A. The pharmaceutical industry can no longer view itself as detached from the well-being of society.
    B. The health and economic costs of chronic diseases have created an impending disaster.
    C. The forces that drive the rise of chronic diseases, including demographic aging, rapid urbanization, and the globalization of unhealthy lifestyles, lie beyond the direct control of the health sector.
    D. Our world is dangerously out of balance. The gaps in health outcomes, within and between countries, are greater now than at any time in recent history.

24. *"As our world becomes increasingly connected, there is a growing realization that public health challenges are global. Disease doesn't respect international borders. Poverty doesn't simply diminish the lives of citizens of underdeveloped nations. In a globally connected world, poverty and disease and underdevelopment threaten us all."*

    This statement contains information about the definitions of the following disciplines of study, EXCEPT

    A. Global health
    B. Community health
    C. Population health
    D. International health

25. The composite measure of global burden of disease used by the World Health Organization DOES NOT include

    A. Years of life lived with disability
    B. Infant mortality rates
    C. Years of life lost due to premature mortality
    D. Disability weights

26. *"In the United States, the healthy life expectancy of 70 for girls and 67 for boys is the lowest of any rich country. As the world grays, the challenge will be to keep citizens healthy even as they live to an ever-riper old age."*

    What is the leading cause of mortality in the United States?

    A. Injuries
    B. Noncommunicable diseases
    C. Communicable diseases
    D. Gun violence

27. In the United States in 2018, the top five leading causes of years of life lived with disability includes

   A. Lower back and neck pain
   B. Ischemic heart disease
   C. Diabetes
   D. Arthritis

28. *"Ageing of the world's population is increasing the number of people living with seque-lae of diseases and injuries. Shifts in the epidemiological profile driven by socioeconomic change also contribute to the continued increase in years lived with disability (YLDs) as well as the rate of increase in YLDs."*

   The current top 10 leading causes of YLD globally DOES NOT include

   A. Iron-deficiency anemia
   B. Depressive disorders
   C. Cancers
   D. Low back pain

29. Pandemic influenza is a good case study for investigating the "One Health" approach to solve global health problems because

   A. It focuses on only one disease at a time.
   B. It focuses on only one solution—vaccination—to the global health problem.
   C. Controlling outbreaks in farm animals is as important as controlling out-breaks in humans.
   D. It is a perfect example of convergence of evidence on genetic risk factors.

30. Natural phenomena such as lightning, earthquakes, and hurricanes can lead to instant death of a large number of people. For example, in 2017, Hurricane Harvey killed about 88 people in Texas, the Sonoma Wildfire killed 44 peo-ple in California, and more than 1,085 people are estimated to have died in Puerto Rico as a result of flooding. Globally, the record for the largest mortality from natural disasters is attributed to the 1931 China floods, which killed up to 4 million people.

   Global health practice includes emergency preparedness and response to nat-ural disasters; the impact of natural disasters on global burden of disease may extend beyond acute mortality to

   A. Mental illness
   B. Obesity
   C. Increased smoking
   D. Diabetes

31. Which of the following disease(s) have been eradicated?

   A. Measles
   B. Polio
   C. Smallpox
   D. Dracunculiasis

32. The potential to eradicate preventable diseases in the future depends on other societal factors that influence coordination and deployment of global health resources. For example, 70 confirmed cases of circulating vaccine-derived poliovirus type 2 (cVDPV2) were reported in Syria, which is embroiled in war. Where else are similar societal challenges preventing the eradication of polio?

    A. Armenia
    B. Nigeria
    C. China
    D. Paraguay

33. When diplomats met to form the United Nations in 1945, one of the things they discussed was setting up a global health organization. The constitution of the World Health Organization (WHO) came into force on April 7, 1948—a date we now celebrate every year as World Health Day. The goal of the WHO is "to build a better, healthier future for people all over the world." Such a healthier future will include focusing resources on priority topics for disease control and prevention. The following are tools, methods, and procedures that the WHO uses to prioritize global health programs, EXCEPT

    A. Global burden of disease assessments
    B. The World Health Assembly, the decision-making body of WHO
    C. Leadership of the WHO director-general
    D. U.S. Department of Health and Human Services

34. Envisioning a world without disease may not be realistic or even desirable, but it is a powerful motivator to eradicate preventable diseases, which are not necessarily infectious diseases for which we have vaccines or antibiotics. For example, theoretically, it should be possible to eradicate lung disease attributable to the human use of tobacco. The following global health strategies are currently being used to discourage tobacco use, EXCEPT

    A. Graphic advertisements about the health impacts of tobacco use
    B. Increasing taxes on tobacco products
    C. Implementing policies to prevent tobacco use in certain locations (e.g., "Smoke-Free Campus")
    D. Enforcing tobacco restriction policies developed by the World Health Organization in all countries

35. The PRECEDE–PROCEED model is

    A. A comprehensive structure for assessing health needs for designing, implementing, and evaluating health promotion and other public health programs to meet those needs
    B. Based on the Sir Austin Bradford Hill's guidelines on causality whereby exposure to the risk factor must precede the symptoms of disease
    C. A government policy that requires approval of a public health intervention plan before proceeding with implementation
    D. A government policy that requires citation of legal precedent before proceeding with implementing a well-established practice for a new population

36. In the PRECEDE–PROCEED model, PRECEDE stands for the following, EXCEPT

    A. Enabling constructs in educational diagnosis and evaluation
    B. Reinforcing constructs in educational diagnosis and evaluation
    C. Predisposing constructs in educational diagnosis and evaluation
    D. Policy constructs in educational and environmental development

37. In the PRECEDE–PROCEED model, PROCEED stands for the following, EXCEPT

    A. Regulatory constructs in educational and environmental development
    B. Policy constructs in educational and environmental development
    C. Organizational constructs in educational and environmental development
    D. Reinforcing constructs in educational diagnosis and evaluation

38. In the PRECEDE–PROCEED model, PRECEDE provides

    A. The structure for implementing and evaluating the public health program
    B. The structure for planning a targeted and focused public health program
    C. The structure and procedure for obtaining permission to implement a public health program
    D. The structure and procedure for postaudit of a public health program

39. In the PRECEDE–PROCEED model, PROCEED provides

    A. The structure for implementing and evaluating the public health program
    B. The structure for planning a targeted and focused public health program
    C. The structure and procedure for obtaining permission to implement a public health program
    D. The structure and procedure for postaudit of a public health program

40. In the PRECEDE–PROCEED model, which of the following is involved in PRECEDE?

    A. Process evaluation
    B. Impact evaluation
    C. Outcome evaluation
    D. Social assessment

41. In the PRECEDE–PROCEED model, which of the following is involved in PROCEED?

    A. Epidemiological assessment
    B. Ecological assessment
    C. Social assessment
    D. Impact evaluation

42. In the Community Readiness Model, communities are motivated by

    A. Total collective financial resources available
    B. Only discretionary financial resources available

    C. Positive outcome of applications for federal or state grants
    D. The difference between current health situations or behaviors and the desire to reach a goal

43. The Community Readiness Model includes the following stages, EXCEPT

    A. Absence of awareness—the community does not recognize the health issue.
    B. Denial or resistance—there is little recognition or concern among community members about the health issue.
    C. Vague awareness—the community may be concerned about the health issue, but the motivation to address it is low.
    D. Developing and maintaining capacity and power to produce lasting change.

44. The Community Organization Model is characterized by the following, EXCEPT

    A. Understanding the context and root causes of health issues
    B. Collaborative decision-making and problem-solving
    C. Denial or resistance—there is little recognition or concern among community members about the health issue
    D. Developing and maintaining capacity and power to produce lasting change

45. Strategies for sustainability planning for public health programs exclude

    A. Maintaining consistent leadership
    B. Forming a highly disciplinary team of staff
    C. Securing stable funding
    D. Connecting with the community

46. The vision statement of a public health organization should

    A. Be developed by only senior leadership within the organization
    B. Communicate the organization's ideal conditions of the population they serve
    C. Communicate the organization's current conditions of the population they serve
    D. Be developed by only external stakeholders who know what is best for the community

47. The vision statement of a public health organization should

    A. Describe the actual activities of the organization
    B. Be developed by only senior leadership within the organization
    C. Communicate the organization's current conditions of the population they serve
    D. Be developed by only external stakeholders who know what is best for the community

48. The stated objectives of a public health organization should

    A. Be developed by only external stakeholders who know what is best for the community
    B. Communicate the organization's ideal conditions of the population they serve

C. Communicate the organization's current conditions of the population they serve

D. Specify personnel, tasks, and due dates of projects

49. The stated strategies of a public health organization should

A. Be developed by only external stakeholders who know what is best for the community

B. Specify the approaches and processes through which each objective will be pursued

C. Communicate the organization's current conditions of the population they serve

D. Specify personnel, tasks, and due dates of projects

50. The action plan of a public health organization should

A. Be developed by only external stakeholders who know what is best for the community

B. Specify the approaches and processes through which each objective will be pursued

C. Communicate the organization's current conditions of the population they serve

D. Specify potential barriers or resistance likely to be encountered in pursuing the organization's mission

51. Program objectives should be the following, EXCEPT

A. Specific
B. Action-oriented
C. Measurable
D. Time unlimited

52. The Planned Approach to Community Health (PATCH) is a planning model that comprises all of the following phases, EXCEPT

A. Predetermined objectives
B. Mobilizing the community
C. Collecting and organizing data
D. Selecting population health priorities

53. The Mobilizing for Action through Planning and Partnerships (MAPP) model consists of the following steps, EXCEPT

A. Visioning
B. Action cycles
C. Identifying strategic topics
D. Doing a program design

54. The intervention mapping model comprises all of the following steps, EXCEPT

A. Developing an implementation plan
B. Developing a logic model

C. Visioning

D. Doing a program design

55. The MAP-IT model was developed to assist communities in implementing Healthy People 2020, and it consists of the following steps, EXCEPT

A. Mobilize

B. Assess

C. Track

D. Consult

56. The following are types of evaluation, EXCEPT

A. Critical

B. Formative

C. Constructive

D. Summative

57. The following are steps in the evaluation process, EXCEPT

A. Engage stakeholders

B. Collect evidence

C. Justify conclusions

D. Give the project a grade

58. The American Evaluation Association's guiding principles for evaluators include the following, EXCEPT

A. Engage stakeholders

B. Competence

C. Integrity and honesty

D. Respect for people

59. An evaluator's respect for people takes into consideration the following, EXCEPT

A. Social and political climate

B. Research ethics

C. Social equity

D. Potential costs of the evaluation

60. Evaluation of public health programs should be informed by social ecological concepts, which emphasize the continuum of influences across the following domains, EXCEPT

A. Individual

B. Family

C. Community

D. Constellation

■ ANSWERS

1. **C.** The Centers for Disease Control and Prevention uses a four-level social-ecological model to better understand social determinants of health and the effect of potential prevention strategies. The model considers the complex interplay between individual, relationship, community, and societal factors. It facilitates understanding of the range of factors that put people at risk for disease and injury.

   See: https://www.cdc.gov/violenceprevention/publichealthissue/social -ecologicalmodel.html

   https://www.unicef.org/cbsc/files/Module_1_SEM-C4D.docx

   https://www.who.int/violenceprevention/approach/ecology/en

2. **D.** Interrogation is not a core public health function.

   The core functions of public health and how they relate to the 10 essential services are the following:

   Assessment

   Policy development

   Assurance

   See: https://www.cdc.gov/nceh/ehs/ephli/core_ess.htm

3. **C.** The 10 essential public health services describe the public health activities that all communities should undertake:

   1. Monitor health status to identify and solve community health problems
   2. Diagnose and investigate health problems and health hazards in the community
   3. Inform, educate, and empower people about health issues
   4. Mobilize community partnerships and action to identify and solve health problems
   5. Develop policies and plans that support individual and community health efforts
   6. Enforce laws and regulations that protect health and ensure safety
   7. Link people to needed personal health services and assure the provision of healthcare when otherwise unavailable
   8. Assure competent public and personal healthcare workforce
   9. Evaluate effectiveness, accessibility, and quality of personal and population-based health services
   10. Research for new insights and innovative solutions to health problems

   See: https://www.cdc.gov/publichealthgateway/publichealthservices/ essentialhealthservices.html

4. **D.** Screening for the criminal record of individuals is not a core function of public health professionals in communities, although collaboration with law enforcement services is important. Wastewater monitoring, disease vector surveillance, and diagnostic screening are part of essential functions.

See: https://www.cdc.gov/violenceprevention/publichealthissue/funded
programs/cardiffmodel/law.html

5. C. Every year the lives of approximately 1.35 million people are cut short
as a result of a road traffic crash. Between 20 and 50 million more people
suffer nonfatal injuries, with many incurring a disability as a result of their
injury. More than 90% of road traffic deaths occur in low- and middle-income
countries. Road traffic injury death rates are highest in the African region.
Even within high-income countries, people from lower socioeconomic backgrounds are more likely to be involved in road traffic crashes.

The design of roads can have a considerable impact on their safety. Ideally,
those designing roads should keep in mind the safety of all road users. This
would mean making sure that there are adequate facilities for pedestrians,
cyclists, and motorcyclists. Measures such as footpaths, cycling lanes, safe
crossing points, and other traffic calming measures can be critical to reducing the risk of injury among these road users.

See: https://www.who.int/news-room/fact-sheets/detail/road-traffic
-injuries

6. A. Participation in "bio-exigency" surveys is not an essential public health
service. Exigency means the demands of an urgent situation, and one can
imagine this to be related to a bioterrorism alert, but in describing essential
functions, it is important to use plain language that is easily understood by
public health professionals and the communities that they serve.

See: https://www.cdc.gov/publichealthgateway/publichealthservices/
essentialhealthservices.html

7. A. One DALY can be thought of as one lost year of "healthy" life. The sum of
these DALYs across the population, or the burden of disease, can be thought
of as a measurement of the gap between current health status and an ideal
health situation where the entire population lives to an advanced age, free of
disease and disability. DALYs for a disease or health condition are calculated
as the sum of the Years of Life Lost (YLL) due to premature mortality in the
population and the Years Lost due to Disability (YLD) for people living with
the health condition or its consequences.

See: https://www.who.int/healthinfo/global_burden_disease/metrics
_daly/en

8. B. Ischemic heart disease (cardiovascular disease) was the leading cause of
mortality globally in 2017.

See: https://www.who.int/gho/mortality_burden_disease/en

http://www.healthdata.org/sites/default/files/files/policy_report/
2019/GBD_2017_Booklet.pdf

http://www.healthdata.org/causes-death

9. A. In 2017, the leading causes of morbidity (Years Lived with Disability) were

Low back pain, headache disorders, depressive disorders, diabetes, hearing
loss

See: http://www.healthdata.org/sites/default/files/files/policy_report/
2019/GBD_2017_Booklet.pdf

10. **C.** Years of Life Lived with Disability for a particular cause in a particular time
period is estimated by the number of incident cases in that period multiplied
by the average duration of the disease and a weight factor that reflects the
severity of the disease on a scale from 0 (perfect health) to 1 (dead).

See: https://www.who.int/healthinfo/global_burden_disease/metrics_
daly/en

11. **D.** The Years of Life Lost due to Premature Mortality is estimated as the number of deaths from a cause multiplied by the standard life expectancy at the
age at which death occurs.

See: https://www.who.int/healthinfo/global_burden_disease/metrics_
daly/en

12. **D.** A disability weight is a weight factor that reflects the severity of the disease
on a scale from 0 (perfect health) to 1 (equivalent to death). Years Lost due to
Disability (YLD) are calculated by multiplying the incident cases by duration
and disability weight for the condition.

Various methods have been used to derive disability weights. The focus
groups needed for person trade-off exercises for estimating the original disability weights implicitly had the socioeconomic, cultural, and severity contexts. Marital status was not an explicit factor.

See: https://www.who.int/healthinfo/global_burden_disease/daly_
disability_weight/en

https://www.who.int/bulletin/volumes/88/12/10-084301/en

https://www.who.int/bulletin/volumes/92/3/13-126227/en

13. **D.** Behavior change index is not included in the models for future projections
of disease burden. The models are based largely on projections of economic
and social development, and the historically observed relationships of these
with cause-specific mortality rates.

See: https://www.who.int/healthinfo/global_burden_disease/projections_
method.pdf?ua=1

14. **D.** Population screening for immigration status of individuals is not traditionally part of the essential services of public health.

See: https://www.cdc.gov/publichealthgateway/publichealthservices/
essentialhealthservices.html

15. **A.** Prioritization of systemic diseases that affect body regions or the whole
body (e.g., high blood pressure) is not essential for a systems view of public
health practice, which is about public health services systems.

"A good health system delivers quality services to all people, when and where
they need them. The exact configuration of services varies from country to
country, but in all cases requires a robust financing mechanism; a well-trained

and adequately paid workforce; reliable information on which to base decisions and policies; well-maintained facilities and logistics to deliver quality medicines and technologies."

See: https://www.who.int/topics/health_systems/en

16. **C.** Life expectancy at birth is not included in the model for estimating attributable risk.

"The contribution of a risk factor to a disease or a death is quantified using the population attributable fraction (PAF). PAF is the proportional reduction in population disease or mortality that would occur if exposure to a risk factor was reduced to an alternative ideal exposure scenario (e.g., no tobacco use). Many diseases are caused by multiple risk factors, and individual risk factors may interact in their impact on overall risk of disease. As a result, PAFs for individual risk factors often overlap and add up to more than 100%."

See: https://www.who.int/healthinfo/global_burden_disease/metrics_paf/en

17. **D.** Lead (Pb) is not used in tooth fillings. Mercury amalgam is used.

In the United States, approximately 4 million households have children living in them that are being exposed to high levels of lead. There are approximately half a million U.S. children aged 1–5 with blood lead levels above 5 micrograms per deciliter (μg/dL), the reference level at which the Centers for Disease Control and Prevention (CDC) recommends public health actions be initiated.

Dental amalgam is a mixture of metals, consisting of liquid (elemental) mercury and a powdered alloy composed of silver, tin, and copper. Approximately 50% of dental amalgam is elemental mercury by weight. The chemical properties of elemental mercury allow it to react with and bind together the silver/copper/tin alloy particles to form an amalgam.

See: https://www.cdc.gov/nceh/lead/default.htm

https://www.fda.gov/medical-devices/dental-amalgam/about -dental-amalgam-fillings

18. **D.** The world has experienced a gradual demographic transition from patterns of high fertility and high mortality rates to low fertility and delayed mortality. The transition begins with declining infant and childhood mortality, in part because of effective public health measures. Lower childhood mortality contributes initially to a longer life expectancy and a younger population. Declines in fertility rates generally follow, and improvements in adult health lead to an older population. These demographic transitions have modified the shape of the global age distribution.

See: https://www.cdc.gov/mmwr/preview/mmwrhtml/mm5206a2.htm

19. **C.** The world has experienced an epidemiologic transition in the leading causes of death, from infectious disease and acute illness to chronic disease and degenerative illness. Developed countries in North America, Europe, and the Western Pacific already have undergone this epidemiologic transition, and other countries are at different stages of progression.

See: https://www.cdc.gov/mmwr/preview/mmwrhtml/mm5206a2.htm

20. **C.** It is not (yet) possible to have a perfectly complete scientific understanding of gene–environment–behavior interactions, and this is not a concern. Most diseases result from a complex interaction between an individual's genetic make-up and environmental agents.

See: https://www.23andme.com/?myg01=true

https://www.niehs.nih.gov/health/topics/science/gene-env/index .cfm

21. **A.** An organizational strategic plan provides a local health department and its stakeholders with a clear picture of where it is headed, what it plans to achieve, the methods by which it will succeed, and the measures to monitor progress.

See: https://www.naccho.org/uploads/downloadable-resources/Pro grams/Public-Health-Infrastructure/StrategicPlanningGuideFinal.pdf

https://www.cdc.gov/program/performance/fy2000plan/2000ii.htm

22. **A.** To be effective, global health security must address multiple disease threats from different parts of the world, not just a single country, or a single disease, or a single risk factor. This is the framework for the global health security agenda. The objective of the World Health Organization (WHO) is the attainment by all peoples of the highest possible level of health. Health, as defined in the WHO Constitution, is a state of complete physical, mental, and social well-being and not merely the absence of disease or infirmity.

The Global Health Security Agenda pursues a multilateral and multi-sectoral approach to strengthen both the global capacity and nations' capacity to prevent, detect, and respond to human and animal infectious disease threats whether naturally occurring or accidentally or deliberately spread.

See: https://healthydocuments.org/appendices/doc49.html

https://www.ghsagenda.org

23. **C.** The forces that drive the rise of chronic diseases, including demographic aging, rapid urbanization, and the globalization of unhealthy lifestyles, lie beyond the direct control of the health sector.

See: https://www.who.int/social_determinants/en

24. **B.** Community health focuses on the health characteristics of populations within a shared geographical area. The World Health Organization has a broader definition of community health, including environmental, social, and economic resources to sustain emotional and physical well-being among people in ways that advance their aspirations and satisfy their needs in their unique environment.

The Centers for Disease Control and Prevention (CDC) views population health as an interdisciplinary, customizable approach that allows health departments to connect practice to policy for change to happen locally. This approach utilizes nontraditional partnerships among different sectors of the community—public health, industry, academia, healthcare, local government entities, and so on, to achieve positive health outcomes.

Goodman, R. A., Bunnell, R., & Posner, S. F. (2014). What is community health? Examining the meaning of an evolving field in public health. *Preventive Medicine, 67* (Suppl. 1), S58–61. doi:10.1016/j.ypmed.2014.07.028

See: https://www.aspph.org/study/community-health

https://www.cdc.gov/pophealthtraining/whatis.html

https://www.healthypeople.gov/2020/topics-objectives/topic/global-health

25. **B.** The World Health Organization uses Disability-Adjusted Life Years (DALYs) as a composite measure of disease burden. The estimates do not include infant mortality rates as an explicit input.

See: https://www.who.int/healthinfo/global_burden_disease/metrics_daly/en

26. **B.** Heart disease (noncommunicable) is the leading cause of mortality in the United States (2016).

See: https://www.cdc.gov/nchs/fastats/leading-causes-of-death.htm

27. **A.** Lower back pain is the leading cause of disability in the United States.

See: http://www.healthdata.org/united-states

28. **C.** Cancers are not one of the top 10 leading causes of disability worldwide.

See: http://www.healthdata.org/gbd

29. **C.** One Health is the idea that the health of people is connected to the health of animals and our shared environment. Learn why One Health is important and how, by working together, we can achieve the best health for everyone.

The Global Influenza Strategy for 2019–2030 provides a framework for the World Health Organization (WHO), countries, and partners to approach influenza holistically through tailored national programs—from surveillance to disease prevention and control—with the goal of strengthening seasonal prevention and control and preparedness for future pandemics. Controlling outbreaks in farm animals is as important as controlling outbreaks in humans.

See: https://www.cdc.gov/features/one-health-connection/index.html

https://www.who.int/influenza/en

https://www.who.int/influenza/global_influenza_strategy_2019_2030/en

https://wwwnc.cdc.gov/eid/article/16/8/10-0673_article

30. **A.** Most people affected by emergencies will experience psychological distress, which for most people will improve over time, but without adequate healthcare, the consequences may be lifelong. Obesity, increased smoking, and diabetes may be secondary outcomes of psychological distress.

See: https://www.who.int/news-room/fact-sheets/detail/mental-health-in-emergencies

31. **C.** Only smallpox has been eradicated from human populations.

See: https://www.who.int/csr/disease/smallpox/en

32. B. Polio has not been eradicated in Nigeria.

Poliomyelitis (polio) is a highly infectious viral disease, which mainly affects young children. The virus is transmitted by person-to-person to spread mainly through the fecal-oral route or, less frequently, by a common vehicle (e.g., contaminated water or food) and multiplies in the intestine, from where it can invade the nervous system and can cause paralysis.

See: http://polioeradication.org/where-we-work/nigeria

https://www.who.int/topics/poliomyelitis/en

33. D. The World Health Organization (WHO) does not use the U.S. Department of Health and Human Services agenda exclusively to prioritize the organization's programs although the United States is a member of WHO.

See: https://www.who.int/dg/priorities/en

34. D. Every year, more than 8 million people die from tobacco use. Most tobacco-related deaths occur in low- and middle-income countries, areas that are targets of intensive tobacco industry interference and marketing. To assist countries in implementing the Framework Convention on Tobacco Control, the World Health Organization (WHO) introduced MPOWER, a package of technical measures and resources, each of which corresponds to at least one provision of the WHO Framework Convention on Tobacco Control (FCTC).

See: https://www.who.int/health-topics/tobacco

35. A. The PRECEDE–PROCEED model is a comprehensive structure for assessing health needs for designing, implementing, and evaluating health promotion and other public health programs to meet those needs. The model applies a medical perspective to public health, even though its focus is health promotion, rather than treatment of disease.

See: http://www.lgreen.net/precede.htm

https://www.cdc.gov/publichealthgateway/cha/assessment.html

36. D. The PRECEDE model does not include policy constructs in educational and environmental development.

PRECEDE is an acronym for Predisposing, Reinforcing, and Enabling Constructs in Educational/Environmental Diagnosis and Evaluation.

See: http://www.lgreen.net/precede.htm

37. D. PROCEED is an acronym for Policy, Regulatory, and Organizational Constructs in Educational and Environmental Development.

See: http://www.lgreen.net/precede.htm

38. B. PRECEDE provides the structure for planning a targeted and focused public health program, and has five phases involving assessment of community factors:

- Social assessment: Determination of the social problems and needs of a given population and identification of desired results
- Epidemiological assessment: Identification of the health determinants of the identified problems and setting of priorities and goals

- Ecological assessment: Analysis of the behavioral and environmental determinants that predispose, reinforce, and enable the behaviors and lifestyles that are identified.
- Identify administrative and policy factors that influence implementation and match appropriate interventions that encourage desired and expected changes
- Implementation of interventions

See: http://www.lgreen.net/precede.htm

   https://www.ruralhealthinfo.org/toolkits/health-promotion/2/program-models/precede-proceed

39. A. PROCEED covers the next steps after comprehensive community assessments, and it includes designing interventions and assessing resources available in the context of logistic considerations for implementing intervention programs.

Green, L., & Kreuter, M. (2005). *Health program planning: An educational and ecological approach* (4th ed.). New York, NY: McGraw-Hill.

See: http://www.lgreen.net/precede.htm

   https://www.ruralhealthinfo.org/toolkits/health-promotion/2/program-models/precede-proceed

40. D. PRECEDE includes the "social assessment" phase where the social problems of a population are identified in the context of its needs, and desired outcomes are specified. The PRECEDE phase does not involve evaluation of process, impact, or outcome.

Green, L., & Kreuter, M. (2005). *Health program planning: An educational and ecological approach* (4th ed.). New York, NY: McGraw-Hill.

See: https://www.ruralhealthinfo.org/toolkits/health-promotion/2/program-models/precede-proceed

41. D. PROCEED includes the "impact evaluation" phase that includes an assessment of the change in behavior resulting from the intervention. PROCEED does not include assessment of ecological, epidemiological, or social factors, which are all associated with PRECEDE.

Green, L.,& Kreuter, M. (2005). *Health program planning: An educational and ecological approach* (4th ed.). New York, NY: McGraw-Hill.

See: https://www.ruralhealthinfo.org/toolkits/health-promotion/2/program-models/precede-proceed

42. D. Communities are motivated in the Community Readiness Model by the difference between current health situations or behaviors and the desire to reach a goal.

See: https://www.ruralhealthinfo.org/toolkits/health-promotion/2/program-models/community-readiness

43. D. The Community Readiness Model does not include developing and maintaining capacity and power to produce lasting change. The stages of community readiness model include awareness levels and resistance.

See: https://www.ruralhealthinfo.org/toolkits/health-promotion/2/program-models/community-readiness

Kelly, K. J., Edwards, R. W., Comello, M. L. G., Plested, B. A., Thurman, P. J., & Slater, M. D. (2003). The Community Readiness Model: A complementary approach to social marketing. *Marketing Theory, 3*(4), 411–426. doi:10.1177/1470593103042006

44. C. The Community Organization Model (COM) is not characterized by denial or resistance, where there is little recognition or concern among community members about the health issue. Rather, COM emphasizes disentangling of risk factors underlying suboptimal health conditions, intersectoral and collaborative decision-making, and capacity building to sustain advances in healthcare.

Eldredge, L. K. B., Markham, C. M., Ruiter, R. A., Fernández, M. E., Kok, G., & Parcel, G. S. (2016). *Planning health promotion programs: An intervention mapping approach.* New York, NY: John Wiley & Sons.

See: https://www.ruralhealthinfo.org/toolkits/health-promotion/2/program-models/community-organization

45. B. An interdisciplinary team of experts is essential for public health systems and their sustainability. Sustainability planning is necessary to withstand shifting health priorities, local economies, and unpredictable funding opportunities.

See: https://www.ruralhealthinfo.org/toolkits/health-promotion/5/sustainability-strategies

https://www.ruralhealthinfo.org/toolkits/health-promotion/5/sustainability

46. B. The vision statement of a public health organization should communicate the organization's ideal conditions of the population they serve. The vision statement should receive input from the hierarchy of the organization and input from all stakeholders.

See: https://www.cdc.gov/eeo/aboutus/mission.htm

47. A. The vision statement of a public health organization should describe the actual activities of the organization. The vision statement should receive input from the hierarchy of the organization, and input from all stakeholders.

For example: A world in which everyone can live healthy, productive lives:

"I envision a world in which everyone can live healthy, productive lives, regardless of who they are or where they live. I believe the global commitment to sustainable development – enshrined in the Sustainable Development Goals – offers a unique opportunity to address the social, economic and political determinants of health and to improve the health and well-being of people everywhere. Achieving this vision will require a strong, effective WHO that is able to meet emerging challenges and achieve the health objectives of the Sustainable Development Goals. We need a WHO – fit for the 21st century – that belongs to all, equally. We need a WHO that is efficiently managed, adequately resourced and results driven, with a strong focus on transparency, accountability and value for money."

See: https://www.who.int/dg/vision

48. D. Objectives are statements describing the results to be achieved, and the manner in which they will be achieved. SMART attributes are used to develop a clearly defined objective.

- Specific: Includes the "who," "what," and "where." Use only one action verb to avoid issues with measuring success.
- Measurable: Focuses on "how much" change is expected
- Achievable: Realistic given program resources and planned implementation
- Relevant: Relates directly to program/activity goals
- Time-bound: Focuses on "when" the objective will be achieved

See: https://www.cdc.gov/std/Program/pupestd/Developing%20 Program%20Goals%20and%20Objectives.pdf

49. B. The stated strategies of a public health organization should specify the approaches and processes through which each objective will be pursued. For example, the Centers for Disease Control and Prevention's (CDC) strategy is based on action plans and detailed measures of success:

Opioids—Reduce U.S. drug overdose mortality by at least 15% by 2021

Opioid data—Reduce data delay from 3 months to 1 week for nonfatal opioid overdoses

Influenza—By 2021, increase flu vaccination coverage rates among children to 65% and among pregnant women to 55%

HIV/AIDS—Eliminate new HIV infections in 10 years

Vaccine-preventable—Increase by 10% up-to-date HPV vaccination coverage rate in 2021 compared to 2017 (48.6%)

Rapid response—By 2022, triple the number of CDC rapid response teams and trained incident managers

Vector-borne—Reduce by 75% cases of Rocky Mountain spotted fever in U.S. tribal communities

Hepatitis C—Reduce hepatitis C-related deaths by 65% in 10 targeted states by 2024, as a first step to a national program

Antibiotics—Reduce by 50% inappropriate antibiotic use in outpatient settings by 2020

Global—Zero countries with wild poliovirus

Diabetes—Reduce the number of new diabetes diagnoses from 1.4 M in 2018 to 1.1 M cases per year by 2025

AMD—Increase the routine use of advanced molecular detection from 37 states (2017) to all states (2019)

See: https://www.cdc.gov/about/organization/strategic-framework/ index.html

50. D. The action plan of a public health organization should specify potential barriers or resistance likely to be encountered in pursuing the organization's mission.

For example, the Centers for Disease Control and Prevention (CDC) created an action plan to improve how the agency creates and shares health information and provides public health services to different audiences.

See: https://www.cdc.gov/healthliteracy/planact/cdcplan.html

https://www.cdc.gov/healthyschools/tths/fus_team-action-plan-template-508.pdf

51. **D.** Program goals and objectives establish criteria and standards against which program performance can be measured. Unless constrained by special circumstances, objectives should not be for an unlimited period of time.

Attributes of SMART objectives:

- Specific: Includes the "who," "what," and "where." Use only one action verb to avoid issues with measuring success
- Measurable: Focuses on "how much" change is expected
- Achievable: Realistic given program resources and planned implementation
- Relevant: Relates directly to program/activity goals
- Time-bound: Focuses on "when" the objective will be achieved

See: https://www.cdc.gov/std/Program/pupestd/Developing%20Program%20Goals%20and%20Objectives.pdf

52. **A.** Predetermined objectives are not included in the PATCH model, as it will be counter-productive.

The PATCH model was developed by the Centers for Disease Control and Prevention (CDC) in partnership with state and local health departments and community groups. Following are the five phases included in PATCH:

- Community members participate in the process.
- Data guide the development of programs.
- Participants develop a comprehensive health promotion strategy.
- Evaluation emphasizes feedback and program improvement.
- The community capacity for health promotion is increased.

See: http://www.lgreen.net/patch.pdf

https://www.cdc.gov/publichealthgateway/cha/assessment.html

53. **D.** The MAPP model was developed by the National Association of County Health Officials to support local health agencies in identifying strategic topics that will make a difference in their populations, visioning outcomes, and informing action cycles. Doing a program design is not a step in the MAPP model.

See: https://www.naccho.org/programs/public-health-infrastructure/performance-improvement/community-health-assessment/mapp

https://www.thecommunityguide.org/content/mapp-mobilizing-action-through-planning-and-partnerships-framework

54. **C.** Visioning is not one of the steps in the intervention mapping model. The model consists of the following:

Needs assessment or problem analysis, identifying what, if anything, needs to be changed and for whom

Matrices of change objectives by combining (sub-) behaviors (performance objectives) with behavior

Identifying which beliefs should be targeted by the intervention

Selecting theory-based intervention methods that match the determinants into which the identified beliefs aggregate, and translate these into practical applications that satisfy the parameters for effectiveness of the selected methods

Integrating methods and the practical applications into an organized program

Planning for adoption, implementation, and sustainability of the program in real-life contexts

Generating an evaluation plan to conduct effect and process evaluations.

See: https://interventionmapping.com

https://www.cdc.gov/globalhealth/healthprotection/fetp/training_modules/17/Program-Planning_PW_Final_09252013.pdf

Kay Bartholomew, L., Parcel, G. S., Kok, G., & Gottlieb, N. H. (2006). *Planning Health Promotion Programs: An Intervention Mapping Approach.* New York, NY: John Wiley and Sons.

55. **D.** Consult is not one of the steps in the MAP-IT model.

Mobilize, Assess, Plan, Implement, and Track are the five steps in MAP-IT model:

- Mobilize partners
- Assess the needs of your community
- Create a plan to reach Healthy People 2020 objectives
- Implement the plan
- Track your community's progress

See: https://www.healthypeople.gov/2020/tools-and-resources/Program-Planning

56. **A.** The most common types of evaluation include the following:

- Formative evaluation ensures that a program or program activity is feasible, appropriate, and acceptable before it is fully implemented. It is usually conducted when a new program or activity is being developed or when an existing one is being adapted or modified.
- Process/implementation evaluation determines whether program activities have been implemented as intended.
- Outcome/effectiveness evaluation measures program effects in the target population by assessing the progress in the outcomes or outcome objectives that the program is to achieve.
- Impact evaluation assesses program effectiveness in achieving its ultimate goals.

See: https://www.cdc.gov/std/Program/pupestd/Types%20of%20Evaluation.pdf

57. **D.** Giving the project a letter grade is not typically one of the steps in an evaluation process. According to the Centers for Disease Control and Prevention (CDC), there is no one "right" evaluation. Rather, a host of evaluation questions may arise over the life of a program that might reasonably be asked at any point in time. Addressing these questions about program effectiveness means paying attention to documenting and measuring the implementation of the program and its success in achieving intended outcomes, and using such information to be accountable to key stakeholders.

See: https://www.cdc.gov/eval/guide/execsummary/index.htm

https://www.cdc.gov/eval/guide/index.htm

https://www.cdc.gov/std/Program/pupestd/Types%20of%20 Evaluation.pdf

58. **A.** The American Evaluation Association's (AEA) guiding principles for program evaluators includes maintaining professional competence as an evaluator, integrity and honesty, and respect for people. Engaging stakeholders is not one of the guiding principles for evaluators according to AEA.

See: https://www.eval.org/p/cm/ld/fid=51

59. **D.** An evaluator of a public health program should take into consideration the social and political context of the program, ethics, and social equity. Potential cost is not included as a guiding principle for respect for people.

See: https://www.eval.org/p/cm/ld/fid=51

60. **D.** Constellation is an astronomical term, and not included in the prevalent social ecological model in public health.

See: https://www.ruralhealthinfo.org/toolkits/health-promotion/2/ theories-and-models/ecological

8

Program Management

INTRODUCTION

The title of "program manager" is often encountered in advertisements of employment opportunities for public health agencies. In a way, this reflects the compartmentalization of public health initiatives into programs that are typically demarcated by population-served, budget-restricted, and time-limited initiatives. A program's success or failure is often defined by achievement of specific goals, for example, the number or proportion of children of a certain age group that are vaccinated over a given period of time. The responsibilities of a program manager vary widely and may include knowledge of principles and practices of management including budgeting, program management and office practices, personnel management including effective supervision and performance management, health administration, and organizational principles and procedures of public health programs, such as chronic diseases, communicable diseases, public health statistics, health education, and nutrition. The required skills may include planning, organizing, coordinating, and implementing public health programs and services on a comprehensive regional level to meet community needs; the ability to communicate effectively both verbally and in writing, with a wide variety of audiences; skills for preparing, analyzing, evaluating, and drawing logical conclusions from data; and selecting appropriate alternatives and implementing recommendations. Public health program managers may also be required to integrate a variety of activities and services to achieve goals, objectives, and priorities; and to establish and maintain effective working relationships with all levels of federal, state, and county employees, public officials, and members of the public. Public health program managers typically have strong analytical and problem-solving skills, and must also be able to establish the roles, responsibilities, and action steps to manage and evaluate the effectiveness of programs. The questions in this section focus on key components of public health program management. These components include opportunities to

- Develop program or organizational budgets with justification
- Defend a programmatic or organizational budget

- Operate programs within current and forecasted budget constraints
- Respond to changes in financial resources
- Develop proposals to secure financial support
- Participate in the development of contracts or other agreements for the provision of services
- Ensure implementation of contracts or other agreements for the provision of services
- Leverage existing resources for program management
- Identify methods for assuring health program sustainability
- Give constructive feedback to others about their performance on the team
- Develop monitoring and evaluation frameworks to assess programs
- Implement a community health plan
- Implement programs to ensure community health

■ QUESTIONS

1. The United States' public health system is a complex network of people, systems, and organizations working at the local, state, and national levels. The U.S. public health system is distinct from other parts of the healthcare system in the following key respect:

   A. Its primary emphasis is preventing disease and disability.
   B. It focuses on individual health rather than population health.
   C. It is cheaper to implement and maintain.
   D. It is decentralized.

2. Bioterrorism is defined as the unlawful release of biologic agents or toxins to kill or sicken people, animals, or plants with the intent to intimidate or coerce a government or civilian population. The following are examples of bioterrorism acts that have been documented in the United States EXCEPT

   A. Intentional contamination of salad bars with *Salmonella* in Oregon (1984)
   B. Intentional contamination of muffins with *Shigella* in Texas (1996)
   C. Intentional contamination of mail by *Bacillus anthracis* in Washington, DC (2001)
   D. Intentional contamination of water by *Legionella* in California (2017)

3. John Snow (March 15, 1813–June 16, 1858) is considered the first to use geographic information science to solve public health problems. What exactly was his accomplishment in this respect?

   A. He mapped the location of factories producing soot and the incidence of asthma.
   B. He mapped the location of swamps and the incidence of malaria.
   C. He mapped the location of water supplies and the incidence of cholera.

    D. He mapped the location of mercury mines and the incidence of Mad Hatter's disease.

4. Which of the following statements is accurate regarding the history of public health?

    A. The miasma theory of disease displaced the germ theory of disease based on evidence.

    B. John Snow was a fervent advocate of the miasma theory of disease.

    C. Jonas Salk developed the hepatitis B vaccine to prevent viral hepatitis infection in the United States.

    D. Robert Koch postulated the germ theory of disease.

5. Natural disasters and war share common threads in terms of public health preparedness. These include which of the following?

    A. Destruction of infrastructure that supports public health

    B. Emergence of chronic diseases due to immobilization of populations

    C. Amelioration of mental health problems

    D. Solutions based on political negotiations

6. There is wide variability among societies across the world in public acceptance of genetically engineered food products. As a public health specialist, which of the following is the best argument in favor of accepting genetically engineered foods?

    A. Although the risks are unknown, the potential benefits are sufficient.

    B. Genetically engineered foods should be adequately labeled so that people are informed about the risks and benefits.

    C. The risks are negligible compared to the benefits of food for all.

    D. Only unreasonable environmental activists complain about such important advances in science that can help people.

7. Basic public health infrastructure includes all of the following EXCEPT

    A. Skilled workforce

    B. Organizational capacity

    C. Information systems

    D. Unlimited resources

8. The application of knowledge, skills, tools, and techniques to project activities to satisfy project requirements is known as

    A. Program management

    B. Project management

    C. Budget management

    D. Requirements management

9. The application of knowledge, skills, tools, and techniques to coordinate several project activities to satisfy program requirements is known as

    A. Program management

    B. Project management

C. Budget management
D. Requirements management

10. A county public health agency has just been awarded the contract for an important community-based project. The agency director has asked you, as the project manager, to create the project charter and send it to her so that she can review and approve it. To create the project charter, you need the project's statement of work (SOW). What should you do?

A. Create the SOW yourself since you are the project manager
B. Look for the SOW in your organizational process assets
C. Ask the funding agency to provide you with the approved SOW
D. Ask your agency director to provide you with the SOW

11. You are overhauling the public website of your public health agency. Your agency director has a great deal of authority regarding project decisions, but you recently discovered that he doesn't have much interest in your project. To complete the project successfully, you need your director's continuous support. What stakeholder management strategy should you use with your director?

A. Keep the director satisfied
B. Manage the director closely
C. Monitor the director's actions
D. Keep the director informed

12. A project manager is leading the construction of a public health laboratory. The project sponsor asks the project manager to email him a project document that was presented during the last project status meeting. The project sponsor states that he has forgotten the name of the document, but he remembers it contained the description, owner, source, priority, and status of construction requirements. Which project document is the project sponsor requesting?

A. The requirements management plan
B. The requirements traceability matrix
C. The scope management plan
D. The work breakdown structure

13. You are managing a public health project in Alaska to control mosquitoes suspected of bringing vector-borne disease associated with climate change. Due to the large scope of the project along with the regulatory and environmental considerations, the development of a detailed project management plan will be critical. As a starting point for initial project planning, what is the first thing you should do?

A. Conduct a project kick-off meeting to inform and engage stakeholders and gain commitment
B. Review the project charter to understand the high-level information about the project
C. Begin the process of identifying stakeholders so they can be engaged as necessary for project planning
D. Share the project scope statement with the project team for a common understanding of project deliverables

14. You are a program manager planning a project to develop a new diabetes prevention strategy, and you are currently in the process of determining, documenting, and managing stakeholder needs and requirements to meet project objectives. A project stakeholder has suggested that it would be helpful to have a visual depiction showing how healthcare providers, patience, and targeted population will interact. You like the idea and want to address it. What is the best way to implement the stakeholder's suggestion?

   A. Develop a context diagram
   B. Design an affinity diagram
   C. Create a fishbone diagram
   D. Build a matrix diagram

15. You are managing the expansion of public health services for your county, and you have asked your project team to calculate the current earned value metrics to determine the project performance. Your team reports back that the project's to-complete performance index (TCPI) is 0.9 based on the budget at completion (BAC). Which of the following is true regarding your project's current situation as reflected by this TCPI value?

   A. The project is within budget.
   B. The project is over budget.
   C. The project is behind schedule.
   D. The project is ahead of schedule.

16. You have just taken over a program to overhaul the public health agency's vaccination campaign. During your first week, you determine that the staff spend at least 80% of their time responding to unexpected requests for information from various stakeholders. Because of these interruptions, your staff cannot focus on their assigned project activities, which is resulting in missed opportunities. What should you do first?

   A. Immediately tell the staff to stop responding to unexpected requests since it is not their responsibility
   B. Push the staff to respond to all the requests faster so that they can perform their assigned project activities
   C. Ask the staff to forward all stakeholder inquiries to you so that they can focus on their originally planned tasks
   D. Review the communications management plan to understand how stakeholder requests should be processed

17. You are working with your suicide prevention team on estimating how much time each activity will take. One of the documents you are using contains information on categories of tasks, materials, and equipment required to complete your project. You are also interested in reviewing the skill levels of your tasks, required certifications, and levels of your supplies. Which of the following documents would you PRIMARILY refer to for this purpose?

   A. Resource distribution structure
   B. Work distribution structure
   C. Risk distribution structure
   D. Skills distribution structure

18. During an inspection of a batch of fliers commissioned for a campaign to pre-vent drunk driving, the team detects the same defect in the flier that has already been identified during a previous inspection. The project manager is confused how this could have happened since a change request was approved to correct the defect. After discussing the issue with the team, the project manager learns that the team never implemented the approved change request. What could have helped prevent this situation?

    A. Holding an approved change requests review
    B. Conducting a retrospective meeting
    C. Performing a root cause analysis
    D. Creating a quality report

19. You are the program manager for diabetes prevention at your healthcare agency, and you are managing a project to update the packaging and digital media for a snack food to promote healthy nutrition and prevent obesity and diabetes. The project is well underway, and you are currently actively collect-ing and storing information about each deliverable team's progress, creating forecasts for your agency director, distributing work performance reports and planning presentations to key stakeholders, and verifying delivery. Which pro-cess are you performing?

    A. Manage communications
    B. Monitor communications
    C. Manage stakeholder engagement
    D. Plan communications management

20. In your role as program manager for cardiovascular disease prevention, you have recently been assigned to lead a project on motivating physical activity. The project is halfway into execution. The project has many stakeholders, and you are trying to determine how to engage them effectively. Which of the fol-lowing will BEST help you in this effort?

    A. Project management plan
    B. Project charter
    C. Work performance reports
    D. Procurement documents

21. Two new M.P.H. practicum students from a nearby university have just joined the project you are leading. The project is large and involves many stakeholders. You want to get the students up to speed with the overall dynamics of the project and engage effectively with the project stakeholders. What should you do?

    A. Ask the students to record any issues they encounter into the issue log
    B. Review the stakeholder register with the students
    C. Schedule a meeting with the students and all project stakeholders
    D. Submit a change request to update the stakeholder engagement plan

22. The county health fair is coming up soon, and a project manager had originally planned to use both of the company's printers simultaneously for a health pro-motion flier but has just learned that one of them will be unavailable. The project manager adjusts the schedule so that the documents are printed sequentially

using the one remaining printer. Unfortunately, this action affects the critical path and delays the planned finish date of the project. What tool or technique has the project manager used in this situation?

A. Fast tracking
B. Resource smoothing
C. Crashing
D. Resource leveling

23. A new global health project is starting, and the team members come from all over the world. The project manager has concerns about communications. What should the project manager do first?

A. Implement an online tool to enable the team members to chat among themselves
B. Enroll the project team members in cultural training to raise cultural awareness
C. Nothing; The business world has been multicultural for so long that there should be no issues
D. Funnel all communications through the project manager to avoid miscommunication

24. An international global health project is entering its final phase. Some work in this phase must be done in a foreign country. Unsure if state policy requires a full-time employee onsite for project work in that country, which project artifact should the project scheduler reference?

A. Team management plan
B. Stakeholder engagement plan
C. Stakeholder register
D. Resource breakdown structure

25. You are leading a project to build a public health clinic, and you are looking for local contractors to outsource some of the construction work. You are in the process of preparing the bid package for prospective contractors. Which of the following documents would you leave out of the package?

A. Request for proposal
B. Statement of work
C. Independent cost estimates
D. Source selection criteria

26. As a program manager for a small university's health promotion and wellness program, you are currently in the process of selecting a vendor to develop a tutorial and other training materials for a new course in student wellness. Several professors are interested in submitting proposals for funds to develop the course. During an information workshop, one of the professors asks about ownership of the intellectual property that will be created from the project. Which project document should have this information at this stage of the project?

A. Request for proposals
B. Requirements documentation

C. Source selection criteria

D. Procurement contract

27. You are managing the development of a new blood pressure cuff for a pharmaceutical company with interests in preventing hypertension, and the company provided you with the objectives and description of the cuff. You and your team are decomposing the company's high-level requirements to the level of detail needed to design the blood pressure cuff and therefore define the scope of the product. In what activity are you involved?

A. Technical performance analysis

B. Statistical analyses

C. Define activities

D. Product analysis

28. You are in charge of a pharmaceutical project, where human trials are to start soon. The director is thrilled about the success of the trials up to this point. She announces that the size of the patient pool for the trials should double from the one originally planned, and results should be tracked in the new system launching this week. What should the project manager do first?

A. Ramp up production to match the demand of the director

B. Consider what might be included in a change request

C. Adjust the scope baseline to reflect the increased trial size

D. Communicate the change of direction with the stakeholders

29. You are managing a program on smoking cessation.
As part of the process to develop the scope statement for the program, you specify the deliverables for the program, include the requirements under which the outcomes will be accepted, and explicitly state what is out of program scope. What should you do next?

A. Obtain approval of the program scope statement

B. Include the acceptance criteria in the scope statement

C. Determine who decides the program is successful

D. Describe outcome scope in the scope statement

30. The Orange County Health Improvement Partnership created a dashboard viewable by all project stakeholders to display various statuses for disease burden, using standard red, yellow, and green colors. Throughout project execution, to meet the needs of the project and some of the project stakeholders, the project manager has been adding more colors to reflect additional statuses. This situation has created confusion among some of the partners over the status naming conventions and meanings. What should the project manager do?

A. Revert the status to the standard of red, yellow, green

B. Explain the meaning of the new statuses to the partners

C. Remove statuses from the dashboard to avoid confusion

D. Add a simpler status for the partners who are confused

31. Imagine that you are managing the social determinants team for the local branch of the American Lung Association.

Up until now, your project team has allowed the use of flextime where project team members may take time off during regular business hours and make up the time during the evening hours or weekends. Recently, excessive use of flextime has become a roadblock as some team members are not available when needed. The team feels they should set a standard that flextime is only to be used for personal emergencies. How should you handle this situation?

A. Contact the human resources department to update the corporate policies to prohibit flextime
B. Submit a change request to update the team charter based on the team's inputs
C. Discuss the issue with the team and update the team charter accordingly
D. Do nothing as the team has already agreed to use flextime for personal emergencies only

32. You are managing the program to prevent opioid addiction for the state. The governor is concerned about possible ethics violations between opioid manufacturers and healthcare providers. What independent review can the governor order?

A. Team assessment
B. Performance review
C. Monte-Carlo analysis
D. Procurement audit

33. Imagine that you direct the public health program for an Alzheimer's Disease Prevention Organization (ADPO). You have completed a 9-month project, and you are in the closing stage. The project was completed on time and under budget and everyone in your department has congratulated you on your achievement. The vice president of ADPO heard about the success of your project and wants a summary overview of project performance so that he can talk about your success at the next board meeting. What should you provide to him?

A. Lessons learned repository
B. Project closure documents
C. Final lessons learned register
D. Final report

34. You are managing the needles exchange project that requires frequent input from the senior management team at your public health agency. Some of the past projects succeeded to engage the team; however, most failed as senior management is notorious throughout the agency for responding slowly and not attending meetings. What is the best strategy for the stakeholder engagement plan of the current project?

A. Patiently wait until management indicates that they are available to provide their input
B. Schedule regular, short update meetings at a constant time and convenient location
C. Review lessons learned from other projects involving the management stakeholders
D. Require one senior management representative to attend meetings or the project will be halted

35. Imagine that you are managing a project to reduce infant mortality in your district, and you are conducting the initial process of identifying stakeholders for a new infrastructure development project. You have just compiled a list of potential stakeholders' names. What should you do next?

    A. Invite the identified stakeholders to the project kick-off meeting
    B. Conduct stakeholder analysis
    C. Complete the project stakeholder management process
    D. Develop the stakeholder engagement plan

36. The John Wayne Airport in Orange County, California, is known for flight paths that prevent excessive noise levels for homeowners living near the airport. You are leading a project to construct a new runway at the airport. After completion of the project, the residents under the flight path of the new runway are complaining about noise levels and want the airport to compensate them for the diminished values of their homes, quality of life, and stress levels. What might you have missed earlier in the project?

    A. Including in the stakeholder register those with a contribution stake in the project
    B. Stakeholder analysis including consideration for those with an interest stake in the project
    C. A thorough review of the agreements prior to the development of the stakeholder register
    D. The inclusion of the affected homeowners in the project charter

37. Imagine that you are in charge of the program to purchase test kits for malaria infection, to be distributed at clinics in the Lower Mekong Delta region. During a bidder conference, a supplier asks why a section is missing from the request for quotation (RFQ). The project manager, realizing that an aspect of the project is indeed missing, becomes flustered and stumbles through a brief reply. When the seller responses were received, all but three fail to address the missing section. What is the best course of action?

    A. Hold the bidder conference again, and explain the importance of the point that was initially missed
    B. Select from the three vendors that submitted complete proposals
    C. Send a revised RFQ to all prospective suppliers and allow them the opportunity to resubmit their proposals
    D. Extend the deadline and allow all of the vendors to resubmit their proposals

38. Imagine that you are leading a project to develop a new online portal on health education. Together with your project team you reprioritize the product backlog, determine velocity for the past iterations, and adapt your work plans accordingly. Additionally, you facilitate retrospectives every 2 weeks. Which of the following processes describes the work you are performing?

    A. Monitor risks
    B. Manage quality
    C. Control schedule
    D. Develop schedule

39. Imagine that you are part of a cross-functional organizational development team with the goal of reducing homelessness as a strategy for improving mental health in your community. The team is piloting an adaptive approach to project management in an organization that has traditionally used a predictive approach. You realize that you have to tailor the template of the schedule management plan. Which of the following components of the template are you likely to tailor the most?

   A. The rules of performance measurement, the summary milestones, and the key deliverables
   B. The organizational procedures links, the units of measure, and the project organization charts
   C. The schedule model development, the release and iteration length, and the reporting formats
   D. The project schedule model maintenance, the level of accuracy, and the level of precision

40. Imagine that you work for an environmental health corporation. Your boss is giving you a rough outline of the scope, constraints, and risks involved in a prospective client's project to test the level of toxic chemicals in consumer products. The project is highly similar to another project you are currently finishing up. The client wants to know how long this project would take your team to complete. You think your team may need 2 months, but what should your answer be?

   A. "Let me run some numbers in a simulation and get back to you tomorrow."
   B. "Give us 2 months. We will knock it out just like the project that we are closing now."
   C. "If it truly resembles this project we are closing, it could be six to ten weeks."
   D. "Considering the uncertainty in scope, I estimate 3 months."

41. The tuberculosis prevention project team performs monthly risk audits for a project in which a large number of identified risks have been realized. So far, the risk responses have been appropriate, and reserves are sufficient. An executive for the requesting organization criticizes the project manager for doing risk audits improperly, stating that like all audits, outside independent resources need to perform risk audits. How should the project manager respond?

   A. Explain that risk audits can be performed either internally or externally as long as they follow the project management plan
   B. Agree with the executive and submit a change request to update the project management plan to have the audits conducted externally
   C. Follow the guidance provided by the executive and hire a team of external auditors to conduct the risk audits going forward
   D. Explain that if the current risk audits are not sufficient, then a comprehensive project audit should be carried out

42. A tuberculosis prevention project manager has just learned that the patients are not showing up to medication compliance meetings, saying they have other more important things to do. Since this behavior has already been identified

as a risk earlier in the project, the project manager escalates the issue to the pharmacy director who is the risk owner responsible for communicating with the patients in such situations. The pharmacy director is shocked to find out she is the assigned risk owner. What most likely went wrong?

A. The stakeholder register had the wrong risk owner.
B. The project manager did not follow the risk management plan.
C. The stakeholder has not read the risk register.
D. The project manager did not notify the stakeholder that he or she was the risk owner.

43. Urine concentrations of illicit drug testing services are still being billed to your program even though no additional services are required or requested. What is the best option for the project manager to take?

A. Confirm that no more services are needed, and the procurement agreements are closed
B. Close all agreements with all service providers engaged with the project
C. Forward the service bills to the project management office for further review and approval
D. Continue paying the bills until the project is formally closed to avoid claims

44. Imagine that you work in a public health organization where sharing of project information is of utmost importance. Project knowledge is shared on multiple systems, services, and Internet applications. The array of locations is becoming overwhelming for some of the project team members. What is the best option for the project manager to manage the project knowledge in this situation?

A. Close down some of the systems that the project team notes as burdensome
B. Consolidate or streamline sharing processes where possible
C. Compromise with the team to allow each to post in the tool they find most productive
D. Coordinate a weekly meeting to post all the team's knowledge at once

45. Imagine that you are managing the urban health program for Los Angeles. A key stakeholder has been resistant to the program's objectives, and the support of this stakeholder is vital to the success of the program. You have employed various engagement strategies that have been ineffective and need to determine the underlying reason that stakeholder engagement is not having the planned effect. What should the program manager do next?

A. Develop a stakeholder engagement assessment matrix
B. Conduct data analysis
C. Submit a change request to update the stakeholder engagement plan
D. Perform an alternatives analysis

46. As the program manager for geriatrics disease and injury prevention, you are planning a project to construct an elderly people's home that will include jacuzzi tubs among its numerous features. Due to technical constraints, it has been decided to eliminate the jacuzzi tubs from the final project requirements for safety and health reasons. You document the jacuzzi tubs as an explicit

scope exclusion in the project scope statement as well as update the requirements documentation to reflect this change. What should you do next?

A. Reflect the scope exclusion in the requirements traceability matrix
B. Document the status of the change in the change log
C. Record the elimination of the jacuzzi tubs as an issue in the issue log
D. Capture the exclusion of the jacuzzi tubs in the exclusion register

47. You are managing the development of a new smartphone-based m-Health initiative. You are planning the must-have features of the smartphone in detail so that work can begin, and the product can be released to the market as early as possible. The future features are unknown at the moment and will depend on what the competitors release. You will plan these features in greater detail later on. As you and your team create the work breakdown structure, what will you use to indicate the future features?

A. Control accounts
B. Rolling wave planning
C. Work packages
D. Planning packages

48. Imagine the project on gun violence that you have been managing for several years is now moving toward completion. Some of the project deliverables have been contracted to vendors. You begin to close the project and want to make sure all activities necessary for project closure are properly completed. Which of the following activities would you NOT perform as part of this process?

A. Reviewing the project exit criteria
B. Measuring stakeholders' satisfaction
C. Ensuring all costs are charged to the project
D. Closing procurements with vendors

49. Imagine that you work for NASA to design population health protocols for an eventual human colony on Mars. While working to determine the budget for an avionics project, NASA decides to hire a highly reputable financial analyst that has worked in the aerospace industry for three decades. Halfway through the project, a series of unanticipated risk events occur, and the project cannot pay its invoices. What is most likely to be the cause?

A. The control accounts were not correctly established.
B. The analyst did not identify risks properly.
C. Funding limit reconciliation was done incorrectly.
D. The management reserves were exhausted.

50. Imagine that you are the program manager for laboratory services at the Centers for Disease Control and Prevention. A new project manager is brought on your team. She wants to understand the process by which her particular project formally accepts deliverables. Which of the following will she have to reference?

A. The scope management plan
B. The stakeholder management plan
C. The quality management plan
D. The requirements management plan

51. Imagine that you are leading a team to upgrade the technology for identifying antibiotic-resistant infections in the community, within a project-oriented organizational structure. You were recently informed that one of your project team members falsified required certification in public health (CPH) on his or her resume, and you have verified the information as accurate. You want to terminate the team member's employment. What should you do first?

   A. Refer the issue to the employee's functional manager
   B. Seek guidance from the resource management plan
   C. Immediately terminate the employee for cause
   D. Review the enterprise environmental factors

52. During the most recent economic downturn in California, a program manager posts a positive risk that in that economic environment, cheaper resources may become available. On the way into work, the program manager hears about a competitor going out of business and contacts the competitor to acquire some equipment, materials, and supplies at a fraction of their normal value. What was the program manager doing?

   A. Executing a mitigation plan
   B. Reacting to a contingency plan trigger
   C. Transferring an identified risk
   D. Sharing a realized positive risk

53. As program manager on breast cancer screening, you are identifying stakeholders for a new product development project. Which of the following activities are you LEAST likely to perform in the creation of the stakeholder register?

   A. Assess any available project documentation and lessons learned from past projects
   B. Perform stakeholder analysis to develop a list of stakeholders with relevant information
   C. Submit a change request to update the stakeholder engagement plan
   D. Categorize the stakeholder's stakes including interest, rights, ownership, and contribution

54. As program manager on skin cancer screening, you are facilitating a first brainstorming session to identify individual risks as well as sources of overall project risk. The meeting attendees are struggling with the task, and the meeting is becoming unproductive. What action might you take to get the meeting back on track?

   A. Consult the risk register
   B. Adjourn the meeting
   C. Call in the project sponsor
   D. Use the "Risk Breakdown Structure" (RBS) as a prompt list

55. As the program manager for community health needs assessment for your public health organization, you are establishing the relative priorities of individual project risks that have been identified earlier in the project. Which of the following tasks are you LEAST likely to perform?

   A. Review the assumption log
   B. Examine the risk register

C. Research the stakeholder register

D. Create the risk report

56. Imagine that you are the program manager responsible for operating the call center for an emergency response agency. A previously unknown risk surfaces on a project and creates an issue that is estimated to cost $50,000. The project manager submits a change request to adjust the schedule baseline and uses the already approved contingency reserves to address the cost. What did the project manager do wrong?

A. Nothing. Sometimes, these risks are unpredictable.

B. The project manager did not account for all possible risks during project planning.

C. The project manager should not have included the schedule baseline in the change request.

D. The project manager used contingency reserves instead of management reserves.

57. Imagine that you are the program manager for a global health initiative with projects that have reached a stage where work is being done in 15 countries. Project team members need to know in which currency they are to report their cost data. Which of the following should they reference?

A. Cost baseline

B. Cost management plan

C. Cost estimates

D. Cost breakdown structure

58. Imagine that you are the program manager overseeing a project that is now 6 months into its 9-month projected duration, and the project manager is reporting that the project is at least 3 months behind schedule because certain key stakeholders were resistant to any changes that might occur as outcomes of the project. What might have been done differently during project planning to have avoided this situation?

A. Development of a stakeholder engagement assessment matrix

B. Creation of a comprehensive stakeholder register

C. Establishment of a more robust communications management plan

D. Better execution of the manage stakeholder engagement process

59. In a steering committee meeting for a project to build a new state-of-the-art electronic health records system, the committee chair reprimands the project manager for not using the company's file sharing system as required by the organization. The project manager explains that the project team chose a newer tool for the project, as it was much better. What most likely caused this situation?

A. The project manager did not research the enterprise environmental factors.

B. The project manager did not review the organizational process assets.

C. The project team did not investigate communication tools.

D. The project manager did nothing wrong.

60. In your Integrative Health Unit, a project manager is meeting with the program manager to review the decomposed deliverables for a new healthcare product. The project manager reviews the work breakdown structure and requests it to be arranged in the order that the work should be performed. Is the project manager correct in saying that the work breakdown structure should be ordered according to how the work will be performed?

A. The project manager is wrong. Work is decomposed and sequenced in the Define Activities process.

B. The project manager is correct. Since she has superiority, the Work Breakdown Structure (WBS) should be ordered the way she wants it to be done.

C. The project manager is wrong. The chronological order of tasks is defined in the Sequence Activities process.

D. The project manager is correct. When decomposing the work, the order of tasks must be considered.

▪ ANSWERS

1. **A.** Public health systems are commonly defined as "all public, private, and voluntary entities that contribute to the delivery of essential public health services within a jurisdiction." This concept ensures that all entities' contributions to the health and well-being of the community or state are recognized in assessing the provision of public health services. The public health system includes the following:

   - Public health agencies at state and local levels
   - Healthcare providers
   - Public safety agencies
   - Human service and charity organizations
   - Education and youth development organizations
   - Recreation and arts-related organizations
   - Economic and philanthropic organizations
   - Environmental agencies and organizations

   See: https://www.cdc.gov/publichealthgateway/publichealthservices/essentialhealthservices.html

   The U.S. healthcare system is the most expensive in the world (per capita). The National Health Expenditure Accounts (NHEA) are the official estimates of total healthcare spending in the United States. Dating back to 1960, the NHEA measures annual U.S. expenditures for healthcare goods and services, public health activities, government administration, the net cost of health insurance, and investment related to healthcare. The data are presented by type of service, sources of funding, and type of sponsor.

   U.S. healthcare spending grew 3.9% in 2017, reaching $3.5 trillion or $10,739 per person. As a share of the nation's gross domestic product, health spending accounted for 17.9%.

   See: https://www.cms.gov/research-statistics-data-and-systems/statistics -trends-and-reports/nationalhealthexpenddata/nationalhealthaccounts historical.html

   Public health governance structures vary from state to state. The relationship between state health agencies and regional/local public health departments also differs across states. These structural differences have important implications for the delivery of essential public health services. Identifying these differences is integral to understanding the roles, responsibilities, and authorities across levels of government for services provided within the community.

   Types of governance health structures:

   - Centralized or largely centralized structure: Local health units are primarily led by employees of the state.
   - Decentralized or largely decentralized structure: Local health units are primarily led by employees of local governments.
   - Mixed structure: Some local health units are led by employees of the state and some are led by employees of local government. No single structure predominates.

- Shared or largely shared structure: Local health units might be led by employees of the state or by employees of local government. If they are led by state employees, then local government has the authority to make fiscal decisions and/or issue public health orders; if they are led by local employees, then the state has authority.

See: https://www.cdc.gov/publichealthgateway/sitesgovernance/index
.html

2. **D.** On September 17, 1984, a disease control expert for the Wasco-Sherman Public Health Department began to receive reports of recent cases of gastroenteritis in persons who had eaten meals in either of two local restaurants in The Dalles several days before symptom onset. The scenario involved the September 1984 outbreak of gastroenteritis (an illness characterized by fever, vomiting, and diarrhea) caused by a specific bacterium, *Salmonella typhimurium.* This specific bacterium is a member of a much larger family of salmonella bacteria. The outbreak occurred among persons living in the community of The Dalles, Oregon. The Dalles (1980 population: 10,500) is the county seat of Wasco County (population: 21,000) and a region of orchards and wheat ranches. The Dalles is located off Interstate 84 and is a frequent stop for travelers. From 1980 through 1983, there had been only 16 isolates of salmonella reported by the local health department (the Wasco-Sherman Public Health Department), and of these, only eight were *Salmonella typhimurium.* In 1981, followers of Bhagwan Shree Rajneesh purchased a large ranch in Wasco County to build a new international headquarters for the guru. Construction of the commune was controversial because of issues involving cultural values and land use. Part of the commune's ranch was incorporated as the city of Rajneeshpuram, but the charter was challenged in the courts, effectively limiting new construction. Commune members believed that the outcome of the November 1984 elections for Wasco County commissioners would have an important impact on further land-use decisions. One measure commune members took to further their interests was to implement a national program to bus hundreds of homeless persons to the commune for the purpose of registering these persons to vote in the election.

See: https://www.cdc.gov/phlp/docs/FE15.pdf

Shigellosis is an infectious disease caused by a group of bacteria called *Shigella* (shih-GEHL-uh). Most who are infected with *Shigella* develop diarrhea, fever, and stomach cramps starting a day or two after they are exposed to the bacteria. Shigellosis usually resolves in 5 to 7 days. Some people who are infected may have no symptoms at all, but may still pass the *Shigella* bacteria to others. The spread of *Shigella* can be stopped by frequent and careful handwashing with soap and taking other hygiene measures.

In September 1996, the Federal Bureau of Investigation (FBI) investigated the theft of rare *Shigella* strains (not usually found in the United States) from a Dallas hospital laboratory that were used to contaminate food that sickened 13 people. While all 13 have since recovered, eight of them suffered from diarrhea and cramps and five were hospitalized. The Texas Department of Health in Austin determined that the bacteria found in the food matched a missing culture of *Shigella dysenteriae* from the microbiology lab at St. Paul Medical Center.

The bacteria were in the lab for testing and research. A former hospital lab employee was sentenced to 20 years in prison.

See: https://groups.google.com/forum/#!topic/alt.true-crime/842
EzFqUHu0

https://www.chicagotribune.com/news/ct-xpm-1996-11-12-961113
0006-story.html

Anthrax is a serious infectious disease caused by gram-positive, rod-shaped bacteria known as *Bacillus anthracis*. Although it is rare, people can get sick with anthrax if they come in contact with infected animals or contaminated animal products.

Soon after the terrorist attacks of 9/11, letters laced with anthrax began appearing in the U.S. mail. Five Americans were killed and 17 were sickened in what became the worst biological attacks in U.S. history. The ensuing investigation by the Federal Bureau of Investigation (FBI) and its partners—codenamed "Amerithrax"—has been one of the largest and most complex in the history of law enforcement.

In August 2008, Department of Justice and FBI officials announced a breakthrough in the case and released documents and information showing that charges were about to be brought against Dr. Bruce Ivins, who took his own life before those charges could be filed. On February 19, 2010, the Justice Department, the FBI, and the U.S. Postal Inspection Service formally concluded the investigation into the 2001 anthrax attacks and issued an Investigative Summary.

The Amerithrax Task Force—which consisted of roughly 25 to 30 full-time investigators from the FBI, the U.S. Postal Inspection Service, and other law enforcement agencies, as well as federal prosecutors from the District of Columbia and the Justice Department's Counterterrorism Section—expended hundreds of thousands of investigator work hours on this case. Their efforts involved more than 10,000 witness interviews on six different continents, the execution of 80 searches, and the recovery of more than 6,000 items of potential evidence during the course of the investigation. The case involved the issuance of more than 5,750 grand jury subpoenas and the collection of 5,730 environmental samples from 60 site locations. In addition, new scientific methods were developed that ultimately led to the break in the case—methods that could have a far-reaching impact on future investigations.

See: https://www.fbi.gov/history/famous-cases/amerithrax-or-anthrax
-investigation

3. **C.** In the year 1854 in London, England, a cramped neighborhood teemed with people and animals living in cramped and filthy domiciles. A deadly outbreak of cholera (*Vibrio cholera*) is spreading. Doctors and scientists believe it's caused by "miasma," or bad air. They theorize that particles from rotting matter and waste are getting into the air and making people sick.

Dr. John Snow, an accomplished physician, becomes convinced that something other than the air might be responsible for the illness. Through carefully mapping the outbreak, he finds that everyone affected has a single connection in common: They have all retrieved water from the local Broad Street pump. On September 8, 1854, Dr. Snow tested his theory by removing the pump's handle, effectively stopping the outbreak, proving his theory, and opening the door to modern epidemiology. Also in 1854, Dr. John Snow was the first to use maps and records to track the spread of a disease back to its source. Today, his ideas provide the foundation for how we find and curb disease all over the world.

See: https://blogs.cdc.gov/publichealthmatters/2017/03/a-legacy-of -disease-detectives

4. D.

- Germ theory replaced miasma theory, not the other way around.
- John Snow's cholera work discredited the miasma theory.
- Jonas Salk developed the vaccine for poliomyelitis.
- Edward Jenner worked on a smallpox vaccine.
- On March 24, 1882, Robert Koch announced to the Berlin Physiological Society that he had discovered the cause of tuberculosis. Three weeks later, on April 10, he published an article entitled "The Etiology of Tuberculosis". In 1884, in a second paper with the same title, he first expounded "Koch's Postulates," which have since become basic to studies of all infectious diseases. He had observed the bacillus in association with all cases of the disease, had grown the organism outside the body of the host, and had reproduced the disease in a susceptible host inoculated with a pure culture of the isolated organism.

See: https://www.cdc.gov/mmwr/preview/mmwrhtml/00000222.htm.

5. A. Every year natural disasters kill around 90,000 people and affect close to 160 million people worldwide. Natural disasters include earthquakes, tsunamis, volcanic eruptions, landslides, hurricanes, floods, wildfires, heat waves, and droughts. They have an immediate impact on human lives and often result in the destruction of the physical, biological, and social environment of the affected people, thereby having a longer-term impact on their health, well-being, and survival.

See: https://www.who.int/environmental_health_emergencies/natural_ events/en

Conflict will inevitably cause loss of lives, physical injuries, widespread mental distress, a worsening of existent malnutrition (particularly among children), and outbreaks of communicable diseases. Internally displaced and refugee populations are at particular risk. Common, preventable diseases, such as diarrhea, threaten life. Chronic illnesses that can normally be treated lead to severe suffering. The dangers of pregnancy and childbirth are amplified.

See: https://www.who.int/features/2003/iraq/briefings/iraq_briefing_ note/en

6. B. The U.S. Food and Drug Administration (FDA) recognizes that many consumers are interested in whether food ingredients are derived from genetically engineered plants and has issued guidance for manufacturers who wish to voluntarily label their foods as containing or not containing such ingredients. If manufacturers wish to label their food as not being produced using genetic engineering, we recommend they use terms such as "not genetically engineered," "not bioengineered," or "not genetically modified through the use of modern biotechnology."

Foods derived from genetically engineered plants must meet the same safety, labeling, and other regulatory requirements that apply to all foods regulated by the FDA.

As articulated in its 1992 "Statement of Policy: Foods Derived From New Plant Varieties," the agency is not aware of any information showing that foods derived from genetically engineered plants, as a class, differ from other foods in any meaningful or uniform way. These foods also don't present different or greater safety concerns than their nongenetically engineered counterparts. However, if a food derived from a genetically engineered plant is materially different from its traditional counterpart, the labeling of that food must disclose such differences.

The FDA has required additional labeling of food derived from a genetically-engineered source where it found that compositional differences resulted in material changes. For example, when the FDA learned during a consultation that a new canola oil had increased lauric acid content compared to conventional canola oil, it required the oil to be labeled "laurate canola oil." Similarly, soybean oil containing higher levels of oleic acid than conventional soybean oil must be labeled "high oleic soybean oil." Also, soybean oil containing significant levels of stearidonic acid must be labeled "stearidonate soybean oil" because stearidonic acid is not found in conventional soybean oil.

On July 29, 2016, the president signed into law the National Bioengineered Food Disclosure Standard (Public Law No. 114-216) which, in part, directs the U.S. Department of Agriculture (USDA) to establish a national standard to disclose certain food products or ingredients that are "bioengineered." As a result, the regulations USDA issues will establish requirements for labeling of human food products derived from biotechnology. Questions regarding such requirements should be directed to the USDA's Agricultural Marketing Service.

See: https://www.fda.gov/food/food-genetically-engineered-plants/labeli ng-foods-derived-genetically-engineered-plants

For national policies, see: http://www.fao.org/food/food-safety -quality/gm-foods-platform/graph/labelling-requirement/en

7. **D.** Public health infrastructure provides communities, states, and the nation the capacity to prevent disease, promote health, and prepare for and respond to both acute (emergency) threats and chronic (ongoing) challenges to health. Infrastructure is the foundation for planning, delivering, evaluating, and improving public health. All public health services depend on the presence of basic infrastructure. Every public health program—such as immunizations, infectious disease monitoring, cancer and asthma prevention, drinking water quality, injury prevention—requires health professionals who are competent in cross-cutting and technical skills, up-to-date information systems, and public health organizations with the capacity to assess and respond to community health needs. Public health infrastructure has been referred to as "the nerve center of the public health system." While a strong infrastructure depends on many organizations, public health agencies (health departments) are considered primary players. Federal agencies rely on the presence of solid

public health infrastructure at all levels to support the implementation of public health programs and policies and to respond to health threats, including those from other countries. Public health infrastructure can best be described by what it is and what it does. It includes three key components:

- A capable and qualified workforce
- Up-to-date data and information systems
- Agencies capable of assessing and responding to public health needs

Public health infrastructure provides the necessary foundation for undertaking the basic responsibilities of public health, which have been defined as the 10 Essential Public Health Services

See: https://www.healthypeople.gov/2020/topics-objectives/topic/public-health-infrastructure

8. **B.** According to the Project Management Institute's *A Guide to the Project Management Body of Knowledge,* Third Edition, a project is defined as a temporary endeavor undertaken to create a unique product, service, or result. Project management is defined as the application of knowledge, skills, tools, and techniques to project activities to meet the project requirements.

Project management knowledge and practices are best described in terms of their component processes. These processes can be placed into five process groups—Initiating, Planning, Executing, Controlling, and Closing—and nine knowledge areas—Project Integration Management, Project Scope Management, Project Time Management, Project Cost Management, Project Quality Management, Project Human Resource Management, Project Communications Management, Project Risk Management, and Project Procurement Management.

See: https://www2a.cdc.gov/cdcup/library/other/about_pm.htm

Project management in the public health sector has some unique challenges that many nongovernment projects do not face. One of the greatest challenges involves the political process including the budgeting processes for public health projects. The budgeting process is initiated several years in advance of the actual project initiation, and often many project factors, including technologies available, change during the time span for the initial funding request and the approval to begin the project. During this time, the elected officials and their agenda may change, which often affects the support and continuation of funding for a project.

Another major area of uniqueness is that the language of public health and project management is very different. For example, the term "program" in public health generally refers to a specific set of activities aimed at addressing a key public health concern, such as the TB prevention program, while in project management the term "program" means a grouping of like projects and operations. In general, project management does apply to public health even in an environment where public health practitioners define themselves frequently in terms of skill sets (epidemiology) and subject matter expertise. The more significant language challenges emerge from separate concepts, such as a work breakdown structure in project management and a data collection protocol in public health. The terms of project management are not routine to public health practitioners, who have deep subject matter expertise in areas such as epidemiology, biostatistics, environmental health, genetic research, and surveillance. Identifying these language differences and agreeing upon the lexicon that will be used in public health projects must be done early on to eliminate confusion and frustrations.

See: https://www2a.cdc.gov/cdcup/library/other/faq.htm

9. **A.** A program may consist of more than one project that features components where the individual objectives contribute to the accomplishment of the program's goal. The term "program" in public health generally refers to a specific set of activities aimed at addressing a key public health concern, such as the tuberculosis prevention program, while in project management the term "program" means a grouping of like projects and operations, for example, screening, medication compliance, and environmental controls.

See: https://www.cdc.gov/eval/tools/programmanagement/index.html

https://www2a.cdc.gov/cdcup/library/other/faq.htm

10. **C.** A statement of work (SOW) is typically used when the task is well-known and can be described in specific terms. Statement of objective (SOO) and performance work statement (PWS) emphasize performance-based concepts such as desired service outcomes and performance standards. Whereas a PWS/SOO establishes high-level outcomes and objectives for performance and the PWS emphasizes outcomes, desired results, and objectives at a more detailed and measurable level, SOWs provide explicit statements of work direction for the contractor to follow. However, SOWs can also be found to contain references to desired performance outcomes, performance standards, and metrics, which is a preferred approach.

See: https://www.gsa.gov/cdnstatic/SOW_Application.Services.and.Component.Framework.pdf

The project charter documents and tracks the necessary information required by decision-maker(s) to approve the project for funding. The project charter should include the needs, scope, justification, and resource commitment as well as the project's sponsor(s) decision to proceed or not to proceed with the project. It is created during the initiating phase of the project.

The intended audience of the project charter is the project sponsor and senior leadership.

See: https://www2a.cdc.gov/cdcup/library/templates/default.htm

11. **D.** The best strategy is to keep the director informed because the director has limited interest but can make decisions based on authority in the agency. Monitoring the director's actions, managing, and guaranteeing satisfaction are likely beyond the scope of the website manager's responsibilities. Stakeholder mapping helps to determine which stakeholders are most useful to engage with to different extents, including communication at a high level, or simply notifying of events.

See: https://doit.maryland.gov/SDLC/Pages/agile-sdlc.aspx

https://www.bsr.org/reports/BSR_Stakeholder_Engagement_Stakeholder_Mapping.final.pdf

https://www.stakeholdermap.com

12. **B.** A Traceability Matrix (TM) is a document that correlates any two-baseline documents that require a many-to-many relationship to check the completeness of the relationship. The TM is used to track the requirements and to check the current project requirements are met. The Requirements Management Plan describes how to elicit, analyze, document, and manage the requirements of a project.

   See: https://www.guru99.com/traceability-matrix.html

13. **B.** The project charter formally authorizes a project, addresses the business need for the project, and describes the product and/or service to be created and/or provided by the project. The project charter summarizes the key aspects of the project and project's scope and identifies the project manager's responsibility and authority to apply organizational resources to project activities. The project charter is developed in the early phases of the project life cycle, often as part of the concept/initiating phase. Creating a project charter is a mutually beneficial process that obtains commitment from all affected groups and individuals within a specific project. The purpose of chartering a project is to document the business need, project justification, customer requirements, the result that is intended, and, at a high level, what is considered in scope and out of scope for the project.

   The initial project charter describes the project at a specific point in time. Every component of the project charter describes characteristics that may, and probably will, change during the life of the project. As the project environment changes, updates in the form of appended change requests, or updates to supporting documentation such as the project management plan, should reflect these changes. Some areas of the initial charter, such as risk, will be expanded upon as the project progresses into the planning phase. However, without a charter, management and the client are not formally obligated to consider requirements before project commitments are made. Not chartering a project has the greater possibility of confusion, rework, change requests, scope modification, and so on. For this reason, a project sponsor at a level that is appropriate to fund the project usually issues and/or approves the project charter.

   Projects are usually chartered and authorized as a result of one or more of the following:

   - Market demand
   - Business need
   - Customer request
   - Technological advance
   - Legal requirement
   - Social need

   Benefits of creating a charter include the following:

   - Giving authority to project teams to commence work with official documented approval
   - Allowing senior management to set boundaries for the project scope
   - Formalizing partnerships
   - Ensuring understanding of what was agreed upon

- Helping project teams identify and plan for risks, increasing the chance of project success
- Serving as a project requirements reference guide

See: https://www2.cdc.gov/cdcup/library/practices_guides/CDC_UP_Project_Charter_Practices_Guide.pdf

14. **A.** Context diagrams depict a project's relationship with external entities as a graphic design that clarifies the interfaces and boundaries among the project components and actors. It shows the project's processes in their context, and is considered the highest level view of a system.

See: https://www.modernanalyst.com/Resources/Articles/tabid/115/ID/1355/Introduction-to-Context-Diagrams.aspx

15. **A.** With a to-complete performance index (TCPI) of 0.9, the project implementation remains within budget. TCPI is calculated according to the equation: TCPI = (BAC – EV) ÷ (BAC – AC), where BAC is "Budget at Completion", EV is "Earned Value," and AC is "Actual Cost." Thus, BAC – EV is equivalent to the value of work remaining, and BAC – AC is equivalent to the amount of work remaining. TCPI of 1.0 is the break-even point.

Scott, W. J. (2012). *TCPI: The tower of power.* Paper presented at PMI® Global Congress 2012—North America, Project Management Institute, Vancouver, British Columbia, Canada. Newtown Square, PA. Retrieved from https://www.pmi.org/learning/library/to-complete-performance-index-tcpi-6009

http://acqnotes.com/acqnote/tasks/to-complete-performance-indexev

16. **D.** The overall objective of a Communications Management Plan (CMP) is to promote the success of a project by meeting the information needs of project stakeholders. The CMP defines the project's structure and methods of information collection, screening, formatting, and distribution, and outlines understanding among project teams regarding the actions and processes necessary to facilitate the critical links among people, ideas, and information that are necessary for project success. The intended audience of the CMP is the project manager, project team, project sponsor, and any senior leaders whose support is needed to carry out communication plans.

Without detailed plans for communications activities that identify the organizational, policy, and material resources needed to carry them out, the <Project Name> will not be able to secure needed resources, coordinate efforts with other groups, or report its activities and results to key oversight stakeholders. Communications planning activities identify the appropriate level of communication for each project stakeholder, what information should be distributed, and the frequency of communications. This plan should also include the vehicle of communications (email, face-to-face meetings, etc). The risk of insufficient planning could result in failure to accomplish key project objectives, duplication of effort, and reduced stakeholder confidence.

See: https://www2a.cdc.gov/cdcup/library/templates/default.htm

17. **A.** Project resource distribution structure in public health agencies is a map of available resources allocated to specific projects based on public health priorities. The structure depends on information, decisions, and implementation. Public health professionals and project managers collect information and send it through the agency's hierarchy to the executive level. Top management decides how to allocate resources to match company goals and priorities.

See: https://www2a.cdc.gov/cdcup/

18. **A.** For any given project, a key management component is the practice of managing change. Change management, also known as change control, is an iterative process that continues throughout the project life cycle. All projects, regardless of type or size, should maintain a change log and regularly manage requested changes. As change requests are submitted and resolved, the updated change log provides historical documentation of requested changes that have been addressed throughout the project's life. The Project Management Institute (PMI) Project Management Body of Knowledge (PMBOK) defines a change management system as a collection of formal documented procedures that define how project deliverables and documentation will be controlled, changed, and approved. This practices guide focuses on change management; however, it is important to distinguish the practice of change management from the practice of configuration management. This practice guide focuses specifically on change management.

The primary purpose of a change management system is to provide a standard process for submitting, documenting, and reviewing changes in preparation for prioritizing those corrections/enhancements. It identifies what changes to make, the authority for approving changes, the support for implementing changes, and the process for formal deviations and waivers from the original agreed upon requirements. The change management process establishes an orderly and effective procedure for tracking the submission, coordination, review, evaluation, categorization, and approval for release of all changes to the project's baselines. The change management system defines the guidelines for the management of project change and describes in detail how changes will be documented, organized, and managed.

When managing competing requirements, evaluate how a change in one constraint affects one or both of the remaining two. Analyze scope, time, and cost to understand the costs and benefits of accepting a requested change.

Each change request is unique and the proper evaluation of each change request is a vital management practice. The way that change requests are evaluated depends on their importance and urgency with the objective of

- Understanding the impact of the changes on all affected parties
- Ensuring that all eventualities are considered
- Consolidating all the individual impact analyses for the purpose of making an informed management decision
- Ensuring that due diligence has been exercised in the evaluation of the change request
- Ensuring that all affected parties have been consulted
- Evaluating the impact of the change being considered and weigh the cost against the benefits of the original change request

See: https://www2.cdc.gov/cdcup/library/practices_guides/CDC_UP_
Change_Management_Practices_Guide.pdf

19. **A.** Effective communication is a key component of successful project management and delivery. It is often estimated that 80% of a project manager's job revolves around communication with the project team, client, and executive management. Without effective communication, vital information may not be exchanged effectively. A lack of communication may even delay or prohibit the execution or completion of scheduled tasks. Project success increases exponentially by avoiding communication issues. The goal of communication management planning is to define the project's structure and methods of information collection, screening, formatting, and distribution. It also outlines understanding among project teams regarding the actions and processes necessary to facilitate the critical links among people, ideas, and information that are necessary for project success. Effective communication planning and management help ensure

- Information needs of project stakeholders are met.
- Project performance is tracked and reported on.
- Project results are formally documented.
- Enthusiasm and support exist for the project.

Most projects will require some form of internal and external communication on a regular basis to sustain momentum on the project and to fulfill organizational reporting requirements. To effectively accomplish and manage this, a Communication Management Plan (CMP) should be developed.

A CMP is a platform for understanding between project participants; it documents the methods and activities needed to ensure timely and appropriate collection, generation, dissemination, storage, and ultimate disposition of project information among the project team and stakeholders. The CMP also defines who will not have access to information and what type of information will not be distributed.

The Project Management Institute's (PMI) Project Management Body of Knowledge (PMBOK) defines CMP as a document that describes the communications, needs, and expectations for the project; how and in what format information will be communicated; when and where each communication will be made; and who is responsible for providing each type of communication. Key elements of a CMP include answers to the following types of questions:

- WHO do you need to talk to?
- WHY are you talking to them?
- WHAT do they need to know?
- WHEN do they need to know it?
- HOW do you communicate with them?
- WHERE do you tell them (communication medium)?

The CMP documents a consistent method for communication and the management of that communication throughout the project's life and should be developed in coordination with, and be accessible to, all project team members and stakeholders.

See: https://www2.cdc.gov/cdcup/library/practices_guides/CDC_UP_
Communication_Management_Practices_Guide.pdf

20. **A.** The Project Management Institute's (PMI) A Guide to the Project Management Body of Knowledge (PMBOK) defines a project management plan (PMP) as a formal approved document that defines the overall plan for how the project will be executed, monitored, and controlled.

The PMP may be a single detailed document or composed of one or more subsidiary planning documents. These additional planning documents provide guidance and direction for specific management, planning, and control activities such as schedule, cost, risk, staffing, change control, communications, quality, procurement, deployment, and so on. Each of the subsidiary planning documents should be detailed to the extent required by the specific project.

A PMP is essential for defining how project integration management will be executed when situations arise where individual processes interact. For example, estimating cost involves not only the cost management process, but also integration of planning, time, risk, scope, and so on.

The PMBOK defines project integration management as the processes and activities needed to identify, define, combine, unify, and coordinate the various processes and project management activities. In the context of project management, integration includes characteristics of unification and consolidation actions necessary for project completion. Project integration management also involves making trade-offs among competing objectives and alternatives. Integration, in the context of managing a project, is making choices about where to concentrate resources and effort on any given day, anticipating potential issues, dealing with these issues before they become critical, and coordinating work. A properly developed PMP outlines how these activities will be conducted, taking into consideration any effect they may have on each other and other management processes and/or activities. As the project environment changes, updates in the form of change requests should reflect any changes to the PMP and/or its subsidiary plans.

Benefits of creating a PMP include the following:

- Clearly defined roles, responsibilities, processes, and activities
- Increased probability that projects will complete on-time, within budget, and with a high degree of quality
- Ensuring understanding of what was agreed upon
- Helping project teams identify and plan for how project activities will be managed (scope, cost/budget, quality, etc.)
- Serving as a project management reference guide

See: https://www2a.cdc.gov/cdcup/library/pmg/concept/pmp_
description.htm

21. **B.** Internships are learning experiences; therefore, proper supervision of interns is essential. The supervisor serves as a teacher, mentor, critic, and boss. Ongoing supervision of the student intern is the key to the success of the internship. This is especially true for students who do not have extensive work experience. Acknowledging and identifying the different expectations

between the workplace and school can help interns make a successful transition to the world of work.

An effective method of intern supervision is to have a set time (bi-weekly is recommended) to meet with the intern to review progress on projects, touch base, and provide feedback. Some supervisors do this over lunch; others choose a more formal setting. The supervisor will oversee and assign the student intern's work. Supervisors will need to monitor the intern's time and submit an intern evaluation form provided by the intern's college for those receiving academic credit. The intern supervisor will also provide the student with a letter of recommendation.

During the orientation period, establish goals and objectives, and clarify these goals and objectives before the intern begins working. Some interns need more guidance than others, and many factors must be taken into consideration. Consider the intern's cultural background, disabilities, learning style, and experience. Evaluate his or her level of maturity and confidence. Is the intern a critical thinker or a creative problem-solver? Take time in the beginning of the internship to introduce the intern to the people in your program. Allow more time for conversation with those employees who are likely to interact with the intern on a regular basis. Some interns, based on personality or culture, may be reluctant to seek out coworkers on their own. By making a special effort to encourage those contacts early on, interns will feel more comfortable asking for advice or support later. Reviewing the external stakeholder register with interns before face-to-face interaction prepares the intern for a focused stakeholder engagement.

See: https://jobs.ca.gov/PDF/Student_Internship_Program_Guide.pdf

22. **D.** The "Guide to the Project Management Body of Knowledge" (PMBOK Guide) defines resource leveling as "a technique in which the beginning and end dates are adjusted based on resource limitation with the goal of balancing demand for resources with the available supply." Resource leveling may be performed when key or shared resources are only available at certain times, or available in limited quantities, or over-allocated to keep resource usage at a constant level by reducing fluctuation in demand for key resources. In contrast, resource smoothing is defined as a technique that adjusts the activities of a schedule model such that the requirement for resources on the project do not exceed certain predefined resource limits.

Project Management Institute. (2013). *A guide to the project management body of knowledge (PMBOK® Guide)* (5th ed., p. 179). Newton Square, PA: Author.

See: https://www.pmi.org/pmbok-guide-standards

23. **B.** At the U.S. Centers for Disease Control and Prevention (CDC), the International Experience and Technical Assistance (IETA) Program was established in response to the increased role in the direct provision of global prevention and prevention research programs. The program was designed to offer Federal Public Health Service employees the opportunity to gain experience overseas, while at the same time providing technical assistance to countries. The program is managed by the CDC's Center for Global Health Overseas Operations Office (CGH/OD/OOO) in Atlanta, Georgia, and follows the same principles upon which it was founded.

Cultural and linguistic competence are part of international engagement in global health, and competence represents a set of congruent behaviors, attitudes, and policies that come together in a system, agency, or among professionals that enables effective work in cross-cultural situations. "Culture" refers to integrated patterns of human behavior that include the language, thoughts, communications, actions, customs, beliefs, values, and institutions of racial, ethnic, religious, or social groups. "Competence" implies having the capacity to function effectively as an individual and an organization within the context of the cultural beliefs, behaviors, and needs presented by consumers and their communities.

See: https://npin.cdc.gov/pages/cultural-competence

https://www.cdc.gov/globalhealth/ieta/overview.htm

24. **A.** Implementation of effective practices to manage staff is essential for the success of public health projects, which are often coordinated across a team of interdisciplinary experts at various stages in their career. Planning for team management demands documentation of team structure (e.g., reporting structure or chain of command and functional teams). An organization chart, if appropriate, expresses the structure and function of each member of the team and his or her relationship to others. External project participants that may support or participate in the project's functional team(s) are included with information on

- Role/responsibility
- Skills required
- Number of staff required
- Time frame needed
- Duration required

The overall approach for team management should include the approach for identifying human resource needs and the approach to determining timing needs for adding and removing project personnel.

See: https://guides.himmelfarb.gwu.edu/c.php?g=365963&p=2473004

https://www.cdc.gov/eval/guide/step1/index.htm

25. **C.** The Independent Cost Estimate (ICE) is the estimate of costs that a contractor/recipient may incur in performing services and/or providing supplies to achieve a public health agency's objective. It serves as the basis for reserving funds during acquisition planning; it provides the basis for comparing costs or prices proposed by offerors/applicants; and it serves as an objective basis for determining price reasonableness in cases in which one offeror/applicant responds to a solicitation.

For examination, the U.S. Agency for International Development refers to the Independent Government Cost Estimate (IGCE) as the USAID Budget because the agency operates mainly through contractual agreements.

See: https://www.usaid.gov/sites/default/files/documents/1868/300maa .pdf

26. B. Some public health projects may encounter severe difficulties because they lack clearly defined and documented requirements. Requirements documentation or management is a systematic approach to finding, documenting, organizing, and tracking requirements and the changes that may occur. Requirements documentation and management helps ensure that the end product meets the needs and expectations of the stakeholders. A key step in requirements management is to determine an agreed upon specific requirements gathering process, documentation of requirements, traceability, and testing expectations. Requirements are defined during the planning phase and are managed throughout the entire process from high-level requirements, through detailed requirements, design, building, and testing.

There is a difference between project and product requirements documentation, meaning that

- Project requirements define how the work will be managed. This includes the budget, communication management, resource management, quality assurance, risk management, and scope management. Project requirements focus on the who, when, where, and how something gets done. Project requirements are generally documented in the project management plan.
- Product requirements include high-level features or capabilities that the business team has committed to delivering to a customer. Product requirements do not specify how the features or the capabilities will be designed.

See: https://www2.cdc.gov/cdcup/library/practices_guides/CDC_UP_ Requirements_Management_Practices_Guide.pdf

27. D. Product analysis is the process of evaluating the fit between the intended and finished products expected as outcomes of a project and can take the form of expert analysis of limited release of post-production projects, including product decomposition, systems analysis, systems engineering, value engineering, value analysis, and functional analysis.

Technical performance analysis is related to product analysis, but forms only one component.

See: https://project-management-knowledge.com/definitions/t/technical -performance-measurement

28. B. The change request procedure is typically included in a Change Management Plan developed to establish an orderly and effective procedure for tracking the submission, coordination, review, evaluation, categorization, and approval for release of all changes to the project's baselines. Communicating change is part of the procedure but comes only after change has been properly documented and approved by the project manager.

See: https://www2a.cdc.gov/cdcup/

29. **D.** Effective project scope management begins with the practice of proper scope planning and documentation of a scope statement. This practice is key to delivering projects successfully. Four primary actions are conducted during the scope planning process. Defining scope planning results in the creation of a project scope management plan that documents how the project scope will be defined, verified, controlled, and how the work breakdown structure will be created and defined.

Scope definition delivers a detailed project scope statement as a basis for future project decisions; Scope verification formalizes a plan for the acceptance of completed project deliverables, whereas scope control establishes a mechanism for controlling changes to the project scope.

Understanding and analyzing project stakeholders is an important early step toward ensuring agreement about project scope and any work expected to be accomplished. To then properly manage this throughout a project's life cycle requires a defined roadmap that outlines product and project direction in-line with stakeholder expectations and associated contractual obligations. Project scope management also includes the processes required to ensure that the project includes all the work required, and only the work required, to complete the project successfully.

Defining project scope involves subdividing major project deliverables, as identified in the project scope statement, into smaller, more manageable components. Scope verification activities include measuring, examining, and testing project deliverables to ensure they comply with agreed upon requirements. How this is accomplished must be documented and agreed upon by key stakeholders during the planning process. The ultimate objective of this process is a documented plan for formally accepting completed project deliverables.

See: https://www2.cdc.gov/cdcup/library/practices_guides/CDC_UP_
Scope_Planning_Practices_Guide.pdf

https://www2a.cdc.gov/cdcup/library/newsletter/CDC_UP_News
letter_v4_i7.htm

30. **B.** Communicating with stakeholders or partners is an important component of stakeholder engagement. The project management strategy should also include procedures for communicating change, when the change is fully justified by potential improvements in project effectiveness.

See: https://www.bsr.org/en/our-insights/report-view/stakeholder-enga
gement-five-step-approach-toolkit

https://www.cdc.gov/eval/guide/step1/index.htm

https://www.cdc.gov/eval/guide/step1/index.htm

https://www.cdc.gov/std/Program/pupestd/Identifying%20and%20
Determining%20Stakeholders.pdf

31. **C.** You should discuss the issue with the team and update the team charter accordingly. The team charter specifies team goals and approaches, while also delineating boundaries. The situation described does not warrant a change in corporate policies to prohibit flextime, or to change the charter. Doing nothing is negligent.

See: https://www.lce.com/Team-Charters-What-are-they-1219.html

32. **D.** Procurement audits are included in project management plans to formally evaluate the performance of suppliers (products or procedures) based on existing contracts. Procurement audits are also used to establish a record that can be used to streamline the procurement practices of a public health agency.

Procurement strategies are described in the project management plan, focusing on how resources should be managed until the project end point. A procurement audit is a project management process that reviews different contracts and contracting processes to determine the completeness, efficacy, and accuracy of the procurement process.

See: https://project-management-knowledge.com/definitions/p/procurement-audits

https://www.gao.gov/new.items/d0487g.pdf

33. **D.** A project's final report is expected to be a stand-alone document that captures essential information about the project, including goals, methods, results, and discussion and/or conclusion. Lessons learned or closure documents may not contain sufficient detail to appreciate the significance of the project and the challenges faced. Essentially, a final report should include sufficient detail for replication of the project, and for those who were not directly involved to be able to build on or extend the project.

See: https://www3.epa.gov/region1/eco/uep/pdfs/HCFinalReport.pdf

34. **C.** The Project Management Institute's (PMI) Project Management Body of Knowledge (PMBOK) defines lessons learned as the learning gained from the process of performing the project. Formally conducted lessons learned sessions are traditionally held during project close-out, near the completion of the project. However, lessons learned may be identified and documented at any point during the project's life cycle. The purpose of documenting lessons learned is to share and use knowledge derived from experience to

- Promote the recurrence of desirable outcomes
- Preclude the recurrence of undesirable outcomes

As a practice, lessons learned includes the processes necessary for identification, documentation, validation, and dissemination of lessons learned. Utilization and incorporation of those processes includes identification of applicable lessons learned, documentation of lessons learned, archiving lessons learned, distribution to appropriate personnel, identification of actions that will be taken as a result of the lesson learned, and follow-up to ensure that appropriate actions were taken.

Lessons learned document the cause of issues and the reasoning behind any corrective action taken to address those issues. When thinking about how to effectively document a project's lessons learned, consider the following types of questions:

- What was learned about the project in general?
- What was learned about project management?
- What was learned about communication?
- What was learned about budgeting?
- What was learned about procurement?

- What was learned about working with sponsors?
- What was learned about working with customers?
- What was learned about what went well?
- What was learned about what did not go well?
- What was learned about what needs to change?
- How will/was this incorporated into the project?

Lessons learned should draw on both positive experiences—good ideas that improve project efficiency or save money—and negative experiences—lessons learned only after an undesirable outcome has already occurred. Every documented lesson learned should contain at least these general elements:

- Project information and contact information for additional detail
- A clear statement of the lesson
- A background summary of how the lesson was learned
- Benefits of using the lesson and suggestions how the lesson may be used in the future.

At any point during the project life cycle, the project team and key stakeholders may identify lessons. The lessons learned are compiled, formalized, and stored through the project's duration. Upon project completion, a lessons learned session is conducted that focuses on identifying project success and project failures, and includes recommendation to improve future performance on projects.

See: https://www2a.cdc.gov/cdcup/library/practices_guides/CDC_UP_ Lessons_Learned_Practices_Guide.pdf

35. **B.** You should conduct stakeholder analysis, which is the second step in a strategic stakeholder engagement protocol, following identification of relevant stakeholders, and followed by mapping stakeholders to program objectives and prioritizing stakeholder relevance.

See: https://www.bsr.org/reports/BSR_Stakeholder_Engagement_Stake holder_Mapping.final.pdf

https://www.cdc.gov/eval/guide/step1/index.htm

36. **B.** Earlier in the project, you might have missed stakeholder analysis including consideration for those with an interest in the project. Stakeholder analysis should reveal the value contributed to each program objective, their legitimate claim (or otherwise) for engagement, willingness to engage, their level of influence, and the necessity of their involvement in the public health project.

See: https://www.bsr.org/reports/BSR_Stakeholder_Engagement_Stake holder_Mapping.final.pdf

https://www.cdc.gov/eval/guide/step1/index.htm

37. **C.** A request for quotation is a solicitation for products or services in which a public health agency such as the Centers for Disease Control and Prevention (CDC) asks suppliers to submit a price quotation and bid on the chance to undertake specific projects.

For example, see: https://www.phi.org/uploads/files/RFQ%20PHI%20CD
C%20GHFP%20Website%20Design%20and%20Development%20Services%
20Final.pdf

38. C. The process of "control schedule" is used to monitor project status in a
task timeline. The control schedule document includes descriptions of project
milestones, any changes made, and progress reports prepared and submitted. Evaluation of control schedules by project managers can inform them
on whether the project activity is on schedule, ahead of schedule, or behind
schedule.

See: https://project-management-knowledge.com/definitions/c/control
-schedule

39. C. Adaptive approaches (also known as agile methodologies) are often con-
trasted with predictive approaches (also known as waterfall methodologies). Adaptive approaches were developed relatively recently in response
to challenges with predictive approaches and are designed to be flexible with
respect to project requirements and specifications, so that the project team can
respond in a timely manner.

Predictive approaches focus on specific milestones to control the project process, and they are sensitive to major changes in project specifications, in which
case they are less flexible. There are different reasons why a team may wish
to change from a predictive to adaptive management approach. Such changes
will need to be accompanied by modifications to the schedule management
plan, including schedule model development, the release and iteration length,
and the reporting formats. Project managers typically are accustomed to either
predictive or adaptive approaches, but either approach may lead to less than
perfect results.

See: https://www.ssipeople.com/2015/10/13/project-management
-adaptive-vs-predictive

40. C. Two guiding points are important in responding to queries such as this.
First, it is important to identify an analogous project based on an archive
of experience; and second, it is important to give a time period rather than
specific date, to allow for variability in the procedures. In both cases, the
response should be reasonable.

41. A. The term "risk audit" is defined in the "Project Management Body of
Knowledge" (PMBOK), Fifth Edition, as a tool that the project manager uses
to control risk during the course of a project. Risks are ubiquitous in public
health projects, and effective project planning aims to avoid and minimize
risks proactively; hence, the need for periodic audits. Both internal and external committees may be charged with risk audits to ensure objectivity, relevance, and absence of conflict of interest.

See: https://project-management-knowledge.com/definitions/p/project
-management-body-of-knowledge-pmbok

https://project-management-knowledge.com/definitions/r/risk-audit

42. **D.** Potential and actual risks should be identified and described in a project management plan including all stakeholders and their role in responding to specific risks or being the sources of the risk. The risk owner should be explicitly notified so that he or she can develop a plan of action before risk events occur. If the system is thorough, the register should not identify the wrong risk owner because that would have been corrected with prompt notification. Project managers should always follow the management plan, and if they are unclear about specific aspects, they should immediately convene the team. Stakeholders that are so disinterested as to not read the plan should be remediated.

See: https://safety.uoregon.edu/erm-risk-owner-roles-and-responsibilities

43. **A.** Procurement closure is the process of completing each procurement, or the acquisition of goods, services, or work from an agent external to an organization. Procurement closure may occur within a project that remains open and continuing, or it may close simultaneously with the end of the project.

See: https://pmstudycircle.com/2012/02/close-procurement-vs-close
-project

44. **B.** Knowledge sharing is the process of exchanging health-related information across multiple sectors or disciplines including situational awareness information among, for example federal, state, local, territorial, and tribal levels of government, and the private sector; or within different branches of a public health agency. Knowledge sharing capability includes the routine sharing of information as well as issuing of public health alerts in preparation for, and in response to, events or incidents of public health significance. Knowledge sharing capability consists of identifying stakeholders to be incorporated into information flow; identifying and developing rules and data elements for sharing; and exchanging information to determine a common operating procedure.

See: https://stacks.cdc.gov/view/cdc/11371/cdc_11371_DS1.pdf

45. **B.** Before reaching a conclusion about why the engagement strategies are not effective, it is important to analyze all available data on the various components of stakeholder engagement. The data analysis should reveal whether or not it is recommended to develop a new stakeholder engagement plan. It is not a good idea to ignore "troublesome" stakeholders. We may disagree with their perspective, but the important thing is to get the variety of input from various stakeholders.

46. **A.** Requirements traceability is an activity that is one part of an overarching requirements management practice and extends from requirements definition through to implementation. Requirements tracing is used to ensure that each step of the product's development process is correct, conforms to the needs of prior and next steps, and conforms to the defined requirements. Requirements tracing is a technique that helps to ensure that the project delivers what stakeholders expect. If applied correctly, requirements tracing is a practice that can greatly increase the quality and reliability of a project's final product while minimizing costly rework resulting from requirements errors.

Requirements traceability can be considered as the backbone of any project and helps ensure correct product delivery that meets the expectations of the client. When verifying project work, using a requirements traceability matrix verifies that the correct functionality is contained within each product module.

See: https://www2.cdc.gov/cdcup/library/practices_guides/CDC_UP_ Requirements_Traceability_Practice_Guide.pdf

47. **D.** A "planning package" is part of the hierarchical decomposition of the total scope of work to be conducted by the project team to accomplish the objectives and required deliverables (work breakdown structure [WBS]). Each descending level of the WBS represents an increasingly detailed definition of the project. The planning package is below the control account with known work content but without detailed schedule activities.

See: https://www.pmi.org/pmbok-guide-standards

48. **D.** The practice of project close-out finalizes all project activities completed across all phases of the project to formally close the project and transfer the completed or cancelled project as appropriate. The purpose of project close-out is to assess the project, ensure completion, and derive any lessons learned and best practices to be applied to future projects. However, in multiphase projects, the close-out practice may be applied at various stages of the project: upon deliverable completion, upon phase completion, upon iteration completion, at designated times during the project's life, or at whatever other juncture represents a completed segment of project work. Applying the close-out practice in this manner closes out only the portion of the project scope and associated activities applicable to that portion of the project.

The practice of project close-out consists of two main activity groups:

Administrative closure—The administrative closure process defines activities, interactions, and related roles and responsibilities of the project team members and other stakeholders involved in executing the administrative closure procedure for the projects.

Performing the administrative closure process includes integrated activities to collect project records, analyze project success or failure, gather lessons learned, transfer the project products or services to production and/or operations, and archive project information for future use by the organization. Among other activities, administrative closure includes

- Confirming the project has met all sponsor, customer, and stakeholder requirements
- Verifying that all deliverables have been delivered and accepted
- Validating exit criteria have been met

Contract Closure—Contract closure includes activities and interactions needed to settle and close any contract agreements established for the project, as well as those related to supporting the formal administrative closure of the project.

Contract closure involves verification that all work has been completed correctly and satisfactorily, updating of contract records to reflect final results, and archiving information for future use. Among other activities, contract closure includes the following:

- Confirming the project has addressed the terms and conditions of the contracts
- Confirming completion of exit criteria for contract closure
- Formally closing out all contracts associated with the completed project

Project close-out should be anticipated and planned as early as possible in the project life cycle even though it is often the last major process of a project's life.

At a high level, the key elements of project close-out are

- Verify acceptance of final project deliverables
- Conduct post-project assessment and lessons learned
- Conduct post-project review and evaluation
- Recognize and celebrate outstanding project work
- Disburse project resources—staff, facilities, and automated systems
- Complete and archive final product records
- Ensure transfer of knowledge

See https://www2a.cdc.gov/cdcup/library/practices_guides/CDC_UP_ Project_Close-Out_Practices_Guide.pdf

A WBS is the cornerstone of effective project planning and is an excellent team collaboration tool for identifying missing deliverables. However, excessive decomposition can actually lead to nonproductive management effort, inefficient use of resources, and decreased efficiency in performing project work. The mistake of excessively subdividing the WBS into too many tasks can actually turn the WBS into an ineffective "to do" list rather than a valuable project planning tool.

A WBS can actually be decomposed to any level of detail. However, three levels are usually adequate unless the work item at that level is still considered to be high cost and/or high risk. Then it may be necessary to further decompose the work of that specific item into additional, more manageable work packages. The WBS should be structured, at its lowest level, into elements that can be when developing a WBS, consider the relationship between WBS elements, project goals, and federal regulations and policies. For example, defining a WBS to the third level may be adequate for the project team to deliver on project goals. However, further decomposition may be necessary to meet federal regulations and/or policies.

See: https://www2.cdc.gov/cdcup/library/practices_guides/CDC_UP_ WBS_Practices_Guide.pdf

49. **D.** Management reserve is an amount of budget earmarked for management control purposes rather than for the accomplishment of specific tasks. The management reserve is not included in the performance measurement baseline, but is included in the total contract budget. Project management reserve is used when risks are realized for identified work within the scope of work.

See: https://www.humphreys-assoc.com/evms/effective-management -reserve-ta-a-60.html

50. **A.** Each project's product and/or service is unique and requires its own careful balance of practices, processes, tools and techniques, and so on, to ensure

the required work is completed as agreed upon by key project stakeholders. The sum of these, along with the product and/or service to be delivered by the project, is known as the project's scope. Getting key parties to agree upon what is the scope of the project's work is known as project scope planning.

The practice of project scope planning is a key management practice for planning and delivering projects successfully. Project scope includes high-level features or capabilities that the business team has committed to delivering to a customer as well as those they have not committed to delivering. Project scope is often defined by executive sponsor, steering committee, project sponsor, and the project's customer with input from other appropriate stakeholders.

Understanding and analyzing who project stakeholders are is an important early step in the scope planning process. Project stakeholders are persons and/or organizations such as customers, sponsors, the public, and so on, that are actively involved in the project, whose interests may be affected by the project, or who exert influence over the project and/or its deliverables.

Diligent scope planning works toward ensuring that key project stakeholders agree upon the project work to be accomplished. Achieving this agreement is facilitated through a process of progressively elaborating and documenting project work and communicating with project stakeholders. This process forms the basis for an agreement between the project team and the customer by relating the work of the project to the project's objectives and ensuring that the project includes all of the work required, and only the work required, to meet the agreed upon project objectives. At a minimum, the scope planning process should consider:

- Project justification—Defining the business need that the project was undertaken to address, such as a customer request, market demand, and so on
- Product description—Documenting the relationship between the created product and/or service and the business need the project was undertaken to address
- Project objective—Outlining criteria the project needs to meet for it to be considered a success. This includes measures of cost, quality, schedule, and so on, to meet the business needs behind why the project was chartered.

Four primary actions are conducted throughout the scope planning process:

1. Scope planning—Creating a project scope management plan that documents how the project scope will be defined, verified, controlled, and how the work breakdown structure (WBS) will be created and defined
2. Scope definition—Developing a detailed project scope statement as the basis for future project decisions
3. Scope verification—Formalizing a plan for acceptance of the completed project deliverables
4. Scope control—Establishing a mechanism for controlling changes to the project scope

See: https://www2.cdc.gov/cdcup/library/practices_guides/CDC_UP_Scope_Planning_Practices_Guide.pdf

51. **D.** Enterprise environmental factors are the conditions in which a public health agency has to perform its functions. These may include political, economic, and cultural environmental factors: Enterprise environmental factors can also represent internal opportunities and constraints:

Organizational culture

Organizational structure

Internal and external political climate

Existing human resources

Available capital resources

Regulatory environment

Financial and market conditions

See: https://www.pmlearningsolutions.com/blog/enterprise-environ mental-factors-versus-organizational-process-assets-pmp-concept-12

52. **B.** Contingency planning can be defined in a number of ways. The National Institute of Standards and Technology (NIST) defines contingency planning as management policies and procedures designed to maintain or restore business operations, including computer operations, possibly at an alternate location, in the event of emergency, system failure, or disaster. The Information Technology Infrastructure Library (ITIL) defines disaster recovery as a series of processes that focus only upon the recovery processes, principally in response to physical disaster, that are contained within business continuity management (BCM). The Department of Health and Human Services (HHS) Enterprise Performance Life Cycle (EPLC) defines a contingency/disaster recovery plan as the strategy and organized course of action that is to be taken if things don't go as planned or if there is a loss of use of the established business product or system due to a disaster such as a flood, fire, computer virus, or major failure.

Contingency planning is one component of a much broader emergency preparedness process that includes items such as business practices, operational continuity, and disaster recovery planning. Preparing for such events often involves implementing policies and processes at an organizational level and may require numerous plans to properly prepare for, respond to, recover from, and continue activities if impacted by an event. Project managers must also consider the impacts of disruptions and plan, in alignment with organizational standards and policies, for such events. As one component of a comprehensive risk management approach, contingency planning should identify potential vulnerabilities and threats and then implement approaches to either prevent such incidents from happening or limit their potential impact. The Centers for Disease Control and Prevention's (CDC) Office of Security and Emergency Preparedness (OSEP) defines a vulnerability as anything that would represent the CDC's susceptibility to harm, be it loss of capability, staff, property, reputation, and so on. OSEP defines a threat as representing an event that can adversely impact CDC personnel, property, or operations. Threats can generally be grouped into three category types:

- *Natural threats* such as floods, tornadoes, earthquakes, hurricanes, ice storms, and so on

- *Technical/humanmade threats* such as radiological, chemical, biological, mechanical, electrical, and so on
- *Intentional acts* such as terrorism, demonstrations, bomb threats, assaults, theft, computer security, and so on

Although contingency planning sometimes is thought of as an operations and maintenance phase activity, contingency measures should be identified and integrated at all phases of the project life cycle. The National Institute of Standards and Technology (NIST) defines a seven-step contingency planning process to developing and maintaining a viable contingency planning program. These seven progressive steps are designed to be integrated throughout a project's life cycle and help guide stakeholders in the planning, development, implementation, key success factors, and maintenance of contingency plans.

1. *Identify any specific regulatory requirements* related to contingency planning. Develop a formal contingency planning policy statement that provides stakeholders the authority and guidance necessary to develop an effective contingency plan. Obtain executive approval and publish such policies
2. *Conduct a business impact analysis* (BIA) to identify and prioritize critical systems, business processes, and components. Include impact of events, allowable outage durations, and recovery priorities
3. *Identify and implement preventive controls and measures* to reduce the effects of disruptions, increase availability, and reduce contingency costs
4. *Develop recovery strategies* ensuring critical systems, business processes, infrastructure, and so on, can be recovered quickly and effectively following a disruption. Integrate them into system architecture
5. *Develop contingency plans* containing detailed guidance and procedures to recover from disruptions
6. *Plan testing, training, and exercises* to reinforce, validate, and test contingency plans to identify gaps and to prepare recovery personnel for unforeseen events. Document lessons learned and incorporate them into updates to contingency plans
7. *Maintain contingency plans* as living documents. Update them regularly to reflect changes in any influencing factors

See: https://www2.cdc.gov/cdcup/library/practices_guides/CDC_UP_ Contingency_Planning_Practices_Guide.pdf

53. C. For any given project, a key management component is the practice of managing change. Change management, also known as change control, is an iterative process that continues throughout the project life cycle. All projects, regardless of type or size, should maintain a change log and regularly manage requested changes. As change requests are submitted and resolved, the updated change log provides historical documentation of requested changes that have been addressed throughout the project's life.

The Project Management Institute's (PMI) Project Management Body of Knowledge (PMBOK) defines a change management system as a collection of formal documented procedures that define how project deliverables and documentation will be controlled, changed, and approved.

This practices guide focuses on change management; however, it is important to distinguish the practice of change management from the practice of configuration management. This practice guide focuses specifically on change management.

The primary purpose of a change management system is to provide a standard process for submitting, documenting, and reviewing changes in preparation for prioritizing those corrections/enhancements. It identifies what changes to make, the authority for approving changes, the support for implementing changes, and the process for formal deviations and waivers from the original agreed upon requirements. The change management process establishes an orderly and effective procedure for tracking the submission, coordination, review, evaluation, categorization, and approval for release of all changes to the project's baselines. The change management system defines the guidelines for the management of project change and describes in detail how changes will be documented, organized, and managed.

When managing competing requirements, evaluate how a change in one constraint affects one or both of the remaining two. Analyze scope, time, and cost to understand the costs and benefits of accepting a requested change.

Each change request is unique and the proper evaluation of each change request is a vital management practice. The way that change requests are evaluated depends on their importance and urgency with the objective of

- Understanding the impact of the changes on all affected parties
- Ensuring that all eventualities are considered
- Consolidating all the individual impact analyses for the purpose of making an informed management decision
- Ensuring that due diligence has been exercised in the evaluation of the change request
- Ensuring that all affected parties have been consulted
- Evaluating the impact of the change being considered and weigh the cost against the benefits of the original change request

There are two types of change to contend with during the life of a project: product change and project change. Within each of these two categories, scope, time, duration, cost, resource, deliverable, product, process, and quality all need to be considered when evaluating a change request.

- **Product change**—PMI PMBOK defines a product as an artifact that is produced, is quantifiable, and can be either an end item in itself or a component item. Product change impacts the product's deliverables, functionality, quality, and so on. A product change may be large enough to also have an impact on project change
- **Project change**—PMI PMBOK defines a project as a temporary endeavor undertaken to create a unique product, service, or result. Project change impacts the project's scope, time, duration, cost, resources, processes, and so on

See: https://www2.cdc.gov/cdcup/library/practices_guides/CDC_UP_
Change_Management_Practices_Guide.pdf

54. D. The work breakdown structure (WBS) organizes and defines 100% of the scope of project work to be accomplished and displays it in a way that relates work elements to each other and to the project's goals. The Project Management Institute's (PMI) Project Management Body of Knowledge (PMBOK) defines a WBS as a deliverable-oriented hierarchical decomposition of the work to be executed by the project team.

A WBS is not a project schedule. The WBS defines the "what" of a project and the project schedule defines the "When" and "Who" of a project. A WBS uses nouns and adjectives to define work, not verbs; it contains no dependencies, durations, activities, or resource assignments. A project schedule uses verbs and nouns to define scheduled activities, outline task dependencies, and note resource assignments.

A WBS provides an efficient format to define project work and for planning and tracking a project's success. The WBS organizes the necessary work by decomposing it into smaller, manageable pieces that can be scheduled, cost estimated, monitored, and controlled. Each descending level of the WBS hierarchy represents an increasingly detailed definition of the project work to be accomplished.

The PMI PMBOK defines decomposition as a planning technique that subdivides the project scope and project deliverables into smaller, more manageable components, until the project work associated with accomplishing the project scope and providing the deliverables is defined in sufficient detail to support executing, monitoring, and controlling the work. This is known as the work package level and is the lowest level in the WBS.

A WBS makes the relationship of work packages clear by decomposing larger work into smaller, more manageable components that outline the work needing to be accomplished for the project to succeed. The process of decomposing project work into a WBS involves the following:

- Identifying project deliverables
- Identifying work related to project deliverables
- Building a high-level WBS based on the previous information
- Decomposing the high-level WBS into work packages

The resulting WBS can take a number of forms such as

- Using major project deliverables and/or subprojects as the first level of the WBS
- Using the phases of the project life cycle as the first level of the WBS with the project deliverables inserted as the second level
- Using a combination of phases and project deliverables within each branch of the WBS
- Managed
- Estimated
- Measured
- CPIC requirements
- Project management
- Project risk
- Enterprise architecture (EA)
- Human resource analysis

- Performance management
- Financial management
- Budgeting/funding
- Acquisition
- System development life cycle (SDLC) management

55. **D.** Project risk must be identified, managed, and addressed throughout the project in order for the project to be successful. Risk management plays an important role in maintaining project stability and efficiency throughout the project life cycle. It proactively addresses potential obstacles that may arise and hinder project success and/or block the project team from achieving its goals. Project risk can be anything that threatens or limits the goals, objectives, or deliverables of a project. Project risk is present in all projects and may have one or more causes and, if it occurs, one or more impacts.

There is often confusion between risk management and issue management and how the activities of each interface and interact with each other. According to the Project Management Institute's (PMI) Project Management Body of Knowledge (PMBOK)

- **A risk** is an uncertain event or condition that, if it occurs, has a positive or negative impact on a project's objectives such as time, cost, scope, quality, and so on.

- **An issue** is a point or matter in question or in dispute, or a point or matter that is not settled and is under discussion or over which there are opposing views or disagreements. Often project issues are first identified as a risk and through the risk management planning process may already have a planned approach to managing the issue.

Project risk management includes the processes for conducting risk management planning, identification, analysis, responses, and monitoring and control of a project. The objectives of project risk management are to increase the probability and impact of positive events and decrease the probability and impact of events adverse to project objectives. Project issue management includes utilizing the outputs from the project risk management planning if the issue was identified as a risk during the risk planning processes.

See: https://www2a.cdc.gov/cdcup/library/practices_guides/CDC_UP_ Risk_Management_Practices_Guide.pdf

56. **D.** The first step in the risk management planning process is to identify sources of risk and then to qualify the risk. The next step is to calculate the contingency and management reserve that provide a margin of operation against known and unknown risks. Project costs and budget depend on these contingency and management reserves.

See: https://pmstudycircle.com/2012/02/contingency-reserve-vs -management-reserve

57. **B.** The Project Management Institute's (PMI) Project Management Body of Knowledge (PMBOK) defines a project management plan (PMP) as a formal approved document that defines the overall plan for how the project will be executed, monitored, and controlled.

The PMP may be a single detailed document or composed of one or more subsidiary planning documents. These additional planning documents provide guidance and direction for specific management, planning, and control activities such as schedule, cost, risk, staffing, change control, communication, quality, procurement, deployment, and so on. Each of the subsidiary planning documents should be detailed to the extent required by the specific project.

A PMP is essential for defining how project integration management will be executed when situations arise where individual processes interact. For example, estimating cost involves not only the cost management process, but also integration of planning, time, risk, scope, and so on.

PMI PMBOK defines Project Integration Management as the processes and activities needed to identify, define, combine, unify, and coordinate the various processes and project management activities.

In the context of project management, integration includes characteristics of unification and consolidation actions necessary for project completion. Integration management also involves making trade-offs among competing objectives and alternatives. Integration in the context of managing a project is making choices about where to concentrate resources and effort on any given day, anticipating potential issues, dealing with these issues before they become critical, and coordinating work. A properly developed PMP outlines how these activities will be conducted, taking into consideration any effect they may have on each other and other management processes and/or activities. As the project environment changes, updates in the form of change requests should reflect any changes to the PMP and/or its subsidiary plans.

Benefits of creating a PMP include the following:

- Clearly define roles, responsibilities, processes, and activities
- Increase probability that projects will complete on time, within budget, and with high degree of quality
- Ensure understanding of what was agreed upon
- Help project teams identify and plan for how project activities will be managed (scope, cost/budget, quality, etc.)
- Serve as a project management reference guide

See: https://www2.cdc.gov/cdcup/library/practices_guides/CDC_UP_ Project_Management_Plan_Practices_Guide.pdf

58. **D.** Stakeholder engagement and stakeholder management are arguably the most important ingredients for successful project delivery, and yet are often regarded as a fringe activity or one that can be outsourced to business-as-usual functions. Project managers depend on people to respond to the outputs and benefits that they deliver. People will only respond if they are engaged. The phrase "stakeholder management" implies that these people can be made to respond positively to a project, but the truth is that a project manager frequently has no formal power of authority and therefore has to rely on engagement to achieve his/her objectives.

See: https://www.apm.org.uk/resources/find-a-resource/stakeholder -engagement/key-principles

59. B. Most likely the project manager did not review the organizational process assets. Organizational process assets provide the foundation for long-term planning benefits to the public health agency. The communication tools and environmental factors are relevant, but not as informative as the overall process assets.

See: https://www.pmi.org/pmbok-guide-standards/foundational/pmbok

60. C. Sequence activities involve the process of identifying and documenting relationships among the project activities. The key benefit of this process is that it defines the logical sequence of work to obtain the greatest efficiency given all project constraints.

Projects often encounter major difficulties because they lack clearly defined and documented requirements. The practice of requirements definition is part of an overarching requirements management practice. This overarching practice is a systematic approach to finding, documenting, organizing, and tracking requirements and the changes that may occur throughout the life of a project, and is described in greater detail in the CDC UP Requirements Management Practices Guide.

According to the Butler Group, ~40% of effort in an average software project is rework. One way of avoiding these issues is to properly define project requirements. The further along the project is in its life cycle, the more costly it becomes to correct requirement errors. The cost of correcting a requirement error increases exponentially as the project matures. For example, to correct a requirement error in the operation stage could cost a multiple of 100 times or more than if that same error was fixed earlier in the project's life. Defining requirements correctly at the start of the project is often the single most important practice that prevents costly errors and increases the potential for project success. The challenge, however, is to get business stakeholders, end-users, and project teams all on the same page in regard to those requirements.

The practice of defining requirements provides a solid foundation for project success and proper delivery of the end product. Properly defined requirements provide the first view of what the intended product must do and how it should perform. They also provide a basis for product design and serve as a foundation for testing and user acceptance of the end product by identifying the goals, needs, and objectives of the project by asking questions such as

- What problem are we trying to solve?
- What do we need to do to solve the problem?
- Why are we trying to solve the problem?
- How do we accomplish solving the problem?

Requirements definition is often the main practice that serves as a bridge between project teams and business stakeholders. The practice should define both product and project requirements as well as related functional and non-functional requirements. Requirements definition should begin early in the planning phase. Requirements should then be managed throughout the life of a project from their high level, through detailed requirements, design, building, and testing. Requirements captured at all business and product levels help to ensure that the project meets its objectives within the agreed upon limitations of time, scope, resources, and quality. Actual requirement types will be dependent upon the project and will also vary based on the methodology used to define them. Some major requirement types include the following:

- **Project requirements** define how the work will be managed. This includes the budget, communication management, resource management, quality assurance, risk management, and scope management. Project requirements focus on the who, when, where, and how something gets done and are generally documented in the project management plan.
- **Product requirements** include high-level features or capabilities that the business team has committed to delivering to a customer. Product requirements do not specify how the features or the capabilities will be designed.
- **Functional requirements** address what the system does. They define any requirement that outlines a specific way a product function or component must perform.
- **Nonfunctional requirements** (also referred to as *Quality of Service* by the International Institute of Business Analysts, Business Analysis Body of Knowledge) address items such as the technical solutions, topics that address the number of people who need to use the product, where the product will be located, the types of transactions processed, and types of technology interactions.

See: https://www.oreilly.com/library/view/a-guide-to/9781935589679/sub6.3.xhtml

https://www2.cdc.gov/cdcup/library/practices_guides/CDC_UP_Requirements_Definition_Practices_Guide.pdf

9

Policy in Public Health

INTRODUCTION

In democratic societies, public health practice sits squarely at the intersection of science and policy. As a population-oriented profession, public health relies on policy making and enforcement to provide the greatest benefit to the largest number of people in society. However, it is often the case that uncertainty exists even in the most secure scientific knowledge about health because there is a myriad combination and interactions of health determinants, including genetics, environmental exposures, human behavior, and societal constraints. Therefore, policies tend to accommodate variability of individuals in a population such that most vulnerable individuals are protected, while also providing benefits to the majority. Ethical guidelines in public health are a way of ensuring fairness in policies that affect everyone. Yet, we do not always get policies right, and there is a continuous process of refining and health-reviewing policies as we learn more about the determinants of health. In some cases, the rights of individuals to make decisions on their own health or risk-taking behavior conflict with attempts to protect populations from individual actions taken under the pursuit of life, liberty, and happiness. The questions in this section focus on key components of policy in public health. These components include opportunities to

- Develop positions on health issues, law, and policy

- Establish goals, timelines, funding alternatives, or partnership opportunities for influencing policy initiatives

- Defend existing health policies, programs, and resources

- Educate policy makers and decision-makers to improve health, social justice, and equity

- Use scientific evidence, best practices, stakeholder input, or public opinion data to inform policy and program decision-making

- Assess positions of key stakeholders for health policies, programs, and resources
- Promote the adoption of health policies, programs, and resources
- Identify the social and economic impact of a health policy, program, or initiative
- Analyze political, social, and economic policies that affect health systems at the local, national, or global levels
- Measure changes in health systems (including input, processes, and output)
- Determine the feasibility and expected outcomes of policy options (e.g., health, fiscal, administrative, legal, ethical, social, political)
- Analyze policy options when designing programs
- Ensure the consistency of policy integration into organizational plans, procedures, structures, and programs
- Implement federal, state, or local regulatory programs and guidelines

■ QUESTIONS

1. The Evidence-Informed Policy Network (EVIPNet) is a network established by the World Health Organization to do the following, EXCEPT

    A. Promote the systematic use of research evidence in health policy making
    B. Strengthen health systems at the national and international levels
    C. Get the right programs, services, and drugs to those who need them
    D. Prioritize healthcare for Executives and Very Important Personalities (EVIP)

2. Which of the following reimbursement methods carry the highest financial risk for medical centers under Managed Care, a healthcare delivery system organized to manage cost, utilization, and quality?

    A. Fee-for-service
    B. *Per diem* (prospective payment)
    C. Percentage co-payment
    D. Capitated

3. In the United States, Medicare is a federal health insurance program authorized in 1966 under the Social Security Administration, and administered through the Centers for Medicare and Medicaid Services. Medicare has several components. Payment for healthcare services of persons over 65 years of age, provided under Medicare Part A, is subsidized in part by the U.S. Government. The financial subsidy is from

    A. Income and employer-based taxes among working age adults
    B. Taxes on consumer products that are also risk factors for disease
    C. Income taxes on the elderly that receive the Medicare benefit
    D. Fees from private hospitals, as well as pharmaceutical and insurance companies

4. The Patient Protection and Affordable Care Act enacted in 2010 specifies some responsibilities for employers depending on the size and structure of the workforce. Employer-based health insurance is characterized by which of the following?

   A. Individuals directly reimburse the provider for the cost of services.
   B. Unemployed persons can qualify if they meet income eligibility requirements.
   C. The federal government subsidizes a portion of the insurance by viewing employer contributions to healthcare as nontaxable income.
   D. The employee has no co-pay for any visits, since the employer assumes all "third-party" risk.

5. The U.S. Centers for Medicare and Medicaid Services (CMS) collects enrollment data from states through multiple reporting channels. The data show that many people who qualify for Medicaid do not enroll. The most likely explanation is

   A. Stigma of poverty implied by participation in a federally funded program
   B. Complicated enrollment rules
   C. Fear of losing Medicaid eligibility if they qualify for employer-based insurance
   D. Medicaid often provides a fragmented healthcare delivery

6. In 2018, the U.S. Bureau of Labor Statistics reported that medical care benefits were available to 69% of private industry workers and 89% of state and local government workers. The most common type of health plan for employed persons covered under private health insurance is

   A. Conventional Insurance
   B. Point of Service (POS)
   C. Preferred Provider Organization (PPO)
   D. Health Management Organization (HMO)

7. In 2017, spending on healthcare in the United States increased 3.9% from the previous year, reaching $3.5 trillion or $10,739 per person. As a share of the nation's gross domestic product, health spending accounted for 17.9%. The most likely reason for the increasing trajectory of healthcare expenditures is

   A. The exorbitant cost of the Managed Care model
   B. Development and purchasing of new technologies (e.g., medical devices, drugs)
   C. Rapid expansion of hospitals operated as businesses for profit
   D. Adverse selection, a state of information asymmetry

8. The distribution, diversity, and organization of healthcare services accessible to a population may influence the quality of care, cost, and comprehensiveness. "Vertical integration" of healthcare services in the organization of healthcare providers means

   A. Multihospital centers serving the same population
   B. Private and not-for profit physicians working together to support the population

    C. Coordination of services across the levels of primary, secondary, and tertiary care

    D. Management of physicians under a "Preferred Provider Organization" (PPO)

9. Managed Care is a healthcare delivery system organized to manage cost, utilization, and quality. Typically, Managed Care Organizations (MCOs) contract with insurers or employers to deliver healthcare using a network of providers offering specific healthcare services. The advantages and disadvantages of MCOs for healthcare outcome have been debated extensively. From the perspective of patients, what is NOT a reported negative characteristic of managed care?

    A. Longer length of visit

    B. Difficulty in directly accessing specialists

    C. Limited choice of providers

    D. Denial of care for some procedures

10. The concept of supply-and-demand is well documented in economics, and its application to healthcare is subject to different interpretations of the relationship between patients and healthcare providers. For example, in some populations, there is a considerable difference in the number of cesarean sections performed in private hospitals compared to public ones. In healthcare, the concept of "supplier-induced demand" means

    A. A healthcare provider ordering more tests, visits, and/or procedures for the patient when the patient may not necessarily need more care

    B. A patient seeking more healthcare because he or she does not pay the full cost of care

    C. Managed Care processes initiated by the federal government based on reimbursable procedures

    D. A healthcare provider acting as the perfect agent for the insurance company

11. As of June 2019, new rules released by the Departments of Labor, Health and Human Services, and the Treasury (collectively, the Departments) permit employers to offer a new "Individual Coverage HRA" as an alternative to traditional group health plan coverage, subject to certain conditions. A consequence of tax subsidies for employer-based health insurance is

    A. Patients seek more healthcare since they had to pay less of its true cost

    B. Expansion of the fraction of the population joining Health Management Organizations (HMOs) and other Managed Care Organizations

    C. Stabilization of healthcare costs

    D. Reduction of overall health insurance premiums

12. U.S. healthcare spending is the highest in the world, and increased 3.9% to reach $3.5 trillion, or $10,739 per person in 2017. The expenditure is not reflected in the health rankings of the U.S. population (e.g., life expectancy of disease burden profile). Cost-effectiveness analysis (CEA) is a strategy that may assist in making the delivery of healthcare resources more efficient. CEA

    A. Represents the basis for the Patient Protection and Affordable Care Act

    B. Measures the net cost of providing a service as well as outcomes obtained

C. Does not relate to persons with disability

D. Resolves the ethical debate between individual versus population benefit

13. In 1960, about 45% of the U.S. population had health insurance coverage compared to more than 80% in 2019. In the same time period, expenditure on healthcare increased from 4% to nearly 18% of gross domestic product. The phrase "moral hazard" is sometimes used in relation to this phenomenon. Moral hazard means

A. Patients request more healthcare procedures if they do not have to pay its full cost.

B. Physicians order more clinical tests to increase their salaries.

C. Individuals seek healthcare only when they are very sick.

D. Insurance companies reject insurance coverage for individuals with preexisting conditions.

14. The increase in access to commercially available genetic testing may provide information of disease susceptibility to individuals who are otherwise healthy. Also, individuals who engage in high-risk lifestyles tend to purchase life insurance or disability insurance, although these genetic predispositions and risky behaviors may not be known by insurance companies; hence, there is information asymmetry. What is the most likely way in which private insurance companies respond to this phenomenon known as "adverse selection"?

A. They assess the health status of potential insurance buyers through extensive interviews or clinical tests.

B. They offer insurance coverage based on preexisting conditions at no additional premium cost.

C. They do not offer disease prevention healthcare costs that target healthy younger people.

D. They offer insurance coverage only to affluent populations.

15. Headache is one of the top 10 contributors to Years Lived with Disability (YLD) worldwide in 2017. In 2019, the U.S. FDA approved Tosymra (sumatriptan) nasal spray for the treatment of acute migraine in adults, expecting that this drug increases the marginal product of health. How will the production function curve unfold?

A. Elevated (shift up)

B. Depressed (shift down)

C. Unchanged

D. Asymptote

16. According to the U.S. Census Bureau, the U.S. population is constantly changing, growing older, and becoming more diverse. The year 2030 will mark an important demographic turning point when all baby boomers will be older than age 65. This will expand the size of the older population so that one in every five residents will be retirement age. In terms of health policy, this aging threatens bankruptcy of

A. Medicare Part A

B. Medicare Part B

    C. Medicare Prescription Drug Coverage
    D. Medicaid

17. In 2018, 30.1 million Americans (11.1%) younger than 65 years do not have health insurance coverage. The concept of health insurance involves

    A. Reduction of out-of-pocket costs for routine purchases
    B. Financial security in the face of uncertainty
    C. An effort to promote social equality
    D. A means to promoting healthy behavior

18. In the United States, employee benefits may include medical, prescription, vision, and dental plans; and dependent care. Most employers did not guarantee health benefits as part of employment contracts before the landmark *Inland Steel Co. v. National Labor Relations Board* lawsuit, settled in 1949. This is a landmark for healthcare policy in the United States because it

    A. Allowed patients to sue physicians for malpractice
    B. Outlawed insurance companies' practice of denying care based on preexisting illness
    C. Gave unions the right to negotiate healthcare benefits, thereby ushering in employer-based health insurance
    D. Validated age 65 as the first year to receive Medicare benefits

19. Co-payments for Medicare Part A are the same amount for all patients, regardless of income. This type of payment structure is referred to as

    A. Equitable
    B. Progressive
    C. Regressive
    D. Proportionate

20. Prohibitive healthcare costs remain a major reason for individuals to declare bankruptcy, even if they have insurance. In the United States, approximately 66% of people who file for bankruptcy cite medical costs as a key reason. What is the purpose of the stop-loss rule in indemnity insurance?

    A. Limits the amount a patient must pay for circumstances in which care is very costly
    B. Limits insurance companies' financial risk
    C. Prevents moral hazard
    D. Provides for an economically fair healthcare provider salary

21. Blockbuster medications generate at least $1 billion in annual revenue for pharmaceutical producers. For example, nearly $20 billion worth of *adalimumab* used for rheumatoid arthritis was sold in 2018. Elimination of patent protection for such blockbuster medications could result in which of the following?

    A. Pharmaceutical companies will reap even larger profits from drug sales.
    B. The manufacture of generic drugs would be outlawed.

   C. A diminished economic incentive for pharmaceutical companies to discover new and innovative drug therapies exists.

   D. Blockbuster drug prices will increase internationally.

22. The World Health Organization defines health as a state of complete physical, mental, and social well-being, and not merely the absence of disease or infirmity. The medical model considers the healthy state as a "product." In this model, the "health production function" describes the relation between

   A. Health inputs (e.g., healthcare, health behaviors) and health outcomes

   B. Health insurance policies and federal expenditures

   C. Healthcare technology and per capita healthcare spending

   D. The population of working age adults and the dependent population of adults older than 65 years

23. In 1990, there were approximately two physicians per 1,000 people in the United States. By 2016, the number was 2.6 physicians per 1,000 people. The increase in physician density presumably led to which of the following phenomena?

   A. The increase in the number of tertiary care specialists

   B. The proliferation of Health Management Organizations (HMOs)

   C. The increase in the number of nursing schools

   D. The strengthening of physician bargaining power with Medicaid and Medicare

24. In the United States, Medicaid is authorized as a collaboration of federal and state agencies to provide healthcare coverage to certain categories of people. The eligibility criterion for Medicaid is

   A. 100 million Americans (~30% of the population)

   B. Low-income families

   C. Adults over 65 years that paid income taxes during their working life

   D. Only children less than 5 years of age

25. The World Health Organization developed an alert system to guide the declaration of an infectious disease outbreak as a "pandemic." Which of the following does NOT satisfy the definition of a pandemic?

   A. Phase 1: No viruses circulating among animals have been reported to cause infections in humans.

   B. Phase 2: Animal influenza virus circulating among domesticated or wild animals is known to have caused infection in humans, and is therefore considered a potential pandemic threat.

   C. Phase 4: This phase is characterized by verified animal-to-animal transmission, but no human transmission.

   D. Phases 5–6: Widespread human infection, in at least two member-countries in at least two different WHO regions.

26. The U.S. agency that is responsible for enforcing policies to protect the health of workers is

  A. Worker Safety and Health Administration
  B. Occupational Safety and Health Administration
  C. Labor Safety and Health Administration
  D. United Workers Union

27. The U.S. agency that is responsible for enforcing policies to protect the environment and human health is the

  A. National Institutes for Health
  B. U.S. Geological Survey
  C. U.S. Environmental Protection Agency
  D. U.S. National Environmental Policy

28. The U.S. agency that is responsible for coordinating all aspects of the health of Americans is the

  A. Department of Health and Human Services
  B. National Institutes of Health
  C. Centers for Disease Control and Prevention
  D. World Health Organization

29. The core function that defines the scope of what will be done by professionals in the public health system is

  A. Assessment
  B. Surveillance
  C. Advocacy
  D. Policy development

30. The policy development core function of public health practice includes which of the following?

  A. Assess, investigate, analyze
  B. Analyze, manage, implement
  C. Advocate, prioritize, plan
  D. Prioritize, investigate, inform

31. Public health advocacy entails the following, EXCEPT

  A. Building constituencies
  B. Identifying resources
  C. Establishing collaborative relationships
  D. Dissolving constituencies to disaggregate the lobbying message

32. Which of the following activities is included in the policy development core function of public health?

  A. Carrying out a toilet inspection in a regional park
  B. Carrying out food inspection in a restaurant

C. Developing goals and measurable objectives for a regional park's role in promoting physical activity

D. Providing health status assessments for a population identified as low income

33. Former United Nations General Secretary Kofi Anan stated, *"It is my aspiration that health will finally be seen not as a blessing to be wished for, but as a human right to be fought for."* Which of the following shows linkages between health and human rights?:

    A. Violations to human rights can have serious health consequences.
    B. Health policies and programs cannot promote or violate human rights in the ways they are designed or implemented.
    C. Vulnerability and the impact of ill health cannot be reduced by taking steps to respect, protect, and fulfill human rights.
    D. Inattention to human rights cannot have serious health consequences.

34. The "right to health" means

    A. Everyone has the right to be healthy.
    B. All governments should establish health services, even if they lack resources.
    C. All governments should establish policies, which will lead to accessible healthcare for all.
    D. All families must have their own physician.

35. Which of the following are criteria for evaluating the right to health?

    A. Availability, accessibility, acceptability, quality
    B. Acceptability, assessment, assurance, accreditation
    C. Accretion, attrition, attribution, allocation
    D. Accreditation, reproduction, qualification, assessment

36. The key steps in the health policy process EXCLUDE

    A. Policy formulation
    B. Policy implementation
    C. Policy modification
    D. Policy compromisation

37. Which of the following is an indirect policy variable used in health policy analysis?

    A. Taxes on tobacco cigarette sales
    B. Incentives to enroll in health insurance
    C. Medicaid eligibility criteria and categories
    D. Private health insurance market reforms

38. The phrase "health in all policies" means

    A. A collaborative approach to improving the health of all people by incorporating health considerations into decision-making across sectors and policy areas

B. All U.S. federal legislation must include a section on public health.
C. All United Nations resolutions must include a section on public health.
D. All state, county, and city hall legislative bills must include a section on public health.

39. Policy instruments exhibit which of the following characteristic(s)?

A. They involve the process of putting a public policy into effect.
B. They are the tools that put a public policy into effect.
C. They are mechanisms to conduct the public policy process in a rational manner.
D. They seek to maximize individual choice.

40. Policy instruments can vary widely in their configuration. An opioid addiction recovery group aims to reduce the societal problems associated with addiction. This could be an example of a

A. Voluntary policy instrument
B. Mixed policy instrument
C. Compulsory policy instrument
D. Indeterminate policy instrument

41. In 2019, California passed a law to make exemptions from mandatory vaccination more difficult to secure. The assessment of public policy concerning mandatory vaccine in terms of the cost of preventable disease management is an example of

A. Positive theory
B. Normative analysis
C. Cost-benefit analysis
D. Cost-effectiveness analysis

42. Policy disagreements are common in public health, particularly when individual freedom and rights appear to conflict with population-level interventions. In the public policy process, satisfying one group's aspirations may mean denying those of another group, which may imply that

A. Government action simply fails to accomplish its intended goals.
B. Gestures, symbols, and words are important components of the political process.
C. Both official claims and concrete action should be looked at carefully.
D. There can be winners and losers in the public health policy process.

43. Voluntary policy instruments in environmental health, for example, allowing manufacturers to voluntarily phase-out potentially toxic chemicals in consumer products, may imply

A. Public policy as government deliberately taking a decision
B. Public policy as government ignoring a public problem it is unaware of
C. Public policy as government, with information, ignoring a public problem
D. Apathetic public engagement

44. As opposed to "command-and-control" policy instruments, "voluntary policy instruments" may be perceived as

    A. Ineffective at addressing complex public health problems
    B. Efficient at addressing complex public health problems
    C. Inconsistent with the notion of a limited state
    D. Effective at addressing complex public health problems

45. Successful implementation of health policy requires clear and consistent communication that includes a combination of

    A. Policy community actors and open government decision-making processes
    B. Normative philosophic arguments and engineering research-obtained facts
    C. Ideological and fiscal explanations
    D. Television and print advertisements

46. Euthanasia is a public health policy issue because

    A. Genetic discrimination is always a public health issue.
    B. Physician-assisted suicide is controversial and only legal in some U.S. states.
    C. Anesthesia is illegal in most U.S. states.
    D. Euthanasia is only a policy issue in Eurasia.

47. Which U.S. government office is responsible for monitoring how other agencies or legislative initiatives regarding public health conduct cost-benefit analyses, for example, of the Patient Care and Affordable Care Act and its implementation?

    A. Department of State
    B. Office of Management and Budget
    C. Council of Economic Advisors
    D. Department of Commerce

48. Which branch of the U.S. government is responsible for ensuring consistency between domestic policies on health and the international policies on public health?

    A. Department of Defense
    B. Department of Homeland Security
    C. Department of Harmonized Policies
    D. Department of State

49. Quarantine policy in public health refers to

    A. Every U.S. citizen having a right to a quart of milk to maintain good health
    B. A byzantine policy that is no longer applicable
    C. Holding individuals suspected of carrying infectious disease in captivity, sometimes against their will
    D. Imprisoning individuals suspected of fraud against the healthcare system

50. Sales tax as a policy instrument (e.g., taxing sugary drinks) can be challenged because of which of the following criteria for evaluating tax policy?

    A. Distributive effects
    B. Buoyancy
    C. Visibility
    D. Collectability

51. Which of the following is NOT an example of an enforceable regulatory public health policy?

    A. Medication quality control
    B. Maximum contaminant levels in water
    C. Air pollutant standards
    D. Dietary intake

52. Many milestone successes in public health result from policies implemented to reduce the impacts, for example, of which of the following risk factor(s)?

    A. Removal of leaded gasoline from use in automobiles
    B. Removal of added sugar in beverages
    C. Removal of saturated fat from food served in restaurants
    D. Removal of salt from snack food items sold in grocery stores

53. The emerging problem of antibiotic resistance is a multifaceted "One Health" issue that is sensitive to public health policies by the following agencies, EXCEPT

    A. The U.S. Environmental Protection Agency
    B. The U.S. Department of Agriculture
    C. The Food and Drug Administration
    D. The U.S. Department of Labor

54. The policy on gun ownership intersects public health policy in the United States because

    A. Injury prevention is not a major task for public health policy.
    B. Cutting costs of running emergency department operations is not a major public health policy issue.
    C. Gun ownership is claimed to be a right guaranteed by the U.S. Constitution, but healthcare is a guaranteed right.
    D. Emergency department visits by gun victims are a major public expenditure.

55. The Centers for Disease Control and Prevention's (CDC) Public Health Law Program has the following strategic goal(s), EXCEPT

    A. To improve the understanding and use of law as a public health tool
    B. To develop the CDC's capacity to apply law to achieve health protection goals
    C. To develop the legal preparedness of the public health system to address all public health priorities
    D. To discover and use loopholes in the legal framework for increasing CDC's budget

56. The United Nations Montreal Protocol on the Ozone Layer is considered a public health policy because

    A. Ultraviolet radiation coming through the ozone hole is a risk factor for skin cancer.
    B. Canadians benefit from having a solid tropospheric ozone layer.
    C. All populations benefit from having a solid tropospheric ozone layer.
    D. The people of Montreal, Canada, were the only population affected by the ozone layer.

57. Many diseases such as vector-borne diseases are sensitive to climate change. The international policy that addresses this risk factor is

    A. The United Nations Framework Convention on Climate Change
    B. The United Nations Climate Pact
    C. The World Health Organization's Framework Convention on Climate Change
    D. The United Nations Environmental Program's Framework Convention on Climate Change

58. In Orange County, California, the Needle-Exchange Program was suspended because of policy disagreements. What is the Needle-Exchange Program?

    A. The gathering of people monthly for needle-work
    B. The supply of injection needles for illicit drug users
    C. The monthly gathering of physicians to teach anyone about vaccination
    D. The free supply of opiods for those in need of relief for existential pain

59. Public health policy processes should include cultural sensitivity at the following stages, EXCEPT

    A. Policy development
    B. Policy implementation
    C. Policy analysis
    D. Policy enforcement

60. U.S. healthcare spending increased 3.9% in 2017, reaching $3.5 trillion or $10,739 per person. As a share of the nation's gross domestic product, health spending accounted for 17.9%, more than any other country. However, healthcare is not considered a typical consumer item because of asymmetric, or imperfect, information, which means which of the following?

    A. Persons in need of treatment having more knowledge about their healthcare needs than health insurance companies
    B. The predictability of healthcare needs and costs
    C. The notion that healthcare is a basic human right
    D. The purchasing of health insurance policies

▪ ANSWERS

1. **D.** The Evidence-Informed Policy Network (EVIPNet) is a network established by the World Health Organization to promote the systematic use of research evidence in health policy making in order to strengthen health systems and get the right programs, services, and drugs to those who need them. EVIPNet does not prioritize healthcare for Executives and Very Important Personalities.

2. **D.** Managed Care is a healthcare delivery system organized to manage cost, utilization, and quality. Medicaid Managed Care provides for the delivery of Medicaid health benefits and additional services through contracted arrangements between state Medicaid agencies and Managed Care Organizations (MCOs) that accept a set per member per month (capitation) payment for these services.

   By contracting with various types of MCOs to deliver Medicaid program healthcare services to their beneficiaries, states can reduce Medicaid program costs and better manage utilization of health services. Improvement in health plan performance, healthcare quality, and outcomes are key objectives of Medicaid Managed Care.

   Some states are implementing a range of initiatives to coordinate and integrate care beyond traditional Managed Care. These initiatives are focused on improving care for populations with chronic and complex conditions, aligning payment incentives with performance goals, and building in accountability for high quality care.

   Capitated refers to participating in, or being a, healthcare system in which a medical provider is given a set fee per patient regardless of the treatment required.

   See: https://www.cdc.gov/mmwr/preview/mmwrhtml/00039850.htm

   https://www.cms.gov/Medicare-Medicaid-Coordination/Medicare-and-Medicaid-Coordination/Medicare-Medicaid-Coordination-Office/FinancialAlignmentInitiative/CapitatedModel.html

   https://www.medicaid.gov/medicaid/managed-care/index.html

3. **A.** In general, Medicare Part A covers

   Inpatient care in a hospital

   Skilled nursing facility care

   Inpatient care in a skilled nursing facility (not custodial or long-term care)

   Hospice care

   Home healthcare

   The U.S. government subsidizes health insurance for most Americans through a variety of programs and tax provisions. In 2017, net subsidies for people under age 65 will total $705 billion, the Congressional Budget Office and the staff of the Joint Committee on Taxation (JCT) estimate.

The federal tax system provides preferential treatment for health insurance that people buy through an employer. That treatment applies to payments and contributions made both by employers and by employees. Unlike cash compensation, employers' payments for their employees' health insurance premiums are excluded from income and payroll taxes. In most cases, the amount that workers pay for their own share of health insurance premiums is also excluded from income and payroll taxes. Contributions made to certain accounts by employers to pay for employees' healthcare costs are excluded from income and payroll taxes as well. In all, that favorable tax treatment cost the federal government about $300 billion in forgone revenues in 2018, and that cost will probably rise over time as the price of healthcare increases. Although a new excise tax will go into effect in 2022, somewhat reducing the tax exclusions' consequences, those exclusions will continue to have significant implications for the federal budget.

See: https://www.cbo.gov/budget-options/54798

https://www.cbo.gov/system/files/115th-congress-2017-2018/reports/53091-fshic.pdf

https://www.medicare.gov/what-medicare-covers/what-part-a-covers

4. **C.** The federal government subsidizes a portion of the insurance by viewing employer contributions to healthcare as nontaxable income. Health Reimbursement Arrangements (HRAs) are a type of account-based health plan that employers can use to reimburse employees for their medical care expenses.

New rules released by the Departments of Labor, Health and Human Services, and the Treasury (collectively, the Departments) permit employers to offer a new "Individual Coverage HRA" as an alternative to traditional group health plan coverage, subject to certain conditions. Among other medical care expenses, Individual Coverage HRAs can be used to reimburse premiums for individual health insurance chosen by the employee, promoting employee and employer flexibility, while also maintaining the same tax-favored status for employer contributions toward a traditional group health plan.

See: https://www.hhs.gov/sites/default/files/health-reimbursement-arrangements.pdf

5. **A.** For the quarter beginning with January 1, 2014, states began reporting Medicaid enrollment data as part of the Medicaid expenditure reporting through the Medicaid Budget and Expenditure System (MBES). The enrollment information is a state-reported count of unduplicated individuals enrolled in the state's Medicaid program at any time during each month in the quarterly reporting period. The enrollment data identifies the total number of Medicaid enrollees and, for states that have expanded Medicaid, provides specific counts for the number of individuals enrolled in the new adult eligibility group, also referred to as the "VIII Group."

In some populations, Medicaid is associated with the welfare system, which is inherently stigmatizing.

See: https://hsrc.himmelfarb.gwu.edu/cgi/viewcontent.cgi?article=1052&context=sphhs_policy_briefs

https://www.medicaid.gov/medicaid/program-information/
medicaid-and-chip-enrollment-data/index.html

https://www.medicaid.gov/medicaid/program-information/
medicaid-and-chip-enrollment-data/enrollment-mbes/index.html

6. C. A Preferred Provider Organization (PPO) is a type of health plan that contracts with medical providers, such as hospitals and doctors, to create a network of participating providers. Individuals pay less if they use providers that belong to the plan's network. Patients can use doctors, hospitals, and providers outside of the network for an additional cost.

Exclusive Provider Organization (EPO): A Managed Care plan where services are covered only if you use doctors, specialists, or hospitals in the plan's network (except in an emergency).

Health Maintenance Organization (HMO): A type of health insurance plan that usually limits coverage to care from doctors who work for or contract with the HMO. It generally won't cover out-of-network care except in an emergency. An HMO may require you to live or work in its service area to be eligible for coverage. HMOs often provide integrated care and focus on prevention and wellness.

Point of Service (POS): A type of plan where you pay less if you use doctors, hospitals, and other healthcare providers that belong to the plan's network. POS plans require you to get a referral from your primary care doctor in order to see a specialist.

Preferred Provider Organization (PPO): A type of health plan where you pay less if you use providers in the plan's network. You can use doctors, hospitals, and providers outside of the network without a referral for an additional cost.

See: https://www.healthcare.gov/choose-a-plan/plan-types

https://www.healthcare.gov/glossary/preferred-provider-organi
zation-ppo

7. B. In 2017, Hospital Care (33% share): Spending for hospital care increased 4.6% to $1.1 trillion in 2017, which was slower than the 5.6% growth in 2016. The slower growth in 2017 was driven by slower growth in the use and intensity of services. Hospital care expenditures slowed among the major payers—private health insurance, Medicare, and Medicaid.

Physician and Clinical Services (20% share): Spending on physician and clinical services increased 4.2% to $694.3 billion in 2017. Growth for physician and clinical services slowed in 2017 and was driven by growth in nonprice factors such as use and intensity of services. Although slowing, growth in clinical services continued to outpace the growth in physician services in 2017.

See: https://www.cms.gov/Research-Statistics-Data-and-Systems/Statis
tics-Trends-and-Reports/NationalHealthExpendData/Downloads/
highlights.pdf

https://www.cms.gov/research-statistics-data-and-systems/statistics
-trends-and-reports/nationalhealthexpenddata/nationalhealthaccounts
historical.html

8. C. Coordination of services across the levels of primary, secondary, and tertiary care is vertical integration that occurs when entities at different levels of the healthcare supply chain combine, such as when hospitals acquire physician practices or health plans acquire pharmacy benefit managers.

See: https://www.ncbi.nlm.nih.gov/pubmed/29613860

9. **A.** Managed Care is a healthcare delivery system organized to manage cost, utilization, and quality. Medicaid Managed Care provides for the delivery of Medicaid health benefits and additional services through contracted arrangements between state Medicaid agencies and Managed Care Organizations (MCOs) that accept a set per member per month (capitation) payment for these services. By contracting with various types of MCOs to deliver Medicaid program healthcare services to their beneficiaries, states can reduce Medicaid program costs and better manage utilization of health services. Improvement in health plan performance, healthcare quality, and outcomes are key objectives of Medicaid Managed Care. Some states are implementing a range of initiatives to coordinate and integrate care beyond traditional Managed Care. These initiatives are focused on improving care for populations with chronic and complex conditions, aligning payment incentives with performance goals, and building in accountability for high quality care. Many states deliver services to Medicaid beneficiaries via managed care arrangements. Federal regulations at 42 CFR 438 set forth quality assessment and performance improvement requirements for states that contract with MCOs and/or prepaid inpatient health plans (PIHPs). These requirements include the development and drafting of a Managed Care quality strategy and the performance of an external quality review (EQR).

Reported quality problems include access to specialists, choice of providers and denial of care, and short visit time periods with providers.

See: https://www.macpac.gov/subtopic/managed-cares-effect-on
-outcomes

10. **A.** Supplier-induced demand (SID) describes the phenomenon where healthcare providers (suppliers) can manipulate patients' demand for healthcare services to create additional demand for these services. It can arise from conflict of interest or vigorous health promotion to improve outcomes.

See: https://www.pc.gov.au/research/supporting/supplier-induced-medi
cal-demand/sidms.pdf

11. **A.** Patients seek more healthcare since they had to pay less of its true cost.

An employer mandate to provide health insurance coverage for employees can be implemented strictly as a mandate requiring compliance without any alternative options, or it can be implemented as a mandate to either provide coverage or pay a "penalty" in the form of a tax or assessment. The premium tax credit is a tax credit that helps eligible individuals and their families pay their premiums for health insurance coverage purchased through the Exchange. The premium tax credit is not available for health insurance coverage purchased outside of the Exchange. Factors that affect premium tax credit eligibility include enrollment in Exchange coverage, eligibility for other types of coverage, and household income.

See: https://aspe.hhs.gov/system/files/pdf/75791/report.pdf

https://www.hhs.gov/sites/default/files/health-reimbursement-arra
ngements.pdf

12. **B.** Cost-effectiveness analysis is a way to examine both the costs and health
outcomes of one or more interventions. It compares an intervention to another
intervention (or the status quo) by estimating how much it costs to gain a unit
of a health outcome, like a life year gained or a death prevented. CEA provides
information on health and cost impacts of an intervention compared to an
alternative intervention (or the status quo). If the net costs of an intervention
are positive (which means a more effective intervention is more costly), the
results are presented as a cost-effectiveness ratio. A cost-effectiveness ratio is
the net cost divided by changes in health outcomes. Examples include cost
per case of disease prevented or cost per death averted. However, if the net
costs are negative (which means a more effective intervention is less costly),
the results are reported as net cost savings.

See: https://www.cdc.gov/policy/polaris/economics/cost-effectiveness
.html

13. **A.** Moral hazard describes the lack of incentive to take precautions against
risk because of protection from consequences, for example, through insurance
coverage. Patients consume more healthcare resources if they do not have to
pay its full cost. For example, the demand for laser ablation to remove spider
veins has increased despite its expense and questionable effectiveness, presumably because the cost is covered by insurance.

See: https://thehill.com/blogs/pundits-blog/healthcare/312035-challeng
ing-the-moral-hazard-in-healthcare-and-insurance

14. **A.** Adverse selection refers to the situation whereby sellers have information
that buyers do not have, or vice versa, about an aspect of product quality.
Insurance companies tend to assess the health of the potential insurance buyers through extensive interviews or tests, and in the past could deny coverage
outright or increase the premium.

See: https://www.naic.org/store/free/ASE-OP.pdf

15. **A.** The production function relates output of a production process to inputs
or factors of production. In this case, the production function curve will be
elevated.

See: https://www.centerwatch.com/drug-information/fda-approved
-drugs/drug/100337/tosymra-sumatriptan-nasal-spray

Schoder, J., & Zweifel, P. (2011). Flat-of-the-curve medicine: A new perspective
on the production of health. *Health Economics Review, 1*(1), 2. doi:10.1186/2191-
1991-1-2

16. **A.** Medicare is a health insurance program for

- People age 65 or older
- People under age 65 with certain disabilities
- People of all ages with end-stage renal disease (permanent kidney failure
  requiring dialysis or a kidney transplant

Medicare Part A (Hospital Insurance)—Part A helps cover inpatient care in
hospitals, including critical access hospitals and skilled nursing facilities (not

custodial or long-term care). It also helps cover hospice care and some home healthcare. Beneficiaries must meet certain conditions to get these benefits. Most people don't pay a premium for Part A, because they or a spouse already paid for it through their payroll taxes while working.

See: https://www.cms.gov/medicare/medicare-general-Information/medicareGenInfo/index.html

17. **B.** Health insurance coverage pays for medical and surgical expenses incurred by the insured. The Center for Consumer Information and Insurance Oversight (CCIIO) is charged with helping implement many reforms of the Affordable Care Act, the historic health reform bill that was signed into law March 23, 2010. CCIIO oversees the implementation of the provisions related to private health insurance. In particular, CCIIO is working with states to establish new Health Insurance Marketplaces. In the first 3 months of 2018, 28.3 million (8.8%) persons of all ages were uninsured at the time of interview—not significantly different from 2017, but 20.3 million fewer persons than in 2010.

See: https://www.cdc.gov/nchs/data/nhis/earlyrelease/Insur201808.pdf

https://www.cdc.gov/nchs/fastats/health-insurance.htm

https://www.cms.gov/cciio/index.html

18. **C.** The *Inland Steel Co. v. National Labor Relations Board* lawsuit gave unions the right to negotiate healthcare benefits, thereby ushering in employer-based health insurance.

See: https://www.courtlistener.com/opinion/1500899/inland-steel-co-v-national-labor-relations-board/

19. **C.** Regressive taxation or co-payment structure is the situation whereby low-income individuals pay a higher amount of their incomes in taxes (or co-pay) compared to high-income earners. So, with the same co-pay regardless of income, Medicare Part A operates with a regressive payment structure.

Medicare Part A is premium-free for people who paid during their employment days. Individuals who buy Medicare Part A pay up to $437 each month. If Medicare taxes are paid for less than 30 quarters, the standard Part A premium is $437. If Medicare taxes are paid for 30–39 quarters, the standard Part A premium is $240.

See: https://www.medicare.gov/your-medicare-costs/part-a-costs

20. **A.** The stop-loss rule in indemnity insurance limits the amount a patient must pay for circumstances in which healthcare is very costly. Under a stop-loss insurance policy, the insurance company is liable for losses that exceed certain limits called deductibles. It does not limit the financial risk or remove moral hazard, nor does it guarantee fair salary for providers.

See: https://www.hcaa.org/page/selffundingstoploss

https://www.cnbc.com/2019/02/11/this-is-the-real-reason-most-americans-file-for-bankruptcy.html

21. **C.** It costs between $600 million and $2.7 billion for a pharmaceutical company to take a medication from discovery to the healthcare market. Therefore, patent protection is desirable for as long as possible, otherwise, there will be

a diminished economic incentive for pharmaceutical companies to discover new and innovative drug therapies.

See: https://khn.org/morning-breakout/facing-the-upcoming-loss-of-block buster-drugs-patent-protections-abbvie-buys-allergan-in-mega-63b -deal

https://www.managedcaremag.com/news/20170914/costs-bring -drug-market-remain-dispute

22. **A.** The production function relates output of a production process to inputs of production.

Health is a state of complete physical, mental, and social well-being and not merely the absence of disease or infirmity. This definition is in the Preamble to the Constitution of WHO as adopted by the International Health Conference, New York, June 19 to July 22, 1946; signed on July 22, 1946, by the representatives of 61 States (Official Records of WHO, no. 2, p. 100) and entered into force on April 7, 1948. The definition has not been amended since 1948.

See: https://www.centerwatch.com/drug-information/fda-approved -drugs/drug/100337/tosymra-sumatriptan-nasal-spray

https://www.who.int/about/who-we-are/frequently-asked -questions

23. **B.** Health Management Organizations (HMOs) are health insurance organizations that charge subscribers a predetermined fee in return for a range of medical services from physicians and healthcare workers registered with the organization.

See: https://data.worldbank.org/indicator/SH.MED.PHYS.ZS?end=2013& locations=XU&start=2013&view=bar

https://www.healthsystemtracker.org/indicator/quality/physicians -per-capita

24. **B.** Medicaid is a healthcare program that assists low-income families or individuals in paying for doctor visits, hospital stays, long-term medical or custodial care costs, and more. Medicaid is a joint program, funded primarily by the federal government and run at the state level, where coverage may vary.

As of 2019, Medicaid provides health coverage to 65.7 million Americans, including eligible low-income adults, children, pregnant women, elderly adults, and people with disabilities. Medicaid is administered by states, according to federal requirements. The program is funded jointly by states and the federal government.

See: https://www.medicaid.gov/medicaid/index.html

25. **C.** In the 2009 revision of the phase descriptions, WHO has retained the use of a six-phased approach for easy incorporation of new recommendations and approaches into existing national preparedness and response plans. The grouping and description of pandemic phases have been revised to make them easier to understand, more precise, and based upon observable phenomena. Phases 1 to 3 correlate with preparedness, including capacity development and response planning activities, while Phases 4 to 6 clearly

signal the need for response and mitigation efforts. Furthermore, periods after the first pandemic wave are elaborated to facilitate postpandemic recovery activities.

See: https://www.who.int/csr/disease/swineflu/phase/en

26. **B.** With the Occupational Safety and Health Act of 1970, the U.S. Congress created the Occupational Safety and Health Administration (OSHA) to ensure safe and healthful working conditions for working men and women by setting and enforcing standards and by providing training, outreach, education, and assistance.

See: https://www.osha.gov/aboutosha

27. **C.** The mission of the U.S. Environmental Protection Agency (EPA) is to protect human health and the environment by ensuring that

Americans have clean air, land, and water.

National efforts to reduce environmental risks are based on the best available scientific information.

Federal laws protecting human health and the environment are administered and enforced fairly, effectively, and as Congress intended.

Environmental stewardship is integral to U.S. policies concerning natural resources, human health, economic growth, energy, transportation, agriculture, industry, and international trade, and these factors are similarly considered in establishing environmental policy.

All parts of society—communities, individuals, businesses, and state, local, and tribal governments—have access to accurate information sufficient to effectively participate in managing human health and environmental risks.

Contaminated lands and toxic sites are cleaned up by potentially responsible parties and revitalized.

Chemicals in the marketplace are reviewed for safety.

See: https://www.epa.gov/aboutepa/our-mission-and-what-we-do

28. **A.** The U.S. Department of Health and Human Services' (DHHS) mission is to enhance and protect the health and well-being of all Americans. The U.S. Department of Health and Human Services fulfills that mission by providing for effective health and human services and fostering advances in medicine, public health, and social services.

See: https://www.hhs.gov/about/index.html

29. **D.** Policy development is a core function of public health with the following essential services:

Inform, educate, and empower people about environmental health issues

Mobilize community partnerships and actions to identify and solve environmental health problems

Develop policies and plans that support individual and community environmental health efforts

See: https://www.cdc.gov/nceh/ehs/ephli/core_ess.htm

30. **C.** Policy development is a core function of public health with the following essential services:

Inform, educate, and empower people about environmental health issues

Mobilize community partnerships and actions to identify and solve environmental health problems

Develop policies and plans that support individual and community environmental health efforts

Analysis, investigation, and implementation are related but tangential to the policy development function, which focuses on advocacy, prioritization, and planning

See: https://www.cdc.gov/nceh/ehs/ephli/core_ess.htm

31. **D.** Dissolving constituencies or sabotaging lobbying messages are the opposite of public health advocacy. For example, the American Public Health Association has a strong advocacy initiative. The group "Public Health Advocates" works to promote health and eliminate health disparities by transforming neighborhoods into places that nurture well-being.

See: https://phadvocates.org/who-we-are

https://www.apha.org/policies-and-advocacy/advocacy-for-public -health

32. **C.** Policy development is a core function of public health with the following essential services:

Inform, educate, and empower people about environmental health issues

Mobilize community partnerships and actions to identify and solve environmental health problems

Develop policies and plans that support individual and community environmental health efforts

Developing goals and measurable objectives for a regional park's role in promoting physical activity is a policy development function. Toilet and restaurant inspections are included in the assurance function, and health status assessment is an assessment core function.

See: https://www.cdc.gov/nceh/ehs/ephli/core_ess.htm

33. **A.** Violations or lack of attention to human rights can have serious health consequences. Overt or implicit discrimination in the delivery of health services—both within the health workforce and between health workers and service users—acts as a powerful barrier to health services, and contributes to poor quality care. Mental ill-health often leads to a denial of dignity and autonomy, including forced treatment or institutionalization, and disregard of individual legal capacity to make decisions. Paradoxically, mental health is still given inadequate attention in public health, in spite of the high levels of violence, poverty, and social exclusion that contribute to worse mental and physical health outcomes for people with mental health disorders. Violations of human rights not only contribute to and exacerbate poor health, but for many, including people with disabilities, indigenous populations, women living with HIV, sex workers, people who use drugs, and transgender and

intersex people, the healthcare setting presents a risk of heightened exposure to human rights abuses—including coercive or forced treatment and procedures.

See: https://www.who.int/news-room/fact-sheets/detail/human-rights -and-health

34. **C.** TThe enjoyment of the highest attainable standard of health is one of the fundamental rights of every human being without distinction of race, religion, political belief, economic, or social condition."

- Statement by Dr. Tedros Adhanom Ghebreyesus, WHO Director-General, December 10, 2017

See: https://www.who.int/mediacentre/news/statements/fundamental -human-right/en

35. **A.** The current discourse on Human Rights and Health is evolving from an exclusive focus on availability of health workers—that is, numbers—toward equal importance accessibility, acceptability, quality, and performance of the health sector.

- Availability—The sufficient supply and appropriate stock of health workers, with the competencies and skill-mix to match the health needs of the population
- Accessibility—The equitable distribution of these health workers taking into account the demographic composition, rural–urban mix, and under-served areas or populations
- Acceptability—Health workforce characteristics and ability (e.g., sex, language, culture, and age) to treat all patients with dignity, create trust, and promote demand for services
- Quality—Health workforce competencies, skills, knowledge, and behavior, as assessed according to professional norms and as perceived by users

See: https://www.who.int/gender-equity-rights/knowledge/aaaq-infogra phic/en

https://www.who.int/workforcealliance/media/qa/04/en

36. **D.** Policy compromisation means breaching or undermining a health protective policy, and it is not supportive of progress.

37. **A.** In 2017, tobacco companies spent $9.36 billion marketing cigarettes and smokeless tobacco in the United States. This amount translates to more than $25 million each day, or more than $1 million every hour. Increasing the price of tobacco products is the single most effective way to reduce consumption. A 10% increase in price has been estimated to reduce overall cigarette consumption by 3% to 5%. Research on cigarette consumption suggests that both youth and young adults are two to three times more likely to respond to increases in price than adults. Taxes are more effective than a direct policy to ban smoking.

See: https://www.cdc.gov/statesystem/excisetax.html

https://www.cdc.gov/tobacco/data_statistics/fact_sheets/ economics/econ_facts/index.htm

38. **A.** Health in All Policies (HiAP) is a collaborative approach to improving the health of all people by incorporating health, equity, and sustainability considerations into decision-making across sectors and policy areas. The approach recognizes that our greatest health challenges—such as chronic illness, climate change, health inequities between populations, and increasing healthcare costs—are highly complex and influenced by policies, programs, and investments across sectors.

    HiAP, at its core, is an approach to addressing the social determinants of health that are the key drivers of health outcomes and health inequities. HiAP supports improved health outcomes and health equity through collaboration between public health practitioners and those nontraditional partners who have influence over the social determinants of health.

    See: https://www.cdph.ca.gov/Programs/OHE/Pages/HIAP.aspx

39. **B.** Policy instruments are interventions made by government agencies in local, national, or international constituencies with the intention to achieve outcomes that conform to the objectives of public policy.

    See: https://www.sciencedirect.com/topics/earth-and-planetary-sciences/policy-instrument

40. **A.** Voluntary policy instruments adopt approaches, for example, in environmental policy, that include agreements on environmental performance negotiated with manufacturing industry, and public programs in which industries can volunteer to participate.

    See: http://www.oecd.org/env/tools-evaluation/voluntaryapproachesforenvironmentalpolicy.htm

41. **D.** Cost-effectiveness analysis is a way to examine both the costs and health outcomes of one or more interventions. It compares an intervention to another intervention (or the status quo) by estimating how much it costs to gain a unit of a health outcome, like a life year gained or a death prevented.

    See: https://www.cdc.gov/policy/polaris/economics/cost-effectiveness.html

    https://www.cdph.ca.gov/Programs/CID/DCDC/pages/immunize.aspx

42. **D.** Public health professionals play an important role in the policy process, for example, by conducting policy analysis, communicating findings, developing partnerships, and promoting and implementing evidence-based interventions. Often, there is a need to debate and negotiate to reach common ground. There can be winners and losers in the public health policy process.

    See: https://www.cdc.gov/policy/analysis/process/index.html

    https://www.nature.com/articles/s41599-018-0121-9

43. **C.** Voluntary policy instruments adopt approaches, for example, in environmental policy, that include agreements on environmental performance negotiated with manufacturing industry, and public programs in which industries can volunteer to participate.

    See: http://www.oecd.org/env/tools-evaluation/voluntaryapproachesforenvironmentalpolicy.htm

44. A. Command-and-control policy refers to environmental policy that relies on regulation (permission, prohibition, standard setting, and enforcement) as opposed to financial incentives, that is, economic instruments of cost internalization. Voluntary policy instruments adopt approaches, for example, in environmental policy, that include agreements on environmental performance negotiated with manufacturing industry, and public programs in which industries can volunteer to participate.

See: https://stats.oecd.org/glossary/detail.asp?ID=383

45. A. Policy implementation requires the translation of the enacted policy into action, monitoring uptake, and ensuring full implementation with the following steps:

Translate policy into practice and define standards for implementation

Implement regulations, guidelines, recommendations, directives, and organizational policies

Identify indicators and metrics to evaluate implementation and impact of the policy

Coordinate resources and train personnel to implement policy

Assess implementation and ensure compliance with policy

Support postimplementation sustainability of policy

Public health professionals build capacity of states, territories, tribes, and communities to implement policy (e.g., education, training, technical assistance, guidance) and support sustainability of policy after implementation (e.g., continued educational efforts)

See: https://www.cdc.gov/policy/polaris/training/policy-cdc-policy-proc ess.html

46. B. Section 1553 of the Affordable Care Act states that the federal government, and any state or local government or healthcare provider that receives federal financial assistance under this Act (or an amendment made by this Act) or any health plan created under this Act (or an amendment made by this Act), may not discriminate against an individual or institutional healthcare entity because the entity does not provide any healthcare item or service that causes, or assists in causing, the death of any individual, such as by assisted suicide, euthanasia, or mercy killing.

See: https://www.hhs.gov/civil-rights/for-individuals/refusal-provide -assisted-suicide-services/index.html

47. D. The Department of Commerce works with businesses, universities, communities, and the nation's workers to promote job creation, economic growth, sustainable development, and improved standards of living for Americans.

See: https://www.usa.gov/federal-agencies/u-s-department-of-commerce

https://www.uschamber.com/report/health-reform-law-101

48. D. To protect the American people, their homes, and their way of life, the United States actively works to prevent, detect, and respond to infectious disease threats. Outbreaks of infectious disease do not respect national boundaries. Halting and treating diseases at their points of origin is one of the best and most economical ways of saving lives and protecting Americans. The U.S. National Security Strategy and U.S. National Biodefense Strategy prioritize U.S. efforts to build global health security capacity. The United States leads internationally, collaborating with countries to invest in basic healthcare systems and address infectious diseases such as HIV/AIDS, malaria, Ebola, Zika, and influenza.

See: https://www.state.gov/policy-issues/global-health

49. **A.** Isolation and quarantine help protect the public by preventing exposure to people who have or may have a contagious disease.

- Isolation separates sick people with a contagious disease from people who are not sick.
- Quarantine separates and restricts the movement of people who were exposed to a contagious disease to see if they become sick.

U.S. Quarantine Stations, located at ports of entry and land border crossings, use these public health practices as part of a comprehensive quarantine system that serves to limit the introduction of infectious diseases into the United States and to prevent their spread.

See: https://www.cdc.gov/quarantine/index.html

50. **A.** Distributive effects address how household incomes and wealth are distributed, what socioeconomic consequences that has, and how the distribution is affected by public policies such as taxation.

See: https://ec.europa.eu/social/main.jsp?langId=en&catId=1196&newsId =2568&furtherNews=yes

51. **D.** Dietary intake by individuals is not an enforceable regulatory public health policy. It may be supported by nutritional guidelines.

See: https://health.gov/dietaryguidelines/2015/guidelines

52. **A.** Dr. Carol Browner, former administrator of the U.S. Environmental Protection Agency, said "the elimination of lead from gas is one of the great environmental achievements of all time" "Thousands of tons of lead have been removed from the air, and blood levels of lead in our children are down 70%. This means that millions of children will be spared the painful consequences of lead poisoning, such as permanent nerve damage, anemia, or mental retardation."

See: https://archive.epa.gov/epa/aboutepa/epa-takes-final-step-phaseout -leaded-gasoline.html

53. **D.** The U.S. Department of Labor is not directly engaged with the One Health approach or antibiotic resistance. The EPA regulates wastewater that may be contaminated with antibiotics, Department of Agriculture regulates antibiotic use in farm animals and plants. FDA regulates antibiotic prescriptions and manufacture. On March 27, 2015, President Obama released the National Action Plan to Combat Antibiotic-Resistant Bacteria.

See: https://obamawhitehouse.archives.gov/the-press-office/2015/03/27/ fact-sheet-obama-administration-releases-national-action-plan-combat- ant

54. D. Each year in the United States, gun violence kills more than 38,000 people and causes about 85,000 injuries. Gunshot victims are typically rushed to emergency departments in hospitals operating at major cost to the public.

See: https://appropriations.house.gov/legislation/hearings/addressing-the-public-health-emergency-of-gun-violence

https://www.apha.org/topics-and-issues/gun-violence

https://www.cdc.gov/nchs/pressroom/sosmap/firearm_mortality/firearm.htm

55. D. The Centers for Disease Control and Prevention (CDC) does not try to discover and use loopholes in the legal framework for increasing the CDC's budget.

The CDC's strategy is based on action plans and detailed measures of success.

Examples include the following:

- Opioids—Reduce U.S. drug overdose mortality by at least 15% by 2021
- Opioid data—Reduce data delay from 3 months to 1 week for nonfatal opioid overdoses
- Influenza—By 2021, increase flu vaccination coverage rates among children to 65% and among pregnant women to 55%
- HIV/AIDS—Eliminate new HIV infections in 10 years
- Vaccine-preventable—Increase by 10% up-to-date HPV vaccination coverage rate in 2021 compared to 2017 (48.6%)
- Rapid response—By 2022, triple the number of CDC rapid response teams and trained incident managers
- Vector-borne—Reduce by 75% cases of Rocky Mountain spotted fever in U.S. tribal communities
- Hepatitis C—Reduce hepatitis C-related deaths by 65% in 10 targeted states by 2024, as a first step to a national program
- Antibiotics—Reduce by 50% inappropriate antibiotic use in outpatient settings by 2020
- Global—Zero countries with wild poliovirus
- Diabetes—Reduce the number of new diabetes diagnoses from 1.4 M in 2018 to 1.1 M cases per year by 2025
- AMD—Increase the routine use of Advanced Molecular Detection from 37 states (2017) to all states (2019)

See: https://www.cdc.gov/about/organization/strategic-framework/index.html

56. A. The international treaty called The Montreal Protocol on Substances That Deplete the Ozone Layer (Montreal Protocol) is gradually eliminating the production and consumption of ozone-depleting substances to limit their damage to the Earth's ozone layer. The Montreal Protocol is signed by 197 countries—the first treaty in the history of the United Nations to achieve universal ratification—and is considered by many the most successful environmental global action. The United States signed the Montreal Protocol in 1987, and has been a leader in guiding the successes of the treaty. Over the past 30 years, the EPA has been a proud contributor to the broad coalition that developed and implemented flexible, innovative, and effective approaches to protect the stratospheric ozone layer. In 1995, the United Nations named September 16 the International Day for the Protection of the Ozone Layer, also known as World Ozone Day.

See: https://www.epa.gov/ozone-layer-protection/international-actions
    -montreal-protocol-substances-deplete-ozone-layer

57. **A.** The United Nations Framework Convention on Climate Change (UNFCCC) entered into force on March 21, 1994. Today, it has near-universal membership. The 197 countries that have ratified the Convention are called Parties to the Convention. The UNFCCC is a "Rio Convention," one of the three adopted at the "Rio Earth Summit" in 1992. Its sister Rio Conventions are the UN Convention on Biological Diversity and the Convention to Combat Desertification. The three are intrinsically linked. It is in this context that the Joint Liaison Group was set up to boost cooperation among the three conventions, with the ultimate aim of developing synergies in their activities on issues of mutual concern. It now also incorporates the Ramsar Convention on Wetlands. Preventing "dangerous" human interference with the climate system is the ultimate aim of the UNFCCC.

See: https://unfccc.int

58. **B.** Since the late 1980s, syringe exchange programs (SEPs) have been operating in California, providing sterile syringes, collecting used ones, and acting as points of access to health education and care for people who inject drugs. SEPs are a critical part of efforts to protect and improve the health of all Californians, and are one of the cornerstones of the efforts to improve the health and well-being of people who inject drugs.

See: https://www.cdph.ca.gov/Programs/CID/DOA/Pages/OA_prev_
    sep.aspx

59. **D.** Policy enforcement should be fair regardless of cultural differences.

Public health is concerned with protecting the health of communities and entire populations. Whether as small as a local neighborhood, or as big as an entire country, policy is one potentially effective way to improve the health of populations. For example, the Centers for Disease Control and Prevention (CDC) policy process includes five domains that often overlap or occur in a different order. However, in an ideal scenario, a problem is defined, potential policy solutions are identified, analyzed, and prioritized, and the best solution is adopted and evaluated.

See: https://www.cdc.gov/policy/polaris/training/policy-cdc-policy
    -process.html

60. **A.** Information asymmetry, or information failure, occurs when one party to an economic transaction possesses greater material knowledge than the other party. In healthcare, patients may know more about their needs than insurance companies.

See: https://www.cms.gov/research-statistics-data-and-systems/statistics-
    trends-and-reports/nationalhealthexpenddata/nationalhealthaccounts
    historical.html

https://www.investopedia.com/terms/a/asymmetricinformation.asp

10 Health Equity and Social Justice

INTRODUCTION

In 1966, Dr. Martin Luther King, civil rights leader and advocate, delivered a remarkable speech at the meeting of the Medical Committee for Human Rights, which was a group of American healthcare professionals organized to provide medical care for civil rights workers, community activists, and volunteers working during the "Freedom Summer" project of 1964. A famous quotation from Dr. King's speech is that *"Of all the forms of inequality, injustice in healthcare is the most shocking and inhumane."* Correcting injustice and inequality in public healthcare remains a major challenge for researchers and practitioners. In fact, increases in health disparities and inequity may be a consequence of human population increases and intranational and international migration. The concentration of wealth in some individuals and transnational characteristics of large corporations, coupled with the rapid expansion of social networks, are relatively new phenomena that may be driving our recognition of gaps in population health status. The root causes of inequality are notoriously associated with social determinants of health, which expands the interdisciplinary and interprofessional scope of public health. It is increasingly important to gain competency in recognizing health equity and social justice issues, with particular attention on the tools and resources needed to prevent problems and to correct problems before they become entrenched. The questions in this section focus on key components of health equity and social justice topics with relevance to the following competencies:

- Application of a social–ecological model to analyze population health issues

- Designing needs and resource assessments for communities or populations

- Assessing how the values and perspectives of diverse individuals, communities, and cultures influence individual and societal health behaviors, choices, and practices

- Using culturally appropriate concepts and skills to engage and empower diverse populations

- Analyzing the availability, acceptability, and accessibility of public health services and activities across diverse populations

- Addressing health disparities in the delivery of public health services and activities

- Conducting culturally appropriate risk and resource assessment, management, and communication with individuals and populations

- Incorporating strategies for interacting and collaborating with persons from diverse backgrounds

- Including representatives of diverse constituencies in partnerships

- Describing the characteristics of a population-based health problem, for example, magnitude, person, time, and place

QUESTIONS

1. Environmental justice is the fair treatment and meaningful involvement of all people regardless of race, color, national origin, culture, or income with respect to the development, implementation, and enforcement of environmental laws, regulations, and policies. Which of the following is true about the environmental justice movements in the United States?

   A. By many accounts, the environmental justice movement began in 1882 in Warren County, North Carolina
   B. In response to growing public concern and mounting scientific evidence, President Clinton issued Executive Order 12898, "Federal Actions to Address Environmental Justice in Minority Populations and Low-Income Populations" in 1994
   C. Global warming is not likely to affect people of color, low-income families, or indigenous communities. Those who are most affected are also responsible for the greenhouse gas emissions that cause the problem—both globally and within the United States
   D. Environmental justice is a European concept, not really applicable to U.S. situations

2. Public health interventions on a large population scale are often controversial because of variations in dose-response among individuals or for political reasons. The following represents examples of such interventions, except

   A. Fluoridation of drinking water
   B. Enrichment of breads with vitamin B3
   C. Genetically engineered rice with vitamin A
   D. Genetically engineered corn with estrogen

3. The concept of "food security" has taken on new meaning and emphasis in public health due to high profile cases such as deceptive practice of adding

melamine to food meant for human consumption. The following include agencies responsible for ensuring the quality and safety of food consumed in the United States, except

A. Food and Drug Administration
B. Department of the Interior
C. Environmental Protection Agency
D. Department of Agriculture

4. The "Healthy People 2020" objectives call on public health professionals to reduce health disparities. As a public health practitioner responsible for developing a plan to reduce disparities in Alzheimer's disease, which of the following areas of disparity should not be of concern?

A. Racial/ethnic
B. Economic income
C. Age
D. Level of education

5. The challenge for public health in changing addictive behavior with respect to harmful drugs is complicated by shifting public attitudes and by the impact of advertising and peer pressure. The following strategies have proven effective in controlling drug abuse at the population level, except

A. Incarceration
B. Education
C. Prevention
D. Early diagnosis

6. Which of the following terms refer to the ability of an individual to understand and respect values, attitudes, and mores that differ across cultures and to consider and respond appropriately to these differences in planning, implementing, and evaluating health education and promotion programs and interventions?

A. Cultural awareness
B. Cultural perspective
C. Cultural competence
D. Cultural relevance

7. The two most important environmental justice components that affect exposure to environmental health and injury risks are

A. Age and race
B. Gender and income
C. Race and gender
D. Race and income

8. Specific disciplines such as cardiology should include training in global health for the following reason(s):

A. Immigrants do not generally have heart diseases
B. Cardiovascular disease is a relevant disease burden only in affluent countries with high life expectancy

C. Research collaborations across countries rarely aid important discoveries
D. Consideration of cultural factors can help cardiologists deliver effective therapies

9. Historical concepts of health usually reflect the means of acquiring knowledge and the depth of knowledge about nature and natural phenomena in different cultures and societies. Which of the following are concepts and theories of health and illness that have been influential in contemporary global health?

   A. Miasma Theory
   B. Shamanism
   C. Transcendental Transition
   D. Germ Theory of Disease

10. Human beliefs about the cause(s) of disease are diverse, influenced by socio-cultural attributes. Consider that historically, the Navajo concept of cancer is understood as part of a larger class of 'sores that do not heal' and 'keep rotting' and disease may result from exposure to animals, natural phenomena, ceremonials, evil spirits, and enemies or aliens, with witchcraft as an additional source of illness. Cultural competence in global health practice instructs that these sorts of believes

    A. Are irrelevant to tackling the Global Burden of Disease
    B. Are inferior to the Miasma Model of Disease Causation
    C. Are inferior to the Germ Theory of Disease Causation
    D. May be important for designing specific strategies to reduce the burden of disease in populations.

11. "Type II diabetes mellitus is currently the leading cause of death in Mexico. Oaxaca is one of the poorest states in Mexico with the largest concentration of indigenous people in the country. Despite the alarming increase of diabetes rates in this region, little is known about the indigenous populations' cultural understandings and related practices for this chronic disease." Research results suggest that younger age and stronger beliefs in punitive and mystical retribution regarding diabetes causality increased the likelihood of using traditional medicine." The research results may be used in what way to reduce the burden of diabetes in Oaxaca?

    A. To aid in the development of culturally tailored programs to address diabetes prevention and management efforts in the region
    B. To provide modern insulin treatment for managing diabetes only to those who do hold strong believe in punitive and mystical retribution regarding diabetes causality
    C. To provide life-style modification programs (e.g., exercise) only to those who do not hold strong believe in punitive and mystical retribution regarding diabetes causality
    D. To campaign against strong believes in punitive and mystical retribution regarding diabetes causality

12. In rural southern Tanzania, special sleeping arrangements are made during funeral ceremonies. "Viewed as a symbol of modernity and a reflection of wealth and individual pride, the bednet becomes physically and symbolically

inappropriate in the more sacred, 'in-between' site of the funeral." This observation provides opportunities to develop interventions against which the following disease burden?

A. Mental illness
B. Diarrheal diseases
C. Malaria
D. Ebola outbreaks

13. In 2015, California passed a law (Senate Bill 277, Pan. Public health; vaccinations) to "eliminate the exemption from existing specified immunization requirements based upon personal beliefs but would allow exemption from future immunization requirements deemed appropriate by the State Department of Public Health for either medical reasons or personal beliefs." This law was passed, despite some citizen protests, in order to more effectively protect Californian's against the resurging global burden of

A. Lung cancer
B. Zika virus
C. Measles
D. Ebola virus

14. Social stigma is one of the risk factors that exacerbate disease burden. Different societies stigmatize various diseases to different extents, thereby complicating efforts to reduce the burden among vulnerable populations. The following diseases are generally considered high on the list of stigmatized diseases internationally, except

A. Mental illness
B. Cardiovascular disease
C. HIV/AIDS
D. Leprosy

15. The U.S. program "Healthy People 2020" defines "health equity" as

A. "Attainment of the highest level of health for all people. Health Equity means efforts to ensure that all people have full and equal access to opportunities that enable them to lead healthy lives."
B. "Preventable differences in the burden of disease, injury, violence, or in opportunities to achieve optimal health experienced by socially disadvantaged racial, ethnic, and other population groups, and communities."
C. "A particular type of health difference that is closely linked with social, economic, and/or environmental disadvantage."
D. "Offering free healthcare, with optional appointments and evening clinic hours to make healthcare more accessible to black men."

16. In the United States, Hispanic and African American patients have been shown to experience organ transplantation programs differently from other racial and ethnic groups. Which of the following is most likely TRUE for Hispanic and African American organ transplant patients?

A. Longer wait times in getting referred to a transplant specialist
B. Shorter wait time on the organ transplant list

    C. Higher rates of graft survival after receiving an organ transplant

    D. Lower mortality after receiving an organ transplant

17. In 2019, an estimated 36,300 homeless people were living in the city of Los Angeles, many in rodent-infested squalid street conditions. If confirmed, higher mortality rates among the homeless population may be due to

    A. Increased likelihood of exposure to *Rickettsia typhi*

    B. Reduced exposure to fine particulate matter

    C. Stress-induced hypotension

    D. Lack of proper education

18. Imagine that you are a public health professional managing a behavior modification project for the county hospital. What approach will you use for an uncooperative, self-abusing opioid-addicted person from a low socioeconomic neighborhood?

    A. Establish an authoritative provider–recipient relationship by using stern language

    B. Refrain from following up on such individuals when possible

    C. Ensure that your personal biases do not taint professional judgment

    D. Allow the addict's self-destructive behaviors to subside before providing preventive information

19. Tuberculosis has always been associated with socioeconomic determinants including housing conditions, labor and employment conditions, and therapy adherence. As a public health professional, how would you guide a tuberculosis-infected person that you suspect is incapable of keeping follow-up appointments?

    A. Encourage the person to educate him- or herself and take responsibility for his or her health

    B. Establish a system of penalties and threats using the fear appeal approach to increase compliance rate

    C. Disregard the person's incapacities and fit them into the schedule anyway

    D. Discuss the importance of personal responsibility before administering follow-up care

20. Poor adherence to antibiotic therapy against tuberculosis infection can result in the incidence of antibiotic-resistant infection. The social determinants of poor adherence include

    A. Inability to take time from multiple jobs to collect pharmaceutical prescriptions

    B. Genetically encoded resistance to antibiotic therapy

    C. Mistrust of the neighbors

    D. Fear of being outed on social network

21. The California Health Information Survey (CHIS; 2011–2012) showed the age-adjusted prevalence of diabetes in Hispanics was 10.5%, more than twice the

rate (4.9%) in non-Hispanic White Californians. As a public health professional, which of the following approaches is most effective in helping patients with type 2 diabetes to lose weight?

A. Advocate the American Diabetes Association's calorie diet limit for all patients
B. Recommend daily exercise and decreased food intake
C. Suggest substituting healthy ingredients for meals and snacks based on the patient's cultural heritage and personal preferences
D. Refer patients to a dietitian for all their diet-related inquiries

22. The use of alternative therapies is common in some populations. How should healthcare providers approach patients with type 2 diabetes who also regularly visit traditional/alternative medicine practitioners?

A. Integrate the alternative therapy by recording the history and current use of alternative medication to avoid drug interactions
B. Warn the patient that alternative medicine and therapies are worthless against diabetes
C. Ask to meet with the traditional medicine practitioner to discuss the best practices
D. Ask to meet with the patient's family members to discourage them from influencing the patient about alternative therapy for diabetes management.

23. Public health professionals may occasionally interact with individuals with misconceptions about the cause of disease or the effectiveness of certain therapies. In such cases, which of the following is the best professional way to respond?

A. Politely agree with the individual about his or her beliefs
B. Politely reject the individual's misconceptions directly and move on
C. Assure the individual that his or her fears are unscientific and based on superstition
D. Explain the scientific basis of the disease and admit to uncertainties in scientific knowledge, if such exist

24. The disparity in morbidity and mortality among populations in various socioeconomic categories is referred to as

A. Health gradient
B. Gender gradient
C. Zipcode gradient
D. Economic gradient

25. The developmental influences of health inequalities is best conceptualized in terms of which of the following approaches?

A. Social Darwinism approach
B. Social Ecological approach
C. Naturalist approach
D. Behaviorist approach

26. In addition to ancestry, individual behavior, families, education, and neighborhoods can explain social inequalities in health according to which of the following explanatory organizational systems?

    A. Megasystem
    B. Mesosystem
    C. Microsystem
    D. Macrosystem

27. Economic factors play roles in defining health status, including but not limited to affordability of insurance and therapies, diet, and access to recreational activities that promote disease prevention. The social gradient in health explains health inequalities as

    A. An artifact
    B. Materialist and structuralist explanations
    C. Natural and social selection
    D. Cultural differences

28. The ecological model of health includes the individual and personal characteristics as one possible explanation for health inequalities. In this model, reckless or irresponsible behavior or incautious lifestyle are explained as

    A. An artifact
    B. Materialist and structuralist explanations
    C. Cultural or behavioral differences
    D. Natural and social selection

29. The relationship between income inequality and health is described by the "health selection" model, which implies that

    A. Healthy people are born, not made.
    B. People are not sick because they are poor. Rather, poor health lowers one's income and limits one's earning potential.
    C. Income inequality erodes social bonds that allow people to work together, decreases social resources, and results in low trust and civic participation, greater crime, and other unhealthy conditions.
    D. Income inequality results in less investment in social and environmental conditions necessary for promoting health among the poorest.

30. Moral philosophers have long debated the theories of fairness and justice. Which of the following principles have featured prominently in the debates?

    A. Assuring people equal basic liberties including guaranteeing the right of political participation
    B. Providing a robust form of class-specific opportunities
    C. Limiting equality to those that benefit the least advantaged
    D. Limiting equality to those that benefit the most advantaged

31. In 1946, the World Health Organization first expressed the right to health as a fundamental human right. Which of the following provides guidance for reconstructing global governance for health by institutionalizing health in the context of human rights?

A. Framework Convention on Global Health
B. Principles of the Global Determinants of Health
C. Framework for Global Governance and Economic Development
D. Global Health Security Agenda

32. Strategic health promotion is one way to address equity issues in health. Which of the following is TRUE of health promotion?

A. Health promotion is any event, process, or activity that facilitates the protection or improvement of the health status of individuals, groups, communities, or populations.
B. Health promotion's objective is to promote commodification of quality of life.
C. Health promotion practice is not sensitive to how health is conceptualized.
D. Health promotion's objective is to promote commodification of preventive measures.

33. Health promotion to improve and promote health by addressing socioeconomic and environmental determinants of health within the community emphasizes which of the following approaches?

A. Behavior modification approach
B. Community-based development approach
C. Biomedical approach
D. Cultural approach

34. The community development approach to health promotion can address health equity and social justice issues by

A. Improving individual attitudes and beliefs, which are key to successful health promotion
B. Working on the close relationship between individual health and its social and material contexts, which are relevant when developing initiatives for change
C. Emphasizing that individuals need to change personal behavior rather than to change the environment to promote health
D. Using the fear appeal to target individual health behavior alone

35. In many societies, the healthcare system consists of nested or overlapping practices. The nonprofessional, nonbureaucratic, specialist sector in healthcare is referred to as

A. The government sector
B. The popular sector
C. The professional sector
D. The folk sector

36. Which of the following is an accepted working definition of social justice?

    A. "Social justice is a political and philosophical concept which holds that all people should have equal access to wealth, health, well-being, justice, and opportunity."

    B. "Social justice is a concept of fair and just relations between the individual and society, as long as individuals carry their weight."

    C. "Social justice is the opposite of jungle justice, whereby nature is perceived as 'red in tooth and nail'."

    D. "Social justice is an individual of good and moral standing capable of being elected to the Supreme Court of the United States."

37. The National Cancer Institute defines complementary medicine as "treatments that are used along with standard medical treatments but are not considered to be standard treatments." One example is using acupuncture to help lessen some side effects of cancer treatment. Which of the following groups describes the majority of users of complementary medicine in the United States?

    A. Poorly educated Chinese Americans

    B. Highly educated Caucasians

    C. Highly educated African Americans

    D. It is prejudicial and too much generalization to define a whole ethnic category as the majority of users of complementary medicine, as the definition varies by cultural and social norms.

38. The National Center for Complementary and Integrative Health states that, "If a non-mainstream practice is used in place of conventional medicine, it's considered alternative." One example is using a special diet to treat cancer instead of anticancer drugs that are prescribed by an oncologist. Which of the following groups describes the majority of users of complementary medicine in the United States?

    A. Poorly educated Native Americans

    B. Highly educated Chinese Americans

    C. Poor African Americans

    D. It is prejudicial and too much generalization to define a whole ethnic category as the majority of users of complementary medicine, as the definition varies by cultural and social norms.

39. Environmental justice is related to health equity and social justice. Environmental justice is best defined as

    A. "The fair treatment and meaningful involvement of all people regardless of race, color, national origin, or income, with respect to the development, implementation, and enforcement of environmental laws, regulations, and policies."

    B. "The fair treatment and meaningful involvement of affluent people regardless of race, color, national origin, or income, with respect to the development, implementation, and enforcement of environmental laws, regulations, and policies."

    C. "Environmental justice is the fair treatment and meaningful involvement of all educated people regardless of race, color, national origin, or income, with respect to the development, implementation, and enforcement of environmental laws, regulations, and policies."

D. "The fair treatment and meaningful involvement of all professional people regardless of race, color, national origin, or income, with respect to the development, implementation, and enforcement of environmental laws, regulations, and policies."

40. The goal of environmental justice will be achieved when

A. Everyone enjoys the same degree of protection from environmental and health hazards.

B. Some people enjoy equal access to the decision-making process to have a healthy environment in which to live, learn, and work.

C. Everyone enjoys some access to the decision-making process to have a healthy environment in which to live, learn, and work.

D. Everyone enjoys some degree of protection from environmental and health hazards.

41. The World Health Organization's Commission on the Social Determinants of Health concluded that

A. "The social conditions in which people are born, live and work are the single most important determinants of good health or ill health, of a long and productive life, or a short and miserable one."

B. "The social conditions in which people are born, live and work are secondary determinants of good health or ill health, of a long and productive life, or a short and miserable one."

C. "The social conditions in which people are born, live and work are tertiary determinants of good health or ill health, of a long and productive life, or a short and miserable one."

D. "The economic conditions in which people are born, live and work are the single most important determinants of good health or ill health, of a long and productive life, or a short and miserable one."

42. "Directly Observed Therapy" (DOT) is the most effective strategy to ensure adherence to a course of treatment. Why might an immigrant be reluctant to participate in DOT?

A. Immigrants are typically not fearful of healthcare professionals, but nobody likes being observed.

B. Immigrants may fear the loss of privacy or cultural misunderstanding.

C. Immigrants may have had unpleasant experiences with physical therapy in other countries.

D. Immigrants may fear repercussions with the Department of Transportation

43. The following may be experienced by individual members of a population perceived as low economic status, EXCEPT

A. Inclusion in all health-supporting infrastructure

B. Self-fulfilling prophecy regarding the outcome of poor health choices

C. Stigma

D. Reduced effort regarding health seeking behavior

44. In the United States as in several countries, considerable stigma may be associated with sexual orientation and behavior, leading to health equity problems. Which of the following reasons is associated with a person's reluctance to reveal sexual orientation in a healthcare setting?

A. Because the person may identify as other than the norm

B. Clarity about how the healthcare provider will react

C. Fear of being stereotyped or stigmatized

D. Clarity about how insurance companies will react

45. HIV infection and AIDS remain major scourges for public health in many countries, in part because of stigmatization and social justice issues. Which of the following statements is correct regarding people at risk for HIV infection?

A. All persons should be considered as being at risk for HIV infection.

B. Only homosexuals should be considered at risk for HIV infection.

C. Only intravenous drug users should be considered at risk for HIV infection.

D. A monogamous heterosexual woman is not considered at risk for HIV infection.

46. Stigma is defined as

A. "The co-occurrence of labeling, stereotyping, separation, status loss, and discrimination in a context in which power is exercised"

B. "A standardized mental picture that is held in common by members of a group and that represents an oversimplified opinion, prejudiced attitude, or uncritical judgment"

C. "An irrational attitude of hostility directed against an individual, a group, a race, or their supposed characteristics"

D. "Preconceived opinion that is not based on reason or actual experience"

47. Delayed acculturation may contribute to health equity problems for immigrants. The adjustment process during the acculturation is characterized by which of the following?

A. Age has no effect on the adjustment process.

B. Older adults tend to experience greater difficulty adjusting to a new culture.

C. Individuals who immigrated early in life have more trouble adjusting.

D. Individuals who immigrated late in life are generally more willing to adjust their behavior or habits.

48. The National Institute of Mental Health's Collaborative Psychiatric Epidemiologic Surveys focus on the cultural and racial influences on mental health. Dr. Thomas Insel, former director of the NIMH, commented that, "Among many intriguing findings, perhaps what is most striking are not the variations in prevalence but the variations in care. Thus, for mental illness in America, the challenge is health equity; that is, achieving equal and optimal healthcare for all

populations." Which of the following is likely to be the MOST important cause on variations in mental healthcare across cultural and racial groups?

A. Lack of a molecular model of mental health
B. Lack of awareness of mental health prevalence
C. Sociocultural stigma about mental health
D. Confusion about mental health therapies

49. In April 2019, the National Academies of Sciences, Engineering, and Medicine hosted a workshop entitled "A Health Equity Approach to Obesity Efforts." Certain ethnic groups exhibit above-average obesity risk in the United States. The following socioecological factor(s) explain disparities in obesity and its consequences at the population level, EXCEPT:

A. Disparities in access to healthy food
B. Individual differences in food intake and physical activity behaviors
C. Lack of opportunities for safe and affordable recreation
D. Disparities in mental capacity of individuals or groups

50. In the United States, civil rights laws have been influential in addressing some health equity issues, including

A. Segregation to entrench traditional access to healthcare services and facilities
B. Prohibition of discrimination on the basis of race and gender
C. American Abilities Act
D. Prohibition of discrimination on the basis of wealth

51. According to the 2010 U.S. Census, approximately 36% of the population belongs to a racial or ethnic minority group. An ethnic group is a category of people who are distinguished, by others or by themselves, on the basis of

A. Cultural or nationality characteristics
B. Their social-political system
C. Physical characteristics
D. Their personalities

52. Health indicators such as life expectancy and infant mortality have improved for most Americans; however, some racial minority groups experience a disproportionate burden of preventable disease, death, and disability compared with non-minorities. A "racialized group" is defined as

A. A category of people distinguished by their political and economic system
B. A category of people distinguished, by others or by themselves, as inferior or superior primarily on the basis of cultural or nationality characteristics
C. A category of people who have been singled out, by others or by themselves, as superior or inferior on the basis of subjectively selected physical characteristics
D. A group that establishes an enclave in a distinct geographic area such as Chinatown

53. Urban planning and zoning laws can produce inequality in access to healthcare, contribute to inequality in exposure to risk factors, and influence public health equity issues. Whether it is perceived as voluntary or manipulated, the spatial and social separation of categories of people by racialization/ethnicity, class, gender, religion, or other social characteristics is known as

    A. Freedom
    B. Discrimination
    C. Colonialism
    D. Segregation

54. Gender inequality damages the physical and mental health of girls and women across the world. In the United States, gender inequality manifests as a public health problem in the following way:

    A. Similar exposures to health-damaging factors
    B. Differential vulnerabilities leading to inequitable health outcomes
    C. Similar economic and social consequences of illness and reproductive health needs
    D. Differential mental and physical capabilities, based on genetic endowment, that are not sensitive to social and environmental conditions

55. Globally, women make up 70% of the health workforce, but only 25% hold senior roles. This means that, in reality, women deliver global health and men lead it. Which of the following is a possible consequence of inequity in the public health workforce?

    A. Shortage of resources to support research and implementation of public health programs occurs to focus on women's health.
    B. There are no demonstrable impacts of workforce demographic pattern on public health outcomes.
    C. The gender inequity in the health workforce reflects different interests in topics related to health and management training. For example, women are more interested in nursing than surgery.
    D. A and B only

56. One of the top priorities of the World Health Organization is "universal health coverage." This means

    A. That all people and communities can use the promotive, preventive, curative, rehabilitative, and palliative health services they need, of sufficient quality to be effective, while also ensuring that the use of these services does not expose the user to financial hardship
    B. That some people and communities can use the promotive, preventive, curative, rehabilitative, and palliative health services they need, of sufficient quality to be effective, while also ensuring that the use of these services does not expose the user to financial hardship
    C. That all people and communities can use the promotive, preventive, curative, rehabilitative, and palliative health services they can afford, and of sufficient quality to be effective
    D. That all people and communities can use the promotive, preventive, curative, rehabilitative, and palliative health services they deserve, of sufficient

quality at the level to which they are accustomed, while also ensuring that the use of these services does not expose the user to financial hardship

57. Universal health coverage (UHC) has the following objective.
    A. Equity in access to health services—everyone who needs services should get them, not only those who can pay for them.
    B. The quality of health services should be good enough to improve the health of those who can pay for the services.
    C. Wealthy people should be protected against financial risk, ensuring that the cost of using services does not put people at risk of financial harm.
    D. Poor people should be protected against financial risk borne by wealthy people, ensuring that the cost of using services does not put people at risk of financial harm.

58. The United States does not have a fully implemented universal health coverage system. As of 2017, approximately 92% of U.S. citizens have health insurance coverage, an increase of nearly 10% over the preceding decade. This increase is attributed to
    A. Increase in economic prosperity
    B. Increase in the gross national product per capita
    C. Patient Protection and Affordable Care Act
    D. Patient Wellness and Insurance Act of 2010

59. The Patient Protection and Affordable Care Act of 2010 and the Healthcare and Education Reconciliation Act of 2010 both promise to reduce the health equity gap in the United States for the following reason:
    A. Restricting the expansion of health insurance coverage only to ethnic minorities
    B. Restricting the expansion of health education provision only to ethnic minorities
    C. Restricting the expansion of health insurance coverage only to those below the poverty line
    D. Promotion of health insurance coverage for all Americans

60. The word "equity" appears once in the text of the "Patient Protection and Affordable Care Act" of 2010: "Sec. 1556. Equity for certain eligible survivors" references the "Black Lung Benefits Act," which refers to
    A. A U.S. federal law that provides monthly payments and medical benefits to coal miners totally disabled from pneumoconiosis arising from employment in or around the nation's coal mines
    B. African Americans who smoked menthol cigarettes
    C. Tobacco settlement funds
    D. A U.S. federal law that provides monthly payments and medical benefits to African American smokers totally disabled from lung cancer

■ ANSWERS

1. **B.** The U.S. Environmental Protection Agency defines environmental justice as the fair treatment and meaningful involvement of all people regardless of race, color, national origin, or income, with respect to the development, implementation, and enforcement of environmental laws, regulations, and policies. This goal will be achieved when everyone enjoys

   - The same degree of protection from environmental and health hazards
   - Equal access to the decision-making process to have a healthy environment in which to live, learn, and work

   See: https://www.epa.gov/environmentaljustice

   A common understanding of key terminology related to an initiative is essential to the success of any partnership. In recognition of this reality, Team—EJ, a working group of the Partnership for Sustainable Communities (PSC), set out to identify relevant terms of environmental justice, sustainability, and health and to assess how each of the three PSC agencies, the U.S. Department of Transportation (DOT), U.S Department of Housing and Urban Development (HUD), and the U.S Environmental Protection Agency (EPA), defines and understands these terms. With input from the Centers for Disease Control and Prevention (CDC), which is a member of the PSC's Team—EJ, health terms and definitions are included in this document. These terms are defined by the relevant federal agencies:

   1. Environmental justice
   2. Sustainability
   3. Affordable housing
   4. Smart growth
   5. Green jobs
   6. Goods movement
   7. Social determinants of health
   8. Health disparity (health equity)
   9. Cumulative impact (cumulative environmental exposure)
   10. Built environment

   See: https://www.epa.gov/sites/production/files/2015-02/documents/team-ej-lexicon.pdf

2. **D.** There are no genetically engineered consumable food products made to produce human hormones such as estrogen. The U.S. Food and Drug Administration (FDA) regulates genetically engineered food products. In response to the question, "Are there long-term health effects of foods from genetically engineered plants?" the FDA states that

   "When evaluating the safety of food from genetically engineered plants, scientists with experience in assessing the long-term safety of food and food ingredients consider several factors, such as information about the long-term safety of the food from traditionally bred crops in combination with information on the food safety of the newly introduced traits. Foods from genetically engineered plants that have been evaluated by FDA through the consultation process have not gone on the market until the FDA's questions about the safety of such products have been resolved."

See: https://www.fda.gov/food/food-new-plant-varieties/consumer-info-about-food-genetically-engineered-plants

3. **B.** The U.S. Food Safety Modernization Act is the most sweeping reform of the Food and Drug Administration's (FDA) food safety authority in more than 70 years. This act gives the FDA new and enhanced mandates and authorities to protect consumers and promote public health. The U.S. Environmental Protection Agency (EPA) is responsible for regulating chemicals such as pesticides used in food production.

The Department of the Interior (DOI) conserves and manages the nation's natural resources and cultural heritage for the benefit and enjoyment of the American people, provides scientific and other information about natural resources and natural hazards to address societal challenges and create opportunities for the American people, and honors the nation's trust responsibilities or special commitments to American Indians, Alaska Natives, and affiliated island communities to help them prosper.

See: https://www.doi.gov/whoweare

https://www.fda.gov/food/guidance-regulation-food-and-dietary-supplements

4. **C.** Alzheimer's disease is the most common type of dementia. It is a progressive disease beginning with mild memory loss possibly leading to loss of the ability to carry on a conversation and respond to the environment. The disease involves parts of the brain that control thought, memory, and language, and can seriously affect a person's ability to carry out daily activities. In 2014, approximately 5 million Americans were living with Alzheimer's disease. The symptoms of the disease can first appear after age 60 and the risk increases with age. Younger people may get Alzheimer's disease, but it is less common. The number of people living with the disease doubles every 5 years beyond age 65. This number is projected to nearly triple to 14 million people by 2060. Age is the best-known risk factor for Alzheimer's disease, and it affects all genders, regardless of level of education, economic income, or ethnicity.

See: https://www.cdc.gov/aging/aginginfo/alzheimers.htm

5. **A.** In 2007, it was estimated that the cost to society of drug abuse was $193 billion, a substantial portion of which—$113 billion—was associated with drug-related crime, including criminal justice system costs and costs borne by victims of crime. The cost of treating drug abuse (including health costs, hospitalizations, and government specialty treatment) was estimated to be $14.6 billion, a fraction of the overall societal costs. Drug abuse treatment is cost effective in reducing drug use and bringing about related savings in healthcare. Treatment also consistently has been shown to reduce the costs associated with lost productivity, crime, and incarceration across various settings and populations. The largest economic benefit of treatment is seen in avoided costs of crime (incarceration and victimization costs). Providing methadone treatment to opioid-addicted prisoners prior to their release,

for example, not only helps to reduce drug use but also avoids the much higher imprisonment costs for drug-related crime.

See: https://www.drugabuse.gov/publications/principles-drug-abuse-trea tment-criminal-justice-populations/providing-drug-abuse-treatment -to-offenders-worth-f

6. **C.** Cultural and linguistic competence involves a set of congruent behaviors, attitudes, and policies that come together in a system, agency, or among professionals that enables effective work in cross-cultural situations. "Culture"'refers to integrated patterns of human behavior that include the language, thoughts, communications, actions, customs, beliefs, values, and institutions of racial, ethnic, religious, or social groups. "Competence" implies having the capacity to function effectively as an individual and an organization within the context of the cultural beliefs, behaviors, and needs presented by consumers and their communities.

Cultural competency is one of the main ingredients in closing the disparities gap in healthcare. It's the way patients and doctors can come together and talk about health concerns without cultural differences hindering the conversation but enhancing it. Quite simply, healthcare services that are respectful of and responsive to the health beliefs, practices, and cultural and linguistic needs of diverse patients can help bring about positive health outcomes.

See: https://www.cdc.gov/nchhstp/socialdeterminants/docs/what_is_cul tural_competency.pdf

7. **D.** Environmental justice is the fair treatment and meaningful involvement of all people regardless of race, color, national origin, or income with respect to the development, implementation, and enforcement of environmental laws, regulations, and policies.

Fair treatment means no group of people should bear a disproportionate share of the negative environmental consequences resulting from industrial, governmental, and commercial operations or policies.

Meaningful involvement means:

- People have an opportunity to participate in decisions about activities that may affect their environment and/or health.
- The public's contribution can influence the regulatory agency's decision.
- Community concerns will be considered in the decision-making process.
- Decision-makers will seek out and facilitate the involvement of those potentially affected.

See: https://www.epa.gov/environmentaljustice/learn-about-environment al-justice

8. **D.** Heart disease affects people worldwide, and, in some cases, children are born with heart defects that need medical intervention. As the global burden of cardiovascular disease continues to increase worldwide, nurturing the development of early-career cardiologists interested in global health is essential in order to create a cadre of providers with the skill set to prevent and treat cardiovascular diseases in international settings. As such, interest in global health has increased among cardiology trainees and early-career cardiologists

over the past decade. International clinical and research experiences abroad present an additional opportunity for growth and development beyond traditional cardiovascular training. The American College of Cardiology International Cardiovascular Exchange Database is a new resource for cardiologists interested in pursuing short-term clinical exchange opportunities abroad, and report some of the benefits and challenges of global health cardiovascular training in both resource-limited and resource-abundant settings.

See: https://www.ncbi.nlm.nih.gov/pmc/articles/PMC4902723

9. **D.** Disease knows no borders. In today's interconnected world, a disease threat anywhere can become a health threat in the United States. We know that disease exploits even the smallest gap to spread and grow. With the ease and speed of global travel, along with rapidly expanding commerce and trade, the need to shut down the expressways available to infectious disease into the United States is more important today than ever before. The most effective—and cost effective—way to protect Americans from known and unknown health threats that begin overseas is to stop them before they spread to our shores. The Centers for Disease Control and Prevention's (CDC) global activities protect Americans from major health threats such as Ebola, Zika, and pandemic influenza. The CDC detects and controls outbreaks at their source, saving lives and reducing healthcare costs. Importantly, the CDC helps other countries build the capacity to prevent, detect, and respond to their health threats through the organization's work. The goal is to stop diseases where they occur as soon as they start. The knowledge and lessons learned from the CDC's work abroad are critical to our public health efforts at home, and to protect Americans.

See: https://www.cdc.gov/globalhealth/what/default.htm

Humans have probably always been aware that invisible, life-like agents influence living and nonliving phenomena, but the attribution of such influences to discrete life forms that we now call bacteria occurred recently—less than five centuries ago. The Italian scholar, Girolamo Fracastoro (1476–1553), is credited as the first to propose, in 1546, an atomistic theory of disease, linking epidemics to particulate contagion. The invention and use of microscopes by Antoni van Leeuwenhoek (1632–1723) initiated an unprecedented era of scientific discoveries in the field of bacterial diversity. However, the appreciation of the consequences of bacterial ecological diversity had to await theoretical and empirical advances, for example, through the works of John Snow (1813–1858) and Louis Pasteur (1822–1895) that finally overturned the prevalent Miasma theory in favor of the "germ theory" of disease causation.

Ogunseitan (2016), O. A. Bacterial diversity, Introduction to. Retrieved from https://www.researchgate.net/publication/303252100_Bacterial_Diversity_Introduction_to

10. **D.** Incorporating cultural competence in public health systems enables professionals to adapt their approaches to benefit individuals and groups from varying cultural backgrounds. Furthermore, improving cultural competence among public health practitioners could help reduce health disparities and improve the quality of care and health for everyone.

Over the years, public health professionals have expanded their approaches to preventing disease, as evidenced by the growing number of practice and translation models designed to meet the needs of multiple cultural groups. Incorporating a thoughtful and consistent emphasis on cultural competence when performing all essential public health functions, including evaluation, creates a necessary foundation for efforts to reduce health disparities.

See: https://www.cdc.gov/dhdsp/docs/cultural_competence_guide.pdf

11. **A.** Diabetes and prediabetes are highly prevalent in adult populations of the United States. This is concerning because diabetes is a risk factor for cardiovascular disease, vision loss, end stage renal disease, disability, and mortality. From 2010 through 2012, African Americans (13.2%), American Indians/Alaska Natives (AI/ANs) (15.9%), Asian Americans and other Pacific Islanders (9.0%), and Latinos (12.8%) were more often diagnosed with diabetes than were non-Hispanic Whites (7.6%). Diabetes is preventable through lifestyle changes that may also assist in diabetes control. The Institute of Medicine (IOM) examined the impact of social and cultural environments on health outcomes and recommends that research advance in this area. According to the IOM report, health behaviors and other social variables occur in a cultural context that must be understood to determine which cultural variables influence adoption of health recommendations.

See: https://www.cdc.gov/diabetes/ndep/pdfs/culturally_competent_
health_provider_communication_webinar_slides.pdf

https://www.cdc.gov/pcd/issues/2015/14_0421.htm

https://www.youtube.com/watch?v=Gr3YQp_P2bM

12. **C.** Malaria is a life-threatening disease caused by parasites that are transmitted to people through the bites of infected female Anopheles mosquitoes. It is preventable and curable. In 2017, there were an estimated 219 million cases of malaria in 87 countries.

The estimated number of malaria deaths stood at 435,000 in 2017. The World Health Organization (WHO) African Region carries a disproportionately high share of the global malaria burden. In 2017, the region was home to 92% of malaria cases and 93% of malaria deaths.

Total funding for malaria control and elimination reached an estimated US$ 3.1 billion in 2017. Contributions from governments of endemic countries amounted to US$ 900 million, representing 28% of total funding. Malaria is caused by Plasmodium parasites. The parasites are spread to people through the bites of infected female Anopheles mosquitoes, called "malaria vectors." There are five parasite species that cause malaria in humans, and two of these species—*Plasmodium falciparum* and *Plasmodium vivax*—pose the greatest threat. In 2017, *P. falciparum* accounted for 99.7% of estimated malaria cases in the WHO African Region, as well as in the majority of cases in the WHO regions of Southeast Asia (62.8%), the Eastern Mediterranean (69%), and the Western Pacific (71.9%).

P. vivax is the predominant parasite in the WHO region of the Americas, representing 74.1% of malaria cases.

Insecticide-treated bed nets (ITNs) are a form of personal protection that has been shown to reduce malaria illness, severe disease, and death due to malaria in endemic regions. In community-wide trials in several African settings, ITNs were shown to reduce the death of children under 5 years from all causes by about 20%. Bed nets form a protective barrier around people sleeping under them. However, bed nets treated with an insecticide are much more protective than untreated nets. The insecticides that are used for treating bed nets kill mosquitoes as well as other insects. The insecticides also repel mosquitoes, reducing the number that enter the house and attempt to feed on people inside. In addition, if high community coverage is achieved, the numbers of mosquitoes, as well as their length of life, will be reduced. When this happens, all members of the community are protected, regardless of whether or not they are using a bed net. To achieve such effects, more than half of the people in a community must use an ITN.

See: https://www.cdc.gov/malaria/malaria_worldwide/reduction/itn.html

https://www.who.int/news-room/fact-sheets/detail/malaria

13. **C.** From January 1 to July 11, 2019, 1,123 individual cases of measles were confirmed in 28 states. This is the greatest number of cases reported in the United States since 1992 and since measles was declared eliminated in 2000. As of July 11, 2019, the states that have reported cases to the Centers for Disease Control and Prevention (CDC) are Arizona, California, Colorado, Connecticut, Florida, Georgia, Idaho, Illinois, Indiana, Iowa, Kentucky, Maine, Maryland, Massachusetts, Michigan, Missouri, New Mexico, Nevada, New Hampshire, New Jersey, New York, Oklahoma, Oregon, Pennsylvania, Texas, Tennessee, Virginia, and Washington.

Immunization requirements for school entry help protect children and communities from vaccine-preventable diseases. Each autumn California schools are required to report to the California Department of Public Health (CDPH) the status of their students under state immunization requirement laws. In recent years there have been changes to these laws and how public health departments assist schools to implement them. In 2014 and 2015 the Assembly Bill (AB) 2109 added requirements for exemptions to required immunizations based on personal beliefs. 2017–2018 is the second full school year that entrants have been subject to Senate Bill (SB) 277, which no longer permits individuals to receive such personal beliefs exemptions (PBEs). Beginning in the 2015–2016 school year, many public health departments in California have assisted schools in correctly identifying and supporting eligible students, described as conditional entrants, who catch up with immunization requirements after entry. The proportion of students attending kindergarten in 2017–2018 reported to have received all required vaccines is 95.1%, a 0.4% point decrease (difference of unrounded values) from the 2016–2017 school year and a 4.7% point increase over the 3 years since 2014–2015. The 2017–2018 rate of 95.1% is the second highest reported for the current set of immunization requirements for kindergarten, which began in the 2001–2002 school year.

See: https://www.cdc.gov/measles/cases-outbreaks.html

https://www.cdph.ca.gov/Programs/CID/DCDC/CDPH%20Document%20Library/Immunization/2017-2018KindergartenSummaryReport.pdf

14. **B.** Complications because of untreated chronic diseases and mental health disorders are the primary cause of missed work and increased presenteeism. Even though there hase been increased attention on mental health in recent years, social stigma and discrimination associated with mental illnesses remains a significant barrier to an individual's health and employment. These issues often affect whether or not an individual will apply for a job or promotion when qualified. Stigma and discrimination may also prevent an employee from seeking help, contributing to presenteeism and absenteeism; if treatment is sought out, it may complicate the transition back to work. Both managers and coworkers alike are often unaware or uncertain how to interact with someone recovering from a mental health disorder. Many employees will not voluntarily disclose that they suffer from a chronic disease or mental health disorder for fear of being stigmatized. This burden leads to added stress that can exacerbate their condition. In addition, not divulging this information prevents the employer from understanding to what extent some of these health issues are problems and subsequently taking action, such as changing the work environment through a workplace health program.

See: https://www.cdc.gov/workplacehealthpromotion/tools-resources/ pdfs/issue-brief-no-2-mental-health-and-chronic-disease.pdf

HIV-related stigma refers to negative beliefs, feelings, and attitudes toward people living with HIV, their families, people who work with them (HIV service providers), and members of groups that have been heavily impacted by HIV, such as gay and bisexual men, homeless people, street youth, and mentally ill people.

See: https://www.cdc.gov/hiv/basics/livingwithhiv/stigma-discrimi nation.html

15. **A.** Health equity is achieved when every person has the opportunity to "attain his or her full health potential" and no one is "disadvantaged from achieving this potential because of social position or other socially determined circumstances." Health inequities are reflected in differences in length of life; quality of life; rates of disease, disability, and death; severity of disease; and access to treatment.

One of the primary goals of the Centers for Disease Control and Prevention's (CDC) National Center for Chronic Disease Prevention and Health Promotion (NCCDPHP) is to achieve health equity by eliminating health disparities and achieving optimal health for all Americans. The NCCDPHP addresses health equity through its programs, research, tools and resources, and leadership.

See: https://www.cdc.gov/chronicdisease/healthequity/index.htm

16. **A.** In the United States, the most commonly transplanted organs are the kidney, liver, heart, lungs, pancreas, and intestines. On any given day there are around 75,000 people on the active waiting list for organs, but only around 8,000 deceased organ donors each year, with each providing on average 3.5 organs. Living donors provide on average only around 6,000 organs per year. In the United States, the most commonly transplanted tissues are bones, tendons, ligaments, skin, heart valves, blood vessels, and corneas. Of around 2 million tissue grafts distributed each year, it is thought that only about

1 million grafts are transplanted. While some organ transplantations are life-saving procedures, serious illness, graft loss, and death can occur from unde-tected infections in donor organs and tissues. Although infrequent, infectious pathogens (i.e., viruses, bacteria, fungi, or protozoa/parasites) have been unknowingly transmitted through transplants.

See: https://www.cdc.gov/transplantsafety/overview/key-facts.html

17. **A.** Flea-borne typhus is a disease caused by *Rickettsia typhi* and possibly *Rickettsia felis* bacteria that are spread by fleas. Human cases of flea-borne typhus are reported worldwide, but mainly in tropical and coastal areas. In the United States, most cases occur in Texas, California, and Hawaii, with an average of about 300 cases every year. In California, flea-borne typhus is con-sidered endemic (always present) in areas of Los Angeles and Orange coun-ties, but cases sometimes are also reported from other parts of California. A person can get typhus by coming in contact with fleas that are infected with the bacteria that causes typhus. Fleas become infected when they bite small animals like rats, opossums, and stray cats. Fleas can then spread typhus to other animals and humans.

See: https://www.cdph.ca.gov/Programs/CID/DCDC/Pages/Typhus
.aspx

18. **C.** The Rx Awareness campaign tells the real stories of people whose lives were torn apart by prescription opioids. The goal of the campaign is to increase awareness that prescription opioids can be addictive and dangerous. The campaign also strives to decrease the number of individuals who use opi-oids recreationally or overuse them. Almost 36% of all U.S. opioid overdose deaths involve a prescription opioid. Overdose deaths involving prescription opioids have increased by about five times since 1999. From 1999 to 2017, more than 200,000 people died from overdoses related to prescription opioids, with more than 17,000 overdose deaths involving prescription opioids occurring in 2017. Whether you are a healthcare provider, first responder, law enforcement officer, public health official, or community member, the opioid epidemic is likely affecting you and your community. No matter who you are, you can take action to end the opioid overdose epidemic ravaging the United States. We all have a role to play on the frontlines of this fight—it starts with address-ing prescription opioid misuse, abuse, and overdose.

See: https://www.cdc.gov/rxawareness/about/index.html

19. **D.** When *Mycobacterium tuberculosis*, the bacterial causative agent of infectious tuberculosis (TB) disease, becomes active and the immune system can't stop the bacteria from growing, this is called TB disease. TB disease will make a person sick. People with TB disease may spread the bacteria to people with whom they spend many hours.

It is very important that people who have TB disease are treated, finish the medicine, and take the drugs exactly as prescribed. If they stop taking the drugs too soon, they can become sick again; if they do not take the drugs cor-rectly, the TB bacteria that are still alive may become resistant to those drugs. TB that is resistant to drugs is harder and more expensive to treat.

TB disease can be treated by taking several drugs for 6 to 9 months. There are 10 drugs currently approved by the U.S. Food and Drug Administration

(FDA) for treating TB. Of the approved drugs, the first-line anti-TB agents that form the core of treatment regimens are

- Isoniazid (INH)
- Rifampin (RIF)
- Ethambutol (EMB)
- Pyrazinamide (PZA)

See: https://www.cdc.gov/tb/topic/treatment/tbdisease.htm

20. **A.** According to the Centers for Disease Control and Prevention (CDC), 20% to 30% of new prescriptions are never filled at the pharmacy.

Medication is not taken as prescribed 50% of the time. For patients prescribed medications for chronic diseases, after 6 months, the majority take less medication than prescribed or stop the medication altogether. Only 51% of patients taking medications for high blood pressure continue taking their medication during their long-term treatment. Many patients do not follow healthcare provider instructions on how to take medications for various reasons, such as not understanding the directions, forgetfulness, multiple medications with different regimens, unpleasant side effects, or the medication doesn't seem to be working. Cost can also be a factor causing medication nonadherence—patients can't afford to fill their prescriptions or decide to take less than the prescribed dose to make the prescription last longer.

See: https://www.fda.gov/drugs/special-features/why-you-need-take-your-medications-prescribed-or-instructed

21. **C.** More than 30 million Americans have diabetes (about 1 in 10), and 90% to 95% of them have type 2 diabetes. Type 2 diabetes most often develops in people over age 45, but more and more children, teens, and young adults are also developing it. Type 2 diabetes symptoms often develop over several years and can go on for a long time without being noticed (sometimes there aren't any noticeable symptoms at all). Because symptoms can be hard to spot, it's important to know the risk factors for type 2 diabetes and to see your doctor to get your blood sugar tested if you have any of them. Type 2 diabetes risk factors include:

- Prediabetes diagnosis
- Overweight
- 45 years or older
- A parent, brother, or sister with type 2 diabetes
- Physically active less than three times a week
- Gestational diabetes (diabetes during pregnancy) or given birth to a baby who weighed more than 9 pounds
- African American, Hispanic/Latino American, American Indian, or Alaska Native (some Pacific Islanders and Asian Americans are also at higher risk)

All interventions should be framed within the cultural context of patients.

See: https://www.cdc.gov/diabetes/basics/risk-factors.html

22. **A.** Complementary and alternative medicine (CAM) are medicines and health practices that are not usually used by doctors to treat cancer. Complementary

medicine is used in addition to standard treatments. Alternative medicine is also used instead of standard treatments.

Cancer patients who are using or considering using complementary or alternative therapy should talk with their doctor or nurse. Some therapies may interfere with standard treatment or even be harmful. It is also a good idea to learn whether the therapy has been proven to do what it claims to do.

Patients, their families, and their healthcare providers can learn about CAM therapies and practitioners from the following government agencies:

- National Center for Complementary and Integrative Health
- National Cancer Institute Office of Cancer Complementary and Alternative Medicine
- Office of Dietary Supplements

See: https://www.cancer.gov/about-cancer/treatment/cam

https://www.cdc.gov/cancer/survivors/patients/complementary-alternative-medicine.htm

23. **D.** The ideas people have about health, the languages they use, the health literacy skills they have, and the contexts in which they communicate about health reflect their cultures. Organizations can increase communication effectiveness when they recognize and bridge cultural differences that may contribute to miscommunication. Culture can be defined by group membership, such as racial, ethnic, linguistic, or geographical groups, or as a collection of beliefs, values, customs, ways of thinking, communicating, and behaving specific to a group. As part of a cultural group, people learn communication rules, such as who communicates with whom, when and where something may be communicated, and what to communicate about. Members of a cultural group also learn one or more languages that facilitate communication within the group. Sometimes, though, language can get in the way of successful communication. When people and organizations try to use their in-group languages, or jargon, in other contexts and with people outside the group, communication often fails and creates misunderstanding and barriers to making meaning in a situation.

See: https://www.cdc.gov/healthliteracy/culture.html

24. **A.** Health inequities are avoidable inequalities in health between groups of people within countries and between countries. These inequities arise from inequalities within and between societies. Social and economic conditions and their effects on people's lives determine their risk of illness and the actions taken to prevent them from becoming ill or treat illness when it occurs.

The poorest of the poor, around the world, have the worst health. Within countries, the evidence shows that in general the lower an individual's socioeconomic position the worse his or her health. There is a social gradient in health that runs from top to bottom of the socioeconomic spectrum. This is a global phenomenon, seen in low-, middle-, and high-income countries. The social gradient in health means that health inequities affect everyone.

For example, if you look at under-5 mortality rates by levels of household wealth, you see that within counties the relation between socioeconomic level and health is graded. The poorest have the highest under-5 mortality rates, and people in the second highest quintile of household wealth have higher mortality in their offspring than those in the highest quintile. This is the social gradient in health.

See: https://www.who.int/social_determinants/thecommission/ finalreport/key_concepts/en

25. **B.** *Theory at a Glance: A Guide for Health Promotion and Practice* frames the ecological perspective as

"...the interaction between, and interdependence of, factors within and across all levels of a health problem. It highlights people's interactions with their physical and sociocultural environments."

Ecological models recognize multiple levels of influence on health behaviors, including

- Intrapersonal/individual factors, which influence behavior such as knowledge, attitudes, beliefs, and personality
- Interpersonal factors, such as interactions with other people, which can provide social support or create barriers to interpersonal growth that promotes healthy behavior
- Institutional and organizational factors, including the rules, regulations, policies, and informal structures that constrain or promote healthy behaviors
- Community factors, such as formal or informal social norms that exist among individuals, groups, or organizations, which can limit or enhance healthy behaviors
- Public policy factors, including local, state, and federal policies and laws that regulate or support health actions and practices for disease prevention including early detection, control, and management

For example, the Centers for Disease Control and Prevention (CDC) uses a four-level social–ecological model to better understand violence and the effect of potential prevention strategies. This model considers the complex interplay between individual, relationship, community, and societal factors. It allows us to understand the range of factors that put people at risk for violence or protect them from experiencing or perpetrating violence. The overlapping rings in the model illustrate how factors at one level influence factors at another level.

Besides helping to clarify these factors, the model also suggests that in order to prevent violence, it is necessary to act across multiple levels of the model at the same time. This approach is more likely to sustain prevention efforts over time than any single intervention.

- Individual: The first level identifies biological and personal history factors that increase the likelihood of becoming a victim or perpetrator of violence. Some of these factors are age, education, income, substance use, or history of abuse. Prevention strategies at this level promote attitudes, beliefs, and behaviors that prevent violence. Specific approaches may include education and life skills training.
- Relationship: The second level examines close relationships that may increase the risk of experiencing violence as a victim or perpetrator.

A person's closest social circle—peers, partners, and family members—influences his or her behavior and contributes to the individual's experience. Prevention strategies at this level may include parenting or family-focused prevention programs, as well as mentoring and peer programs designed to reduce conflict, foster problem-solving skills, and promote healthy relationships.

- Community: The third level explores the settings, such as schools, workplaces, and neighborhoods, in which social relationships occur and seeks to identify the characteristics of these settings that are associated with becoming victims or perpetrators of violence. Prevention strategies at this level impact the social and physical environment—for example, by reducing social isolation, improving economic and housing opportunities in neighborhoods— as well as the climate, processes, and policies within school and workplace settings.
- Societal: The fourth level looks at the broad societal factors that help create a climate in which violence is encouraged or inhibited. These factors include social and cultural norms that support violence as an acceptable way to resolve conflicts. Other large societal factors include the health, economic, educational, and social policies that help to maintain economic or social inequalities between groups in society.

See: https://www.ruralhealthinfo.org/toolkits/health-promotion/2/theories-and-models/ecological

https://www.cdc.gov/violenceprevention/publichealthissue/social-ecologicalmodel.html

26. **C.** The microsystem of social organization can explain inequalities, according to Urie Bronfenbrenner's ecological systems theory, which holds that we encounter different environments throughout our life span that may influence our behavior in varying degrees. These systems include the microsystem, the mesosystem, the exosystem, the macrosystem, and the chronosystem.

Bronfenbrenner, U. (2009). *The ecology of human development: Experiments by nature and design.* Cambridge, MA: Harvard University Press.

27. **B.** There is scholarly consensus about descriptive aspects of health inequalities and equity; however, there is no agreement on the explanation or root causes. Competing hypotheses include natural or social selection, cultural or behavioral explanation, and materialist or structural explanation. Materialist or structuralist explanations refer to a range of factors determined by the class or income structure and that have an impact on health and well-being. Under this explanation, there remains confusion between the "hard" version, in which physical aspects of the environment are the key determinants of health, and the "soft" version in which "social" as well as economic capital (e.g. education) are dominant.

See: http://www.sphsu.mrc.ac.uk/library/other%20reports/OP_Sept-1998.pdf

28. **C.** The Social Ecological Model (SEM) is a theory-based framework for understanding the multifaceted and interactive effects of personal and environmental factors that determine behaviors, and for identifying behavioral and organizational leverage points and intermediaries for health promotion

within organizations. There are five nested, hierarchical levels of the SEM: individual, interpersonal, community, organizational, and policy/enabling environment. The most effective approach to public health prevention and control uses a combination of interventions at all levels of the model.

See: https://www.unicef.org/cbsc/files/Module_1_SEM-C4D.docx

29. **B.** Socioeconomic status (SES) can be a root cause of ill health, whereas poor health can also cause low SES (health selection).

According to the Centers for Disease Control and Prevention (CDC), SES measures a person's social, economic, and work status. Social status is measured by how many years a person spent in school. Economic status is measured by how much money a person earns each year. Work status is measured by whether a person has a job. For example, a person with a high SES may have a college degree, earn an above-average income, and have a full-time job that pays well. A person with a low SES may not have finished high school, doesn't earn enough money to live comfortably, and may be unemployed or have a low-paying job. A person's SES affects his or her ability to get healthcare. A person with more education is more likely to get a job that pays well and provides health insurance and paid sick leave. For example, people who have higher incomes and health insurance are more likely to get tests that can find cancer early, and get the right treatment if cancer is found. So people with a higher SES often have higher cancer survival rates, and may allow them to work, earn income, and purchase health insurance (health selection). People with a low SES are less likely to get cancer screening tests. So their cancer is often found at a later stage, when it causes symptoms. Even if their cancer is treated, patients are less likely to survive cancer that's found after it has advanced.

See: https://link.springer.com/article/10.1007/s11205-018-1871-x

  https://www.cdc.gov/cancer/healthdisparities/basic_info/challenges
  .htm

30. **A.** Public health ethics deals primarily with the moral foundations and justifications for public health, the various ethical challenges raised by limited resources for promoting health, and real or perceived tensions between collective benefits and individual liberty (Stanford Encyclopedia of Philosophy). The Centers for Disease Control and Prevention (CDC) defines public health ethics as "a systematic process to clarify, prioritize, and justify possible courses of public health action based on ethical principles, values, and beliefs of stakeholders, and scientific and other information." A public health ethics lens ensures a uniquely expanded focus on population health opportunities and challenges.

See: https://www.cdc.gov/healthequity/forums/phe/2017/index.html

31. **A.** The World Health Organization (WHO) Constitution was the first international instrument to enshrine the enjoyment of the highest attainable standard of health as a fundamental right of every human being ("the right to health"). The right to health in international human rights law is a claim to a set of social arrangements—norms, institutions, laws, and an enabling environment—that can best secure the enjoyment of this right.

It is an inclusive right extending not only to timely and appropriate healthcare but also to the underlying determinants of health, for example, access to health information, water and food, housing, and so on.

The right to health is subject to progressive realization and acknowledges resource constraints. However, it also imposes on states various obligations that are of immediate effect, such as the guarantee that the right will be exercised without discrimination of any kind and the obligation to take deliberate, concrete, and targeted steps toward its full realization.

See: https://www.who.int/topics/human_rights/en

In 2015, Lawrence Gostin and colleagues asked, "What will it take to eliminate the gross health inequities that continue to plague the world, the unconscionable health gaps between the rich and poor?"

See: https://www.who.int/bulletin/volumes/91/10/12-114447/en

32. **A.** Chronic diseases—such as heart disease, cancer, and type 2 diabetes—are the leading causes of death and disability in the United States. They are also leading drivers of the nation's $3.3 trillion in annual healthcare costs. Many chronic diseases are caused by a short list of risk behaviors: tobacco use, poor nutrition, lack of physical activity, and excessive alcohol use. The Centers for Disease Control and Prevention's (CDC) National Center for Chronic Disease Prevention and Health Promotion works to improve health for adults by

- Helping smokers quit and promoting smoke-free public spaces
- Increasing access to healthy foods and physical activity opportunities
- Promoting lifestyle change and disease self-management programs
- Promoting women's reproductive health
- Promoting clinical preventive services
- Promoting oral health through community water fluoridation
- Promoting healthy sleep

See: https://www.cdc.gov/chronicdisease/resources/publications/factsheets/promoting-health-for-adults.htm

33. **B.** In response to the 1979 Surgeon General's Report on Health Promotion and Disease Prevention, Healthy People, the Center for Health Promotion and Education was created at the Centers for Disease Control and Prevention (CDC) in 1981. This center was established as a broad-based entity that focused on health issues including reproductive health, nutrition, smoking, alcohol use, physical fitness, stress, violence, accidents, and other risk factors of public health significance. In subsequent years, the center's scope expanded to include important infant and maternal health initiatives, the widely used Planned Approach to Community Health, and the Behavioral Risk Factor Surveillance System and other key surveillance programs. By 1988, the CDC established the National Center for Chronic Disease Prevention and Health Promotion (NCCDPHP), which became increasingly disease-specific, spreading the expertise in health education and community health promotion across diversified programs. Consequently, no one unit within NCCDPHP is the primary resource for public health practitioners seeking to improve the efficacy and effectiveness of community health promotion.

See: https://www.cdc.gov/chronicdisease/pdf/community_health_promo
tion_expert_panel_report.pdf

34. **B.** Health equity is achieved when every person has the opportunity to "attain his or her full health potential" and no one is "disadvantaged from achieving this potential because of social position or other socially determined circumstances." Health disparities or inequities are types of unfair health differences closely linked with social, economic, or environmental disadvantages that adversely affect groups of people. Achieving health equity, eliminating disparities, and improving the health of all groups is an overarching goal for *Healthy People 2020* and a top priority for the Centers for Disease Control and Prevention (CDC). The CDC's Healthy Communities Program supports eliminating socioeconomic and racial/ethnic health disparities as an integral part of its chronic disease prevention and health promotion efforts. To improve health on the local, state, and national level, communities are encouraged to identify and address social determinants of health and improve these conditions through environmental changes.

See: https://www.cdc.gov/nccdphp/dch/programs/healthycommunities
program/overview/healthequity.htm

35. **D.** The World Health Organization's (WHO) Traditional Medicine Strategy 2014–2023 was developed and launched in response to the World Health Assembly resolution on traditional medicine (WHA62.13). The strategy aims to support member states in developing proactive policies and implementing action plans that will strengthen the role traditional medicine plays in keeping populations healthy. The strategic objectives are

- To build the knowledge base for active management of traditional and complementary medicine (T&CM) through appropriate national policies
- To strengthen the quality assurance, safety, proper use, and effectiveness of T&CM by regulating products, practices, and practitioners
- To promote universal health coverage by integrating T&CM services into healthcare service delivery and self-healthcare

The WHO global report on traditional and complementary medicine 2019 was developed to address the gap in reliable, credible, and official data from member states in the area of T&CM. This report reviews global progress in T&CM over the past two decades and is based on contributions from 179 WHO member states. It provides valuable information for policy makers, health professionals, and the public for capitalizing on the potential contribution of T&CM to health and well-being.

See: https://www.who.int/traditional-complementary-integrative-
medicine/en

36. **A.** The United Kingdom's government policy on "social justice: transforming lives" states that social justice is about making society function better—providing the support and tools to help turn lives around. This is a challenging new approach to tackling poverty in all its forms. It is not a narrative about income poverty alone: This Government believes that the focus on income over the last decades has ignored the root causes of poverty, and in doing so

has allowed social problems to deepen and become entrenched. The new set of principles that inform the approach are

1. A focus on prevention and early intervention
2. Where problems arise, concentrating interventions on recovery and independence, not maintenance
3. Promoting work for those who can as the most sustainable route out of poverty, while offering unconditional support to those who are severely disabled and cannot work
4. Recognizing that the most effective solutions will often be designed and delivered at a local level
5. Ensuring that interventions provide a fair deal for the taxpayer

See: https://assets.publishing.service.gov.uk/government/uploads/ system/uploads/attachment_data/file/49515/social-justice-trans forming-lives.pdf

> In her book entitled *Health and Social Justice*, Jennifer Prah Ruger defines a theory of health and social justice, which she calls the "health capability paradigm"—whereby she says that all people should have access to the means to avoid premature death and preventable morbidity. Hers is a vision that incorporates the philosophical, economic, and political to make a compelling case that all societies (through public–private partnerships) can design and build effective institutions and systems to achieve health capabilities. Although she focuses (perhaps overly so) on the provision of medical care, Ruger offers a rich explanation of the essential drivers of health, such as surveillance, preventive measures, clean air, safe drinking water, and nutritious food.

See: https://www.who.int/bulletin/volumes/89/1/10-082388/en

37. **D.** In December 2008, the National Center for Complementary and Integrative Health (NCCIH) and the National Center for Health Statistics (part of the Centers for Disease Control and Prevention) released new findings on Americans' use of complementary and alternative medicine (CAM). The findings are from the 2007 National Health Interview Survey (NHIS), an annual in-person survey of Americans regarding their health- and illness-related experiences. The CAM section gathered information on 23,393 adults aged 18 years or older and 9,417 children aged 17 years and under. A similar CAM section was included in the 2002 NHIS, providing the opportunity to examine trends in CAM use, too.

In the United States, approximately 38% of adults (about 4 in 10) and approximately 12% of children (about 1 in 9) are using some form of CAM. People of all backgrounds use CAM. However, CAM use among adults is greater among women and those with higher levels of education and higher incomes. Nonvitamin, nonmineral natural products are the most commonly used CAM therapy among adults. Use has increased for several therapies, including deep breathing exercises, meditation, massage therapy, and yoga.

See: https://nccih.nih.gov/research/statistics/2007/camsurvey_fs1.htm

38. **D.** People use complementary and alternative medicine (CAM) for an array of diseases and conditions. American adults are most likely to use CAM for musculoskeletal problems such as back, neck, or joint pain. The use of CAM therapies for head or chest colds showed a substantial decrease from 2002 to 2007. People of all backgrounds use CAM. However, CAM use among adults is greater among women and those with higher levels of education and higher incomes.

See: https://nccih.nih.gov/research/statistics/2007/camsurvey_fs1.htm

39. **A.** Environmental justice is the fair treatment and meaningful involvement of all people regardless of race, color, national origin, or income, with respect to the development, implementation, and enforcement of environmental laws, regulations, and policies. This goal will be achieved when everyone enjoys

- The same degree of protection from environmental and health hazards
- Equal access to the decision-making process to have a healthy environment in which to live, learn, and work

See: https://www.epa.gov/environmentaljustice

40. **A.** Environmental justice will be achieved when everyone enjoys

- The same degree of protection from environmental and health hazards
- Equal access to the decision-making process to have a healthy environment in which to live, learn, and work

See: https://www.epa.gov/environmentaljustice

41. **A.** The social determinants of health are the conditions in which people are born, grow, live, work, and age. These circumstances are shaped by the distribution of money, power, and resources at global, national, and local levels. The social determinants of health are mostly responsible for health inequities—the unfair and avoidable differences in health status seen within and between countries.

See: https://www.who.int/gender-equity-rights/understanding/sdh
-definition/en

42. **B.** In 2017, 70% of tuberculosis (TB) cases were diagnosed in foreign-born persons in the United States, as opposed to 30% in 1993. In cities that are home to many newly arriving immigrants and refugees, rates of TB can be well above the national average. Additionally, the prevalence of drug-resistant TB or extrapulmonary TB cases, which are more challenging to diagnose and manage, is higher among foreign-born persons.

The most effective strategy to ensure adherence to treatment is Directly Observed Therapy (DOT). With DOT, a patient meets with a healthcare worker every day or several times a week. The patient takes the TB medicines while the healthcare worker watches. The healthcare worker also asks the patient about any problems or side effects with the medication. DOT should be done at a time and place that is convenient for the patient. DOT should be used for ALL patients with TB disease, including children and adolescents. There is no way to accurately predict whether a patient will adhere to treatment without this assistance.

See: https://www.cdc.gov/tb/webcourses/tb101/page 3832.html

https://www.cdc.gov/immigrantrefugeehealth/guidelines/domestic/tuberculosis-guidelines.html

43. A. Systemic bias against populations defined by low economic status often means exclusion from health-supporting infrastructure such as recreational parks, healthy food stores, and healthy homes in safe neighborhoods. These conditions are further exacerbated by the stigma of poverty, which in turn drives lack of self-confidence.

The *Healthy People 2020* program defines social determinants of health as conditions in the environments in which people live, learn, work, play, worship, and age that affect a wide range of health, functioning, and quality-of-life outcomes and risks. Conditions (e.g., social, economic, and physical) in these various environments and settings (e.g., school, church, workplace, and neighborhood) have been referred to as "place." In addition to the more material attributes of "place," the patterns of social engagement and sense of security and well-being are also affected by where people live.

Healthy People 2020 developed a "place-based" organizing framework, reflecting five key areas of Social Determinants of Health:

Economic stability

Education

Social and community context

Health and healthcare

Neighborhood and built environment

Resources that enhance quality of life can have a significant influence on population health outcomes. Examples of these resources include safe and affordable housing, access to education, public safety, availability of healthy foods, local emergency/health services, and environments free of life-threatening toxins.

See: https://www.cdc.gov/socialdeterminants/faqs/index.htm#faq7

44. C. People who are lesbian, gay, bisexual, or transgender (LGBT) are members of every community. They are diverse, come from all walks of life, and include people of all races and ethnicities, all ages, all socioeconomic statuses, and from all parts of the country. The perspectives and needs of LGBT people should be routinely considered in public health efforts to improve the overall health of every person and eliminate health disparities.

Many healthcare providers do not routinely discuss sexual orientation or gender identity (SO/GI) with patients, and many healthcare facilities have not developed systems to collect structured SO/GI data from all patients. Without this information, LGBT patients and their specific healthcare needs cannot be identified, the health disparities they experience cannot be addressed, and the provision of important healthcare services may not be delivered. Such services include appropriate preventive screenings, assessments of risk for sexually transmitted diseases and HIV, discussions about parenting, and effective interventions for behavioral health concerns that can be related to the experiences of anti-LGBT stigma. An opportunity for transgender people to share information about their SO/GI in a welcoming and patient-centered environ-ment opens the door to a more trusting patient–provider relationship.

See: https://www.cdc.gov/actagainstaids/campaigns/transforming health/healthcareproviders/collecting-sexual-orientation.html

https://www.cdc.gov/nchs/nhis/sexual_orientation/statistics.htm

45. **A.** HIV-AIDS disproportionately affects various populations in the United States. Differences in HIV burden, by sex and race/ethnicity (i.e., Blacks/African Americans, Hispanics/Latinos, and Whites), have long been high-lighted through HIV surveillance data in the United States. Such disparities may not be directly related to sex, race/ethnicity, or behavioral risk factors but may instead be related to the social determinants that affect the health of populations.

See: https://www.cdc.gov/hiv/pdf/statistics_2005_2009_HIV_Surveil lance_Report_vol_18_n4.pdf

https://www.cdc.gov/nchhstp/dear_colleague/2018/dcl-061818 -AtlasPlus.html

https://www.hiv.gov/topics/socialdeterminants

46. **A.** Stigma is shame and disgrace that result from prejudice associated with something regarded as socially unacceptable. Stigma around HIV includes certain words, beliefs, and actions that have negative meaning for those at high risk for getting HIV or those already living with HIV. Here are a few examples:

- Referring to people as HIV positive
- Believing that only certain groups of people can get HIV
- Refusing casual contact with someone living with HIV
- Making moral judgments about people who take steps to prevent HIV transmission
- Socially isolating a member of a community because he or she is HIV positive
- Refusal by a healthcare professional to provide high-quality care or ser-vices to a person living with HIV

Ongoing stigma in our communities leads to perceived discrimination, fear, and anxiety.

See: https://www.cdc.gov/stophivtogether/index.html?CDC_AA_refVal =https%3A%2F%2Fwww.cdc.gov%2Factagainstaids%2Findex.html

47. **B.** Many immigrant populations assimilate to the prevalent U.S. culture, but full assimilation is more difficult with the increasing age of arrival in the United States. Instead, acculturation is more realistic as a process of integrat-ing native and traditional cultural values with dominant cultural ones.

See: https://www.cdc.gov/nccdphp/dch/programs/healthycommunities program/tools/pdf/hispanic_latinos_insight.pdf

48. **C.** Attitudes and beliefs about mental illness are shaped by personal knowl-edge about mental illness, knowing and interacting with someone living with mental illness, cultural stereotypes about mental illness, media stories, and

familiarity with institutional practices and past restrictions (e.g., health insurance restrictions, employment restrictions, adoption restrictions). When such attitudes and beliefs are expressed positively, they can result in supportive and inclusive behaviors (e.g., willingness to date a person with mental illness or to hire a person with mental illness). When such attitudes and beliefs are expressed negatively, they may result in avoidance, exclusion from daily activities, and, in the worst case, exploitation and discrimination. Stigma has been described as - a cluster of negative attitudes and beliefs that motivate the general public to fear, reject, avoid, and discriminate against people with mental illnesses. When stigma leads to social exclusion or discrimination (experienced stigma), it results in unequal access to resources that all people need to function well: educational opportunities, employment, a supportive community including friends and family, and access to quality healthcare. These types of disparities in education, employment, and access to care can have cumulative long-term negative consequences.

See: https://www.cdc.gov/hrqol/Mental_Health_Reports/pdf/BRFSS_Full%20Report.pdf

49. **D.** Obesity is not linked to mental capacity in the general population. Obesity has been on the rise in the United States over the past two decades and is at high levels. In addition to population-wide trends, it is clear that obesity affects some groups more than others and can be associated with age, income, disability, education, gender, race and ethnicity, and geographic region.

See: https://www.cdc.gov/nccdphp/dnpao/state-local-programs/health-equity/index.html

50. **B.** Section 601 of the Title VI of the Civil Rights Act of 1964 42 U.S.C. Section 2000d et. seq. states that "No person in the United States shall, on the grounds of race, color or national origin, be excluded from participation in, be denied the benefits of, or be subjected to discrimination under any program or activity receiving Federal financial assistance." Minority health determines the health of the nation—The United States has become increasingly diverse in the last century. According to the 2010 U.S. Census, approximately 36% of the population belongs to a racial or ethnic minority group. Though health indicators such as life expectancy and infant mortality have improved for most Americans, some minorities experience a disproportionate burden of preventable disease, death, and disability compared with nonminorities.

See: https://www.cdc.gov/healthequity/timeline/index.htm

https://www.cdc.gov/minorityhealth/index.html

https://www.hrsa.gov/sites/default/files/grants/apply/Technical Assistance/patientcivilrights.pdf

51. **A.** The U.S. Office of Management and Budget's (OMB) minimum categories for data on race are American Indian or Alaska Native, Asian, Black or African American, Native Hawaiian or other Pacific Islander, and White. There are two OMB minimum categories for data on ethnicity: Hispanic or Latino, and Not Hispanic or Latino. More information on the U.S. Office of Management and Budget minimum categories and federal standards for classifying data on race and ethnicity is available at http://www.whitehouse.gov/omb/

See: https://www.cdc.gov/mmwr/PDF/rr/rr4210.pdf

https://www.cdc.gov/phin/resources/vocabulary/documents/cdc-race--ethnicity-background-and-purpose.pdf

52. **C.** Racialization is the process of assigning racial identities to a group that did not identify itself as such. It often results from the interaction of a group with another group that it dominates and ascribes identity to keep the status quo.

See: https://www.cdc.gov/socialdeterminants/neighborhood/index.htm

53. **D.** Social, cultural, and economic factors influence where and how many resources and opportunities are available in a metropolitan area. One of the factors most prominent in U.S. metropolitan areas is racial/ethnic residential segregation. Research has found it is not only linked to health, but to the differences in resources and opportunity availability where people live. For example, the more segregated a metropolitan area is, the poorer the health outcomes are among Blacks. While many studies of metropolitan area segregation and health have focused on Blacks, a particular focus is paid on the impact of neighborhood-level residential segregation on Blacks.

See: https://www.cdc.gov/dhdsp/pubs/docs/sib_may2015.pdf

54. **B.** Health equity is when everyone has the opportunity to be as healthy as possible. Health disparities are differences in health outcomes and their causes among groups of people. For example, African American children are more likely to die from asthma compared to non-Hispanic White children. Reducing health disparities creates better health for all Americans. Reducing and eliminating health disparities is fundamental to reaching health equity and building a healthier nation. The Centers for Disease Control and Prevention's (CDC) Office of Minority Health and Health Equity (OMHHE) advances health equity and women's health issues across the nation through the CDC's science and programs. OMHHE also increases the CDC's capacity to leverage its diverse workforce and engage stakeholders to this end. OMHHE is composed of three units: Women's Health, Diversity and Inclusion Management, and Minority Health and Health Equity.

See: https://www.cdc.gov/healthequity/index.html

https://www.cdc.gov/women/index.htm

55. **A.** 200 million workers contribute to the health and social sector, one of the biggest and fastest growing employers of women (70% of the workforce). Yet, half of women's contribution to global health is unpaid. Without action, health coverage expansion may be thwarted by a shortfall of 18 million health workers. The International Labor Organization-Organization for Economic Cooperation and Development-World Health Organization Working for Health program in collaboration with the Global Health Workforce Network Gender Equity Hub aims to accelerate the expansion and transformation of the health and social workforce. This infopoint session will explore the gender dividend and the Sustainable Development Goals (SDG) gains within grasp through investments into the health and social workforce.

See: https://www.who.int/hrh/events/2018/women-in-health-workforce/en

56. A. Universal health coverage (UHC) means that all people and communities can use the promotive, preventive, curative, rehabilitative, and palliative health services they need, of sufficient quality to be effective, while also ensuring that the use of these services does not expose the user to financial hardship. This definition of UHC embodies three related objectives:

- Equity in access to health services—everyone who needs services should get them, not only those who can pay for them.
- The quality of health services should be good enough to improve the health of those receiving services.
- People should be protected against financial risk, ensuring that the cost of using services does not put people at risk of financial harm.

UHC is firmly based on the World Health Organization (WHO) constitution of 1948 declaring health a fundamental human right and on the Health for All agenda set by the Alma Ata declaration in 1978. UHC cuts across all of the health-related Sustainable Development Goals (SDGs) and brings hope of better health and protection for the world's poorest.

See: https://www.who.int/health_financing/universal_coverage_definition/en

57. A. Universal health coverage (UHC) has three related objectives:

1. Equity in access to health services—everyone who needs services should get them, not only those who can pay for them.
2. The quality of health services should be good enough to improve the health of those receiving services.
3. People should be protected against financial risk, ensuring that the cost of using services does not put people at risk of financial harm.

UHC is firmly based on the World Health Organization (WHO) constitution of 1948 declaring health a fundamental human right and on the Health for All agenda set by the Alma Ata declaration in 1978. UHC cuts across all of the health-related Sustainable Development Goals (SDGs) and brings hope of better health and protection for the world's poorest.

See: https://www.who.int/health_financing/universal_coverage_definition/en

58. C. The Prevention and Public Health Fund was established under Section 4002 of the Patient Protection and Affordable Care Act of 2010 (ACA). Also known as the Prevention Fund or PPHF, it is the nation's first mandatory funding stream dedicated to improving the United States' public health system. By law, the Prevention Fund must be used "to provide for expanded and sustained national investment in prevention and public health programs to improve health and help restrain the rate of growth in private and public healthcare costs."

See: https://www.cdc.gov/funding/pphf/index.html

https://www.healthcare.gov/glossary/patient-protection-and-affordable-care-act

59. **D.** Together with the Patient Protection and Affordable Care Act, the Health-care and Education Reconciliation Act will ensure that all Americans have access to quality, affordable health insurance and put students ahead of private banks. The Congressional Budget Office has determined that together, these two bills are fully paid for; will ensure more than 94% of Americans have access to quality, affordable healthcare; will bend the healthcare cost curve; and will reduce the deficit by $143 billion over the next 10 years with further deficit reduction in the following decade. Historic investments in our economic future will make college more affordable and accessible through a transformation in student loan programs.

See: https://www.dpc.senate.gov/healthreformbill/healthbill61.pdf

https://www.healthcare.gov/glossary/patient-protection-and-afforda ble-care-act

60. **A.** On December 20, 2000, the Department of Labor published a final rule amending the regulations implementing the Black Lung Benefits Act. This compliance guide explains some of the procedures that will be followed under the amended rules for processing Black Lung Benefit claims filed after January 19, 2001. The final rule and an extensive preamble discussion are published at 65 Federal Register 79920-80107 (Dec. 20, 2000). The Black Lung Benefits Act provides monthly payments and medical benefits to coal miners totally disabled from pneumoconiosis (black lung disease) arising from their employment in or around the nation's coal mines. The Act also provides monthly benefits to a miner's dependent survivors. Unless the miner was awarded benefits pursuant to a claim filed before 1982, a survivor must establish that pneumoconiosis was a substantially contributing cause of the miner's death to be entitled to benefits.

The program provides two types of medical services related to black lung disease: diagnostic testing for all miner–claimants to determine the presence or absence of black lung disease and the degree of associated disability and, for miners entitled to monthly benefits, medical coverage for treatment of black lung disease and disability. Diagnostic testing includes a chest x-ray, pulmonary function study (breathing test), arterial blood gas study, and a physical examination. Medical coverage includes (but is not limited to) costs for prescription drugs, office visits, and hospitalizations. Also provided, with specific approval, are items of durable medical equipment, such as hospital beds, home oxygen, and nebulizers; outpatient pulmonary rehabilitation therapy; and home nursing visits.

See: https://www.dol.gov/owcp/dcmwc/regs/compliance/blbenact.htm

Index